SO-CFI-636

Advance Praise for *The Headache Alternative*

"Dr. Mauskop, a leader in the treatment of headache, has written a comprehensive guide to alternative therapies in headache care. This is a tremendously valuable volume, both for the physician and the layperson."

—Dr. Glen Solomon, Cleveland Clinic Foundation

"THE HEADACHE ALTERNATIVE looks refreshingly at complementary medicine and headache. It will serve as an excellent resource guide."

—Dr. Steven Graff-Radford, director of The Pain Center,
Cedars Sinai Medical Center, and adjunct associate professor,
UCLA School of Dentistry

"*The Headache Alternative* is an exhaustive guide of new and established treatments. It is an important book for headache sufferers of all kinds."

—Dr. R. Michael Gallagher, D.O., F.A.C.O.F.P.,
University of Medicine and Dentistry of New Jersey,
School of Osteopathic Medicine

"Few doctors have extensive knowledge about the nonpharmacologic approaches to headache, and the advice offered to patients who seek this information is often limited. From this perspective, Dr. Mauskop's effort to create sources of unbiased information about the full range of these approaches is laudable. Dr. Mauskop, a respected headache specialist, first emphasizes the critical medical issue, the need for proper diagnosis, then lucidly describes the issues related to diet and many drug-free approaches to headache now in use. His book will be a valuable resource for both patients and doctors."

—Dr. Russell K. Portenoy, co-chief, Pain and Palliative Care Service,
Memorial Sloan-Kettering Cancer Center

QUANTITY SALES

Most Dell books are available at special quantity discounts when purchased in bulk by corporations, organizations, or groups. Special imprints, messages, and excerpts can be produced to meet your needs. For more information, write to: Dell Publishing, 1540 Broadway, New York, NY 10036. Attention: Special Markets.

INDIVIDUAL SALES

Are there any Dell books you want but cannot find in your local stores? If so, you can order them directly from us. You can get any Dell book currently in print. For a complete up-to-date listing of our books and information on how to order, write to: Dell Readers Service, Box DR, 1540 Broadway, New York, NY 10036.

THE HEADACHE ALTERNATIVE

A Neurologist's Guide to Drug-Free Relief

Alexander Mauskop, M.D.,
and
Marietta Abrams Brill

Illustrations by Michael Reingold

A DELL TRADE PAPERBACK

Research about headaches is ongoing and subject to interpretation. Although every effort has been made to include the most up-to-date and accurate information in this book, there can be no guarantee that what we know about this complex subject won't change with time. The reader should bear in mind that this book should not be used for self-diagnosis or self-treatment, and he or she should consult appropriate medical professionals regarding all health issues.

A DELL TRADE PAPERBACK
Published by
Dell Publishing
a division of
Bantam Doubleday Dell Publishing Group, Inc.
1540 Broadway
New York, New York 10036

If you purchased this book without a cover you should be aware that this book is stolen property. It was reported as "unsold and destroyed" to the publisher and neither the author nor the publisher has received any payment for this "stripped book."

Excerpt appears on page: 174
From *Acupressure's Potent Points* by Michael Reed Gach. Copyright © 1990 by Michael Reed Gach. Used by permission of Bantam Books, a division of Bantam Doubleday Dell Publishing Group, Inc.

Excerpt appears on page: 99
From *Headache Free* by Roger Cady, M.D., and Kathleen Farmer, Psy.D. Copyright © 1993 by Roger Cady and Kathleen Farmer. Used by permission of Bantam Books, a division of Bantam Doubleday Dell Publishing Group, Inc.

Excerpt appears on page: 116
Reprinted from the January 1996 issue of the *Harvard Women's Health Watch.* Copyright © 1995 President and Fellows of Harvard College.

Excerpt appears on pages: 124–133
From *Prescription for Nutritional Healing* by James Balch, M.D., and Phyllis Balch, C.N.C. Copyright © 1990. Published by Avery Publishing Group, Inc., Garden City Park, New York. Reprinted by permission.

Excerpt appears on page: 15
From *Healing Wise,* Ash Tree Publishing, Woodstock, NY. Copyright © 1989 and used with permission of Susun S. Weed.

Excerpt appears on pages: 19–21
Used with permission of Sterling Publishing Co., Inc., 387 Park Ave. S., NY, NY 10016 from *Ayurveda: The Gentle Healing System* by Hans H. Rhyner. Copyright © 1992 by BLV Verlag, English Translation © 1994 by Sterling Publishing Co., Inc.

Excerpt appears on pages: 65–66
Reprinted with permission from *Conquering Headache,* by Alan Rapoport, M.D., and Fred Sheftell, M.D. Empowering Press, 1995.

Copyright © 1997 by Alexander Mauskop and Marietta Abrams Brill

All rights reserved. No part of this book may be reproduced or transmitted in any form or by any means, electronic or mechanical, including photocopying, recording, or by any information storage and retrieval system, without the written permission of the Publisher, except where permitted by law.

The trademark Dell® is registered in the U.S. Patent and Trademark Office.

Library of Congress Cataloging in Publication Data
Mauskop, Alexander.
The headache alternative : a neurologist's guide to drug-free
relief / Alexander Mauskop and Marietta Abrams Brill :
illustrated by Michael Reingold.
p.   cm.
Includes bibliographical references and index.
ISBN 0-440-50820-7
1. Headache—Alternative treatment.   I. Abrams-Brill, Marietta.
II. Title.
RB128.M35   1997
616.8'49106—dc21   97-5769
CIP

Printed in the United States of America
Published simultaneously in Canada
November 1997
10 9 8 7 6 5 4 3 2 1
BVG

For Karen, my love and guiding light.
—A.M.

Acknowledgments

My thanks go to Drs. Burton Altura, Bella Altura, and Roger Cracco, without whom none of my magnesium research could have happened.

—A.M.

Heartfelt thanks go out to the many people who helped make this book happen. To Peter for his patience and encouragement, to our agent Judith Riven for her support and persistence, to my family for their ongoing belief, to my friends for their insights and eternal good humor, and to Addy, who never left my side.

We would also like to thank the following professionals for generously sharing their expertise:

Roger Jahnke, OMD, Health Action Press, Santa Barbara, Calif.; Jan Balkam, aromatherapist, Lexington, Mass.; Beryl Bender Birch, yoga instructor and therapist, New York, N.Y.; Al Bumanis, National Association for Music Therapy, Silver Spring, Md.; Roger Cady, M.D., The Shealy Institute for Comprehensive Healthcare; Jay Cardinale, Hellerwork practitioner, Brooklyn, N.Y.; Rosemary Feitis, D.O., Structural Integration therapist, New York, N.Y.; Barry Gruber, M.D., biofeedback specialist, Medical Illness Counseling Center, Annapolis, Md.; Julia Kendall, co-chair, Citizens for a Toxic-Free Marin, San Rafael, Calif.; Nancy Ford-Kohne, M.A., director, Yoga and Health Studies

Center, Alexandria, Va.; Michelle Larson, PhysicalMind Institute, Santa Fe, N.M.; Harriet Miller, body-mind therapist, New York, N.Y.; Charles Millman, Kushi Institute, Becket, Mass.; Ann Naylor, Bonnie Prudden Myotherapist, San Francisco, Calif.; Aurora S. Ochampo, nurse practitioner/Reiki practitioner, Beth Israel Hospital, New York, N.Y.; David Rowe, chiropractor, New York, N.Y.; Alison Rapp, Feldenkrais instructor, W. Va.; Simon Sinnett, applied kinesiologist, New York, N.Y.; Judith Stern, Alexander Technique practitioner, New York, N.Y.; Dana Ullman, director, National Center for Homeopathy, Alexander, Va.; Enid Whitaker, Bonnie Prudden Institute, Tuscon, Ariz.; Richard Wong, M.D., University of Maryland, Divison of Complementary Medicine, Bethesda, Md.; Janet Xenos, D.O., osteopathic physician (cranial manipulation), Santa Ana, Calif.

—M.A.B.

Contents

INTRODUCTION:
A Neurologist's New Perspective
on Headache Treatment

If you suffer from frequent headaches, you have probably become painfully aware of how often modern medicine falls short of giving you what you really seek: safe, reliable control over your pain. Today's typical medical response to pain is drugs. And while prescribed drugs have been "clinically proven" to provide relief, I do not think you would be reading this book if you were satisfied with the results. Either the drugs failed to ease your pain or you felt uncomfortable with the risk of side effects that virtually every drug carries. Or you simply believed, as I do, that there are alternatives to conventional medicine that can help *prevent* the headache before treatment is necessary—or that might provide treatment that is safer, more effective, and in the long run less expensive.

Know that you are not alone in your desire to explore beyond conventional Western medicine: A recent survey in *The New England Journal of Medicine* showed that 34 percent of us have sought out alternative therapies.[1] And most people sought these treatments for chronic conditions, including headache. It's clear that many of the healing methods we once thought of as peripheral or antiquated are now becoming central.

As a neurologist who was educated at modern medical institutions, I believe that some pharmaceuticals have their place in the treatment of headaches. As the director of the New York Headache Center, I have prescribed these drugs to headache patients in my care, many of whom have found relief. But many have not. However, rather than close the door on modern medicine and blame it for its failures, it seems more positive, and logical, to open the door to alternatives.

One of the options that opened my eyes to alternative methods is the success of magnesium in preventing certain types of headaches. Through many years of research in this area, I became convinced that the treatments for headache relief and prevention are not limited to the pharmacy counter at your local drugstore.

TODAY'S COMPLEMENTARY MEDICINE: WHERE THE AGE-OLD AND THE NEW AGE MEET

You might have heard about alternative treatments. Whether they are age-old remedies such as acupuncture or "new age" approaches like guided imagery, they all seem new—especially in light of modern society's single-minded reliance on drugs. And, to many of you, alternative treatments might appear exotic and almost magical.

In fact not only have many of these remedies been used successfully for hundreds or thousands of years (acupressure and herbal remedies, for example) but many have very logical—*physio*logical—bases for success. We know, for example, that vitamins and minerals are important to life. An imbalance of these nutrients can cause the body to work improperly. In some cases this imbalance might cause headache. By paying close attention to the foods we eat and, when necessary, taking nutritional supplements, we may be able to correct the problem.

In the same way the medical benefits of herbs have been known for centuries. Through ancient Roman, Hebrew, and Egyptian medical records we see that herbs were used to treat virtually every known illness. The pharmaceutical industry got its start by purifying and processing these natural ingredients—and there is a renewed effort today among some pharmaceutical companies to explore the value of herbs.

Acupressure and acupuncture, both ancient Chinese practices, operate on the concept that there are key junctures in the body: the application of pressure or hair-thin needles to these specific points is thought to release the blockages and tension that can cause pain and provide pain relief.

Even the newer alternative treatments are rooted in age-old concepts of medicine. For example homeopathy, which was developed in the late eighteenth century, uses the essences of plants (and other substances) to stimulate and strengthen the body's own natural defenses. Chiropractors, and some osteopathic physicians, specialize in the manipulation of joints and other tissues to reduce nerve irritation and release muscle tension that might cause headaches. Other "bodywork" therapies—methods such as massage, osteopathic manipulations, Alexander Technique, craniosacral therapy, and Rolfing—also manipulate the body to relieve muscle tension and in some cases to release emotional sources of muscle or connective-tissue contraction. Modern mind-body techniques—such as biofeedback, autogenic training (self-hypnosis), relaxation, imagery, and visualization—are simply formalized ways of helping the body to release pain-causing tension.

Ironically, advances in modern medicine are indirectly providing scientific proof for some of these "unproven" methods. In an effort to uncover cures of diseases of the immune system, for example, scientists have discovered more about the powerful and complex workings of our own natural defenses—and how these defenses can be strengthened by the foods we eat and the way we live our lives. In fact the National Institutes of Health (NIH), a research branch of our nation's public-health service, has acknowledged the possible validity of alternative approaches by funding the Office of Alternative Medicine, a department of the NIH dedicated to research into nondrug treatments and preventive approaches. More than twenty-five major medical colleges and universities offer courses in alternative medicine. Medical journals directed at physicians seeking knowledge about alternative approaches are now available. Insurance providers are even beginning to offer plans that cover preventive and alternative treatments. In short even modern science is opening up to age-old and new age treatments.

HOW TO USE THIS BOOK

This book is written for those who want to take an active role in their health. Consider it a resource guide of drug-free treatments for the prevention and relief of headache. But before embarking on your journey of self-healing, it is important to keep some things in mind.

Though each human being shares the same basic physical makeup, each person is also unique. Your lifestyle, the food you eat, your genetic heritage, and even your profession and where you live can influence your health—and your reasons for having chronic headache.

Similarly, even though medical experts have been able to identify categories for headache—migraine, cluster, and tension-type, to name the top three—we also know that the "triggers" that set off a headache are often as unique as the people who experience them. For example, while cigarette smoke might trigger one person's migraine, stress might set the migraine in motion for someone else.

In short it is very difficult to generalize about the causes of headache and the proper treatment for each individual. The first step toward finding the right relief is understanding the source or sources of your headache—of which there may be more than one. Those causes will be described in Part I.

Once you gain an understanding of what causes your headache, you will be better prepared to understand the logic behind the drug-free methods available to treat it. No single treatment is right for every person. You might even want to try a combination of approaches. To help you find the one that's right for you, the drug-free methods will be described in Part II.

Some of the approaches described in this book have been medically proven. However, the success of many drug-free regimens is, in the vocabulary of conventional modern medicine, "anecdotal." This means that these methods might not have undergone the rigors of formal clinical study as we know it. Rather, the proof of their success is based on a collection of positive results. (For an explanation of clinical study designs, see the Glossary.) I say this certainly not to scare you away but, as with any approach you take—whether it be modern pharmaceutical methods or alternative, drug-free methods—to urge that you exercise caution.

In addition many of the approaches described in this book require a personal commitment to your health. As a culture most of us living in the United States today have become accustomed to taking a passive role in the care of our bodies. We are referred to as ''patients'' patiently (or impatiently) waiting for someone else to fix us. We expect miracle cures and fast relief; take a pill and feel better. For life-threatening illness—such as raging infections, heart attacks, or stroke—we are often *unable* to take an active role. In the realm of acute disease, modern medical tools, such as antibiotics and surgical innovations, have made true heroes out of doctors. But with chronic illnesses such as headache, our commitment to drug-free approaches may need to be even greater.

Holistic approaches engage the whole individual, with the belief that the mind and spirit play integral roles in generating the body's self-healing abilities. As patients waiting for a quick cure, we deprive the body of the chance to engage its own natural healing ''intelligence.'' But this takes active persistence and commitment. For example, while a change in diet might ''miraculously'' cure your headache, the cure lasts only as long as you stick with the regimen. Similarly, a typical acupuncture session lasts twenty to thirty minutes; many herbal teas need to be brewed at home for several hours. Repeated sessions/doses are often required before you feel relief.

This effort need not be viewed as a chore. On the contrary the rewards of becoming actively involved in your own health can extend beyond pain relief, bringing you to a renewed sense of overall health and respect for your body's innate power.

Keep in mind that some of the approaches described in this book reflect a life philosophy or belief system. While you don't need to adopt Taoist practices, for example, in order to benefit from Chinese herbs, you might gain *more* by understanding how other aspects of your lifestyle contribute to imbalances in your energy flow. To help in your exploration of these belief systems, you'll find suggested readings in the "Resources" section at the end of this book.

Finally, no one knows your pain better than you and your physician. If you are lucky enough to have a doctor who is open-minded about drug-free approaches, rely on him or her as a partner in your exploration of them. If not, we have listed some organizations at the end of this book (see "Resources") to help you along the way.

A WORD ABOUT WORDING

It has been a challenge to find comfortable and accurate terms for so-called alternative methods and, for that matter, modern medical practices. As people who receive medical care in late-twentieth-century United States or Europe, most of us regard our drug-based medicine as "traditional" medicine. This is a misnomer—especially in the context of this book. While the term reflects our current tradition, a more appropriate term might be *conventional*. Comparatively speaking, modern Western medicine has a very short history or tradition. Modern medicine as we know it is just a few centuries old. And many of the early concepts guiding modern medical care were remarkably similar to those we regard as nontraditional or alternative. The so-called nontraditional healing approaches, such as Oriental medicine and Ayurveda, have very long traditions, sometimes thousands of years old. For much of the world these methods are traditional.

As alternatives to pharmaceutical-based treatments become more accepted by today's physicians and nurses, the term *complementary medicine* has gained popularity. *Complementary* implies the use of nondrug approaches in conjunction with—to complement—pharmaceuticals. This indeed is my perspective, and therefore that is the term I feel comfortable using.

We reveal these semantic difficulties not as an excuse for awkward phrasing but to illustrate the great shifts now under way in medicine. It is my hope that many of the approaches we describe in the following pages will soon be regarded by the prevailing medical community not as alternatives but as viable, primary options in the treatment of headache.

PART I

A Look at Headaches

CHAPTER 1

How Headaches Happen

Divine is the work to subdue pain.
—HIPPOCRATES

━━━━━━

Virtually everyone can sympathize with the headache sufferer. At some point in their lives 90 percent of the population has endured a headache of one type or another. For most people the pain is acute—which, in terms of headache, means that it doesn't last long and happens only occasionally. But for forty million Americans, the pain is chronic, severe or recurrent, like a dreaded visitor who barges rudely into our homes with confounding frequency to make our lives miserable. For more than twenty million the pain is so all-consuming that we can do nothing—neither work, play, nor sometimes even sleep—until it decides to leave.

There are dozens of different types of headache. For many of these headache types, such as true sinus headache, the causes are clear. But for the top three—tension-type, migraine, and cluster headaches—modern Western medicine can't agree on the causes.

SCHOOLS OF THOUGHT ABOUT THE ORIGIN OF HEADACHE PAIN

Pain by any name feels the same for the headache sufferer. But concepts about the *mechanism of pain*—how pain happens in the body—can differ greatly depending on the therapeutic approach. An understanding of how different healing disciplines view pain is an important step in understanding the logic behind the treatment.

I employ aspects of several alternative disciplines in my practice—mostly those that have been studied and supported by some scientific evidence. This is my orientation. It does not mean that I dismiss the potential benefit of other approaches. For example I have not used Therapeutic Touch in my practice, but it is used, with success, in major hospitals across the country. Similarly I am not an Ayurvedic physician, but this traditional system of medicine has endured for thousands of years. I believe conventional Western medicine has much to learn from these traditions. So, while I do not use all of the approaches I will describe, I do encourage their exploration and study.

Conventional Western Medicine

Background

For as long as people have been practicing medicine, concepts of health and disease were guided by the idea that by observing nature one could identify what was healthy (and normal) and what was unhealthy (not normal). This older worldview embraced all aspects of human "nature"—states of health or disease were described in terms of an intricate linking of mind, body, and spirit. With roots in Greek culture, Western medical practice required schooling not only in anatomy and physiology but also in philosophy. Hippocrates, the founder of Western medicine, believed that there were four humors that regulated the body—and that any imbalance could result in pain. Plato, the Greek philosopher, thought that pain originated not only from physical influences but also from emotions. In these respects even early Western medicine bore similarities to other traditional medical practices, such as Ayurveda and traditional Oriental medicine.

With technological advances and philosophical shifts came a change in medical thinking. By the mid eighteenth century matters of the spirit and the mind were no longer the domain of medical healers but were relegated to the church. The emergence of rationalism gave rise to scientific disciplines that focused on specific parts of the body in order to better understand specific disease processes. For the first time medical science split away from medical practice. Medical theory began to isolate the physiological parts that make up the whole, with less emphasis on how the parts interact—and with little regard for factors that could not be observed, such as spiritual and emotional influences.

As a result practitioners of conventional Western medicine are not taught to view our bodies as being connected with our mental, spiritual, and emotional selves. In its approach Western medicine looks for signs and symptoms as indicators of disease: Their absence is strongly indicative of the absence of disease. One could say that our view of health is an absence of disease.

This is not to minimize some of the extraordinary healing tools that have resulted from recent medical research, particularly those used for the treatment of acute disorders. Today's doctors are highly skilled at coping with the body in trauma due to acute clinical problems, such as severe injury and infection.

In addition in recent years Western medicine has been using its sophisticated research methods to confirm the role of anxiety, stress, and other "nonphysical" factors on body health. Landmark studies conducted in the early 1960s confirmed that major life changes (good or bad) that produce emotional stress also cause physical stress. Another example: In the study of heart disease (Americans' leading cause of death), a very large population survey was designed to look at the lifestyles of a huge number of people—both with and without heart disease. The study, known as the Framingham Heart Study, found conclusively that diet and emotional stress play an important role in determining whether or not an individual will suffer from heart disease. These findings have brought the medical community to another level of awareness of how nutrition and stress influence the pathology of disease. So it seems that conventional medicine is slowly making its way back to a more holistic view of disease and health. But until medical school curricula put more emphasis on these lifestyle factors, most of today's Western physicians remain ill equipped to diagnose and treat vital factors that contribute to chronic disease.

Approach to Headache

Based in the concept that health is the absence of disease, conventional Western medicine aims to reverse or eliminate disease or symptoms. This approach is often described as *allopathic*—which means a system of treating disease that is antagonistic to the disease process. For example, to treat infection (caused by microbes), doctors prescribe antimicrobials. For viruses we recommend antiviral agents. And so on—you get the idea. Often this approach mandates use of aggressive methods that are invasive or toxic to the body. When considering a certain treatment, physicians evaluate its "risk-to-benefit ratio": Are the benefits worth the potentially toxic effects of this powerful treatment? It is not difficult to see that when potent weapons are being used against disease, doctors want to make certain that they've made an accurate diagnosis.

In the case of chronic headache, an accurate diagnosis is not easily ascertained. In general we can feel a source of our pain. If we scrape our knees, we feel pain in the knees. But with headache the source of pain is often less obvious. Ironically the pain that causes headache rarely originates from inside the brain. (Uncommon exceptions include *organic* causes of headache, such as brain tumors, bleeding from stroke or trauma, and meningitis, to be discussed in Chapter 2.) The brain itself is numb to pain—it does not contain nerve endings. Rather it *perceives* pain signals transmitted by nerve endings from the muscles, blood vessels, and tissue around the skull, the face, and other parts of the body. Headache is a common symptom of many underlying conditions, ranging from muscle tightness and hormonal imbalances to sensitivities to food and other environmental substances, as we'll discover in the next few chapters.

The diagnosis of headache also stumps medical doctors because, unlike many other conditions, there are no specific diagnostic tests for chronic headache. If you have an ulcer, for example, there are tests available to confirm its diagnosis. But the mechanisms of chronic headache seem to evade detection by available medical tests. And because headache pain can derive from so many sources, the symptoms are not very specific. As many of you are all too well aware, headache sufferers often go from doctor to doctor, and from test to test, without finding a medical explanation for the source of their pain.

There are several theories about the mechanisms of the different types of chronic headache, but experts have not reached a consensus. Recently for example, research has revealed that the neurotransmitter *serotonin* could play a central role in the development of migraine. Serotonin is a naturally occurring amine which, among other functions, transmits pain messages in the brain. As a result several new drugs have been designed to counteract the presumed dysfunction in serotonin.

In the treatment of other types of chronic headache—cluster and tension-type headache—the target of treatment is less well defined, as you will see in Chapter 2. Not knowing the specific cause of pain, doctors cannot prescribe specific treatment; instead we recommend ways to reduce the primary symptom—pain. It is not a cure but a relief of symptoms.

Traditional Oriental Medicine

Background

As with many holistic disciplines, the goal of traditional Oriental medicine is to stimulate the body's own healing abilities rather than treat specific diseases.

Many of the practices that evolved from theories of Oriental medicine—including acupuncture, acupressure, qigong, nutrition, and herbal treatments—date back more than five thousand years. These techniques have their roots in the same concept: Pain and disease emerge when there is an obstruction in the free flow of life energy, known as *chi* or *qi* (pronounced ''chee'') and of ''Blood'' and ''Body fluids.'' It is the power of qi that moves Blood and Body Fluids, with all their nutrients, through the body. It is the force of qi that connects everything we do and feel—our physical actions, thoughts, and emotions. In traditional thought qi is the foundation for all life.

The medical concepts guiding Oriental medicine are an extension of a broader spiritual cosmology of *Tao* (pronounced "dow"). Tao is "the Way of nature," the intrinsic order of the universe, which is expressed as the balance of the polar but complementary forces of yin and yang. The harmonious workings of the universe, including everything in it from planetary movement to the functioning of the smallest human cell, rely on a balance of yin and yang.

In Taoist philosophy the qualities of yang are dry, active, and hot— the creative, "heaven," action. Yin is wet, passive, and cold—the receptive, "earth," matter.

Yet, according to Taoist theory, these forces are interdependent. Yang does not exist without yin, and vice versa. Yang is the force that moves and motivates yin. Yin nurtures and anchors yang. Health is the balance of yin and yang as modulated by qi. These characteristics have meaning for every aspect of health; different parts of the body are predominantly yin or yang; foods, climates, activities, and herbs have yin and yang qualities—and can be prescribed to help restore harmony to physical imbalances.

The interplay of yin and yang is constant; matter is continually transforming to energy, and energy to matter. One can see how this works in daily life: The more energy we expend, the more physical weight we lose. Similarly when we expend too much energy—emotionally or physically—we become depleted and ill. The goal of traditional Oriental medicine is to maintain a healthful balance.

One can also see how traditional Oriental medicine views all aspects of our beings as part of an integrated continuum, with no single part playing more important a role than the other.

Approach to Pain

Oriental medicine maintains that, in the body, qi is yang; it is the life force. Its tendency is to rise upward. Qi circulates through the body by way of twelve invisible main *meridians* or *channels*. Any imbalance of qi—due to a blockage, deficiency, or excess—can result in pain.

The twelve meridians are all connected to a major organ and are named after that organ. The meridians traverse the body from foot to hand, crossing over the self-named organ. It should be noted that problems related to the bladder meridian, for example, do not necessarily mean you have a bladder problem. They are names to describe the channel of energy that connects with that organ—and its function. The bodywide function of an organ confers greater importance than the organ itself.

Yin Organs	Function
Heart	Governs blood
Liver	Controls movement of qi
Lungs	Governs breath and distributes qi
Kidneys	Governs reproductive system and bones; stores qi
Pericardium	Protects heart—from emotions and other factors
Spleen	Governs all other organs and transforms fluids to nutrients

Yang Organs	Function
Bladder	Helps kidney; distributes fluids
Colon (large intestine)	Governs waste; absorbs nutrients
Gallbladder	Helps liver; stores waste
Small Intestine	Governs change, aiding heart and digestive system
Stomach	Stores and distributes qi to the spleen
Triple Heater (Triple Burner)	Controls heat, protects other organs

Approach to Headache

According to traditional Chinese medicine, the diagnosis of headache involves identifying the part of the head that hurts, which in turn is linked with *pairs of meridians.* Pain results when the flow of qi is impaired in the meridian. In general this happens for one of three reasons: due to a *blockage* of qi, an *excess,* or a *deficiency.* Both blockage and excess may cause pain due to an imbalance in the accumulation of qi in the meridians. Deficiency, on the other hand, causes a narrowing or breakdown of the meridian, which can also result in pain. Each circumstance can be caused by a variety of mechanisms. For example headache could be caused by a blockage resulting from allergies (referred to as *Wind Evil* invasions). Excess may result from congestion of qi caused by emotional upsets and stress. Deficiency can produce headaches related to hunger or fatigue (in this case the body has literally used up too much energy without being refueled). These are just a few examples. Because Oriental medicine maintains that every part of the body is interdependent, the ways in which qi can become imbalanced are many.

A variety of methods are used to free the flow of qi in the body, including dietary approaches (page 106), acupuncture (page 163), acupressure (page 173), qigong (page 182), and herbal therapies (page 298).

Nutritional and Environmental Medicine

Background

Egyptian records of dietary cures for diseases date back to 1500 B.C. Hippocrates put great emphasis on diet as a way to prevent or ease illness. And certainly many ancient traditional systems of medicine, such as Oriental medicine and Ayurveda, focus on the importance of diet in maintaining health.

Over the past four centuries nutritional research has isolated many of the vitamins, minerals, and other nutrients (referred to as *micronutrients*) found in foods that are indispensable to life—and deficiencies of which lead to disease.

Nutritional and environmental medicine share a few guiding principles. Both are health disciplines based on the belief that substances (chemicals, foods, and inhalants in the environment) are primary causes of many health problems—and that removing these "stressors" can relieve symptoms. Both assert that a substance that causes symptoms in one person may not produce problems in another, and that each individual has a unique susceptibility *threshold* to different substances. For some people who are very sensitive, intolerant, or actually allergic to a specific substance, their threshold, or their ability to cope with the "toxic load," may be very low. It will take very little of that substance to cause a reaction. In addition one substance can cause different symptoms in different individuals. Furthermore the effects of environmental or dietary toxicity can be cumulative; you might not react immediately to low-level toxicity but may reach a point where your body can no longer cope with the accumulated toxicity. Headache is a common response to internal or external stressors.

Approach to Headache

Many traditional and newer complementary therapies emphasize good nutrition as a fundamental step in preventing and treating illness. But modern Western medical research has also confirmed the roles of many environmental and dietary *triggers* of headache. It is apparent that at least some people are genetically predisposed to having a lower threshold to headache, and react to certain foods or changes in the environment. In many individuals, stress- or disease-related deficiencies in important vitamins or minerals, such as magnesium, may set off a cascade of biochemical events that lead to headache. There is some evidence that headaches can be due exclusively to allergies. We'll discuss these factors in more detail in Chapter 3.

Mind-Body Methods

Background

The idea that the mind, or consciousness, exerts a powerful influence over physical health has been central to almost every traditional healing system. Most complementary healing methods are based on the concept that the mind and body are part of an integrated whole and that each has the power to affect the other.

Evidence of the mind-body connection abounds in recent medical literature. Studies have shown significant health benefits among people who focus their beliefs and wishes on healing—through meditation, prayer, psychotherapy, and other methods.

Recent research in people with multiple personalities vividly illustrates the power of the mind to influence the body. Candace Pert, Ph.D., biochemist at the Center for Molecular and Behavioral Neuroscience at Rutgers University, reveals that some people with multiple personalities have specific physical signs and symptoms that change with each personality.[1] For example one personality might be diabetic and have insulin levels that reflect the disease; a short time later a different personality emerges without any abnormalities. Did this individual *will* the change in insulin levels to match her desired personality—or did the insulin levels change due to the emotional stress of her condition, as is often seen in people with diabetes? Either way the implication of these results is that the individual exerts profound biochemical changes that have a source either in the subconscious will or in the emotions or both.

The placebo effect is a more commonplace example of the mind-body connection. A placebo is a substance or procedure without any inherent therapeutic value. It is literally translated as "to please." In studies of many diseases, including headache, about one third of people taking placebo treatments show improvement.[2] The placebo effect points again to the power of an individual's belief in or desire for a specific response. In spite of these dramatic and widespread results, the modern Western medical community is generally dismissive of the placebo's therapeutic value. But viewed from a holistic standpoint, it is eloquent testimony of the power of the mind to affect, or even heal, the body.

There is also growing scientific evidence to support the concept of a biochemical basis for emotion. For example research shows that groups of amino acids known as *peptides* act as the biochemical messengers communicating important information from one body system to another. Dr. Pert's studies suggest that peptides and their receptors are biochemical units of emotions, which serve as the elusive link between the mind and the physical body[3] (*Healing and the Mind,* Doubleday).

But even Dr. Pert is dissatisfied with modern science's tendency to reduce this mind-body connection to a string of amino acids. The ability of mental stimuli to generate spontaneous and simultaneous body-wide responses still defies physiological or biochemical explanation—and suggests that the mind's domain straddles both the physical plane, with responses that can be measured, and a nonphysical plane, where responses cannot yet be measured.

In spite of accumulating clinical support for the effectiveness of the mind in healing the body, conventional Western medicine remains skeptical of this approach.

Arguably most holistic health approaches—from Ayurveda to yoga—would appear to be mind-body therapies. But in Chapter 8 we focus on methods that work directly with the mind to cope with physical problems. The following mind-body approaches will be discussed:

- Autogenic training
- Biofeedback
- Guided imagery and visualization
- Hypnosis
- Meditation
- Prayer
- Progressive relaxation
- Psychotherapy (behavior therapy and cognitive restructuring)
- Reiki
- Therapeutic Touch

Approach to Headache

The approach to pain in general, or headache specifically, depends on the mind-body technique. Overall, most methods have been shown to induce relaxation. The *relaxation response* is a term coined by Herbert Benson, M.D., in the late 1960s to describe a series of complex, healthful biochemical reactions that result from reduced stress.[4] Benson, and others, suggest that an overactive nervous system is at the root of many diseases and that relaxation helps the body to retune the nervous system.

However, some mind-body methods go beyond the general relaxation response. Through biofeedback, for example, the headache sufferer not only benefits from overall relaxation but can learn to willfully alter specific mechanisms of headache, such as constricted blood vessels, that normally cannot be consciously changed.

Physical Approaches

Background

As we just discussed, most alternative approaches embrace the idea that the body and mind are parts of an integrated whole and that imbalances in either part will affect our health. In this way the physical approaches we'll discuss in this book are similar to mind-body approaches. Physical approaches differ, however, in their focus on the body as the main tool for change (as opposed to mind-body approaches, which mainly engage the mind to effect changes in the body).

The spectrum of physical approaches ranges from those that work almost exclusively to correct presumed structural misalignments (such as chiropractic and osteopathy) to methods which intimately connect physical activities with conscious awareness (such as Rolfing, Alexander Technique and Feldenkrais Method). Also, the traditional systems of medicine, such as Ayurveda and traditional Oriental medicine, maintain that chronic headaches, like other illness, derive from an imbalance in the flow of vital life energy, which can be corrected by physical interventions, such as yoga, breathing, acupuncture, and so on.

Approach to Headache

Some traditional and modern physical approaches have developed specific therapeutic tools aimed at directly relieving specific conditions, such as headache. These include chiropractic, osteopathy, craniosacral therapy, massage, as well as traditional Oriental techniques such as acupressure, acupuncture, qigong, shiatsu (and related therapies), and Myotherapy.

With other physical approaches, relief of headache or other symptoms comes as a secondary benefit from work on the entire body. The relief of chronic muscle contractions—and a newfound awareness of how postural or emotional "habits" create that tension—helps reduce or eliminate pain that results from stresses in the muscles and/or connective tissues. Methods based on this concept include Alexander Technique, Feldenkrais, Trager Psychophysical Integration, and PhysicalMind Therapy, among others.

In Chapter 7 we'll look more closely at these and other approaches, and how they can help relieve headache.

Botanical Remedies

Background

The word *drug* has its roots in the German *drooge,* which means "dry"—and has been historically applied to describe any dried plant used for therapeutic (or harmful) effect. Plants have been used for thousands of years by healers in almost every culture for healing disease. Many of the drugs used today have been synthesized from plants. The medicine-chest standby, aspirin, for example, was originally derived from willow bark. New drugs are currently being developed based on botanical substances.

Today there is a revived interest in the traditional use of plants in their many forms—dried into tablets (Chinese herbs), diluted in water or alcohol (homeopathy and Bach Flower Remedies), infused or decocted for teas (herbal remedies), or distilled to pure essential oils for massage and diffusion into the air (aromatherapy). Though the beneficial effects of many herbs were discovered by trial and error, ongoing research has been under way to scientifically "prove" their biochemical effects.

Why use herbs instead of drugs? Many herbalists believe that plants contain nutrients that enable the body to better ingest the active ingredient, with fewer side effects. They are "whole" foods with multiple, complementary nutritional and healing properties. In theory, plants (properly prepared) constitute a gentler, more adaptable form of the active ingredient. Susun Weed, author of many books about herbalism, says that "herbalists see the whole herb, the physical forces and the subtle forces, and respect this wholeness . . . using it as a whole, not dividing it into parts and seeing power only in the 'active' principle."[5] (*Healing Wise,* Ash Tree).

Beware: Herbs are not by definition safe. While they may be natural, and perhaps *safer* than most drugs, they should still be considered potent chemicals. At high doses, or when used carelessly, some herbs can cause serious side effects. They should be prepared and taken with great care, especially by children and pregnant women and by people with coexisting conditions such as heart, kidney, or liver disease.

Approach to Headache

Some herbs are prescribed for immediate relief of symptoms, while others can be taken over long periods to gently regenerate the body's own healing abilities. Often an herb will be recommended to treat an underlying problem that is causing headache.

In Chapter 9 we will review specific botanical approaches to headache, including herbal medicine and aromatherapy. We will look at homeopathy in Chapter 10.

Macrobiotics

Background

Most people view macrobiotics as a way of eating, but it is much more: For many it is a way of life rooted in an all-embracing and complex cosmology devised first by George Ohsawa, a protégé of the Japanese physician Sagen Ishikuzuka in the early 1900s. Ohsawa espoused a traditional Japanese diet of brown rice, miso soup, and sea vegetables. His teachings were interpreted by Michio Kushi, who brought them to the United States in the 1970s. The practices that arise from this belief system focus strongly on dietary measures, but also embrace other lifestyle factors.

According to macrobiotic belief, everything in the universe is in a state of flux. At the center of this action is infinity (God, Universal Will, Spirit, etc.), which is pure motion directed outward in all directions. The motion creates currents that intersect, causing contraction (*yang* force) and expansion (*yin* force). The world is a symphony of interacting yang and yin, and each living being manifests some qualities of both. By learning how yang and yin relate to each other, we can begin to understand the workings of life itself, according to macrobiotic thought. (Because an explanation of macrobiotic cosmology is beyond the scope of this book, we refer those who are interested to the ''Resources'' section beginning on page 340 for further reading. However, it isn't necessary to embrace the spiritual aspects of macrobiotic thought in order to benefit physically.)

Every muscle and organ in our body expresses tendencies of both yang and yin. When moving inward in a *yang,* or contracting, direction energy increases in speed, heightens in temperature, and becomes denser and heavier. When moving in a *yin,* or expanding, direction, energy is cooler, more expanded, and lighter. Our heart, lungs, blood vessels, and even our brains contract (yang) and expand (yin) to maintain life.

At the same time, each part embodies its own distinct combination of yang and yin. For example, compared with other body parts the head is comparatively dense and compact—it is structurally yang. Yet it functions with less motion than other body organs; thus energy-wise it is more yin. On the other hand, the heart is comparatively hollow and light; it is yin in structure. But the heart's energy is ceaseless and therefore more yang. The challenge in living a healthy life is to maintain a balance of yang and yin. One of the most effective ways of meeting this challenge is through proper diet, which will be discussed in more detail in Chapter 6.

Approach to Headache

From the macrobiotic point of view, imbalances of yang and yin in one part of the body produce biochemical changes that result in symptoms of pain in the head.

As mentioned, the head, in general, is yang in structure: compact and dense. The torso and extremities, the complementary opposite of the head, are more yin: rounder and more expansive. However, some *parts* of the head are more yin, others are more yang. For example the front of the head is more yin than the back. An overconsumption of yin foods, such as sugar or fruit, could therefore be the cause of a headache in your forehead or eyes. An excess of yang foods, such as protein-rich meats and legumes, might result in pain in the back of the head.

Although the underlying principles of macrobiotics are relatively straightforward, the interplay of influencing factors can be complex and highly individualized. For these reasons it is often helpful to consult a macrobiotic counselor who will help you evaluate your unique needs.

Ayurveda

Background

Ayurveda is a science from India that is over six thousand years old. The word comes from the Sanskrit *ayus* ("life") and *veda* ("knowledge"—or the science of life). It is so-called because it emerged from the deep contemplations of *rishis,* or seers. According to Ayurvedic history, the rishis intuited the teachings from the cosmic consciousness. In its current form, Ayurvedic medicine is the result of a strong master-student tradition where information is carefully tested and recorded.

Ayurvedic philosophy holds that all consciousness is energy, and all energy is expressed as five primary elements: Ether, Air, Fire, Water, and Earth. In the beginning the world was pure consciousness. Very subtle vibrations in consciousness produced Ether, or space. As Ether moved, Air was created—and from the friction of that ethereal movement came heat and Fire. The heat of Fire liquefied Ether, producing Water, and solidified into Earth. And, finally, from Earth, all organic life was born.

All matter, including humankind, embodies the five basic elements, which influence different functions. In different combinations, the five elements express themselves in humans as three different bio-energies, or *doshas,* known collectively as *tridoshas.*

- Vata = ether and air
- Pitta = fire and water
- Kapha = earth and water

The tridoshas describe categories that regulate biological and psychological functions of the body. In health the tridoshas are in balance; conversely all physical expressions of disease are caused by an imbalance of these three doshas. Each individual manifests different proportions of vata, pitta, and kapha—and everyone can be described as being constitutionally one or the other. No person is made up solely of any single dosha, but is a combination of all three. To determine your dosha, or bio-type, you can seek out an Ayurvedic physician or take a bio-type test. Hans H. Rhyner, in his book *Ayurveda: The Gentle Healing System,* has compiled the one that appears below.

Ayurvedic Bio-Type (Dosha) Test

Check off the appropriate answer for each question. Afterward, add up the ones you marked in each column. Your bio-type is the column that has the most number of answers checked.

	Vata	Pitta	Kapha
Do you tend to be	Underweight	Ideal with good muscles	Overweight
Is your frame	Small-boned	Normal	Large-boned
Are you	Very short	Normal	Small and stout
	Very tall	Medium height	Large and stout
Are your hips	Narrow	Medium	Wide
Are your shoulders	Narrow	Medium	Wide
Is your chest	Flat	Normally developed	Fully developed
Is your hair	Normal	Balding, prematurely gray	Full
Has your face	Irregular features	Prominent features	Round features
Are your eyes	Small	Medium	Large
	Dry	Red	Moist
Is your nose	Small	Medium	Large
	Small, long	Straight, pointed	Wide
Are your lips	Small, rather dark	Medium, red, soft	Wide, velvety
Are your teeth	Not straight	Medium, straight	Large, straight
Are your fingers	Small, long	Regular	Wide, angular
Are your nails	Brittle	Soft	Strong, thick
Are your feet	Small, narrow	Medium	Large, wide
Are your hands and feet	Cold, dry	Warm, pink	Cool, damp
Is your skin	Dry	Freckled	Soft and smooth
	Brownish	Radiant	Light, white
Are your veins	Easily visible	Evenly distributed	Not visible
Where is your fat	Around the waist	Evenly distributed	Around thighs and buttocks
Are you	Hyperactive	Active	Somewhat lethargic
Do you walk	Rather fast	Normally	Rather slowly

	Vata	**Pitta**	**Kapha**
Is your sleep	☐ Light and interrupted	☐ Short and even	☐ Long and deep
Is your thirst	☐ Variable	☐ Good	☐ Not noticeable
Is your appetite	☐ Variable	☐ Strong	☐ Moderate
Is your perspiration	☐ Sparse, odorless	☐ Heavy with a strong odor	☐ Heavy with a pleasant odor
Is the amount of your urine	☐ Little but frequent	☐ Normal but often	☐ Profuse, infrequent
Is your stool	☐ Hard, dark ☐ Constipation	☐ Loose, yellowish ☐ Diarrhea	☐ Soft, well formed
Is your creativity	☐ Distinct and rich in ideas	☐ Inventive and technical or scientific	☐ In the area of business
Is your memory	☐ Average	☐ Excellent	☐ Good
Is your decision-making ability	☐ Problematic	☐ Quick, decisive	☐ Well thought out
Is your speech	☐ Fast	☐ Loud	☐ Melodic
When handling money, are you	☐ Wasteful	☐ Methodical	☐ Thrifty
Are you	☐ Shy ☐ Nervous ☐ Insecure ☐ Intuitive	☐ Jealous ☐ Ambitious ☐ Egotistical ☐ Practical	☐ Solicitous ☐ Lethargic ☐ Self-satisfied ☐ Resilient
Is your sexual drive	☐ Extreme or the opposite	☐ Passionate and domineering	☐ Constant and loyal
Do you love	☐ Travel ☐ Art ☐ Esoteric subjects	☐ Sports ☐ Politics ☐ Luxury	☐ Quiet ☐ Business ☐ Good food
Do you dislike	☐ Cold, wind, and dryness	☐ Heat and midday sun	☐ Cold and dampness

From *Ayurveda: The Gentle Healing System*

Approach to Headache

Evaluation of the three doshas is the first step toward treating any physical, mental, or emotional problem. Diagnosis involves evaluating the tongue, feeling the pulse, and assessing other vital signs through a complex process known as *nadi vigyan*.

Dosha imbalance is just one factor evaluated by the Ayurvedic physician; mental issues, lifestyle, and the accumulation of toxins in the body tissues are also important. Headache could result from imbalances in one, or a combination, of these factors. Treatments include herbs, massage, yoga postures, meditation, dietary recommendations, and elimination therapies—all individually designed to improve both physical health and personal consciousness.

Extensive studies of the Ayurvedic practices have demonstrated their effectiveness in conditions ranging from high blood pressure to diabetes. In one recent study performed in Holland, 79 percent of people with chronic diseases, including headache and chronic sinusitis, showed improvement using a combination of Ayurvedic therapies.[6]

In North America today there are ten Ayurveda clinics; more than two hundred physicians have received training as Ayurvedic practitioners through the American Association of Ayurvedic Medicine. An estimated twenty-five thousand people have received Ayurvedic treatment since 1985.

Ayurveda is a complex, systematic medical discipline. We will try to address some of its general guidelines throughout Part II. But we refer interested readers to the "Resources" section for more information.

Naturopathy

Background

Naturopathy means "nature cure." It is an eclectic system of medicine that has beginnings tracing back to Hippocrates, sharing the Hippocratic view that the body has the ability to heal itself. The term *naturopathy* was first coined by the New York physician John Scheel, M.D., and the discipline formalized by Benedict Lust.

Lust described naturopathy as a natural system of curing disease that encompasses not only lifestyle habits but numerous healing approaches aimed at allowing the individual to thrive in a vital state of health, even in the face of environmental, physical, and mental stress.

This *vitalistic* approach to healing, as it is known, is shaped by the belief that the body has an innate intelligence that is always striving for health. Also, disease occurs not from outside influences but from the body's inability to defend itself against these invasive stressors (bacteria, toxins, etc.). And symptoms are seen as the body's natural way of coping with these stressors.

Like many modern alternative disciplines, naturopathy shares much with conventional medical approaches. Naturopathic practitioners are often up-to-date on new medical findings about disease processes, and make ample use of modern diagnostic technology. They diverge, however, in their philosophy of how to treat their "patients."

The naturopathic physician may employ a variety of natural therapies to help individuals prevent and cope with disease. Some specialize in a specific area, while others have skills in many areas. These therapeutic modalities include (but are not limited to) nutrition, homeopathy, botanical medicine, acupuncture, hydrotherapy, physiotherapy, minor surgery, and lifestyle counseling.

A visit to a naturopathic doctor involves a complete review of your medical history and questioning about your lifestyle.

Approach to Headache

As mentioned, the naturopathic physician may employ one or more of a variety of natural ways to prevent headache's recurrence, or to encourage the body to heal itself. For example naturopaths adhere to the theory governing scientific medicine today that migraine is caused by serotonin disorders. But rather than prescribe a drug, the naturopath will look into dietary factors (such as food allergy), chiropractic, relaxation, and other natural treatments that aim to stimulate the body's own healing abilities. In Part II, we'll look at these approaches in more detail.

CHAPTER 2

What Type of Headache Do You Have?

What a head have I!
It beats as it would fall
in twenty pieces.
—*WILLIAM SHAKESPEARE*, Romeo and Juliet

Headache is a general symptom for an astonishing variety of conditions. It can be pounding, stabbing, or dull. It can last minutes, hours, or days. Headaches may appear along with other symptoms. Usually people who have chronic headaches are all too familiar with the distinct patterns of their individual pain.

In this chapter we'll examine the major categories of headache as seen by Western medicine. Keep in mind that some headache symptoms may overlap with other disease symptoms, leading to possible misdiagnosis and, in the worst-case scenario, improper treatment. For example people with cluster headaches can also have nasal congestion, which may mistakenly lead to a diagnosis of sinus headache.

In the next few chapters of Part I we'll explore in depth some of the more common underlying causes for headache symptoms, such as diet, environment, and female hormonal imbalances. Many of these proposed mechanisms not only guide modern medical treatments but form the basis for alternative treatments as well. For example the idea that muscle tension causes some headache types gives credibility to physical approaches (see Chapter 7). The concept that emotional stress plays a role in headache helps us understand how relaxation and mind-body techniques work (Chapter 8). That certain foods or chemicals trigger headache in some people forms the rationale for nutritional or environmental medicine (Chapter 6). And so on.

Chronic head pain rarely occurs as an isolated event. People can have headache along with nausea, for example. For this reason some headache types are regarded as *syndromes*—groupings of symptoms that include headache. Taken on their own, many of these symptoms are *nonspecific,* meaning that they could be shared by other physical or psychological conditions. This is one reason why chronic headaches are often difficult to diagnose.

The first appearance of a severe headache can be a frightening event. Most doctors will first try to rule out the rare but potentially life-threatening causes (see below). These dangerous types of headache are part of a group of *organic* headaches, which account for less than 1 percent of headaches. Much more common are *nonorganic* headaches, or so-called *benign* headaches, which originate from conditions in other parts of the body that affect the muscles and blood vessels near the head, causing pain.

FIRST: RULE OUT DANGEROUS HEADACHES

Most of the chronic-headache types described in this chapter are not life-threatening. But sometimes a headache can signal a serious condition that requires immediate medical attention. If you have any of the symptoms described in the box on page 27, I strongly urge you to see your doctor or visit an emergency room as soon as possible.

Aneurysm Headache

Aneurysm is caused by a ballooning blood vessel that can burst and cause a headache. The pain is often severe, occurs very suddenly, and may be accompanied by neck stiffness, nausea, confusion, and/or loss of consciousness.

Brain Tumor

Brain tumors are very rare but potentially very serious. With brain tumors head pain becomes increasingly more severe and frequent over time. Other symptoms are more "diagnostic" of brain tumors, such as double vision, slurred speech, personality changes, seizures, and lack of coordination.

Head Injury

Headaches caused by head injury usually appear soon after the trauma. In rare cases, head pain may be due to hydrocephalus, which may appear weeks or months after injury. In some cases preexisting headaches become worse after a head injury.

Hypertension Headache

This type of headache usually announces itself in the morning by pain that has a throbbing quality of pressure. It usually occurs suddenly, and only in cases of very high blood pressure.

Lupus Headache

Systemic lupus erythematosus is an autoimmune disease; this means that the immune system mistakes the body's own tissues for foreign invaders, somewhat like an allergen, and launches an attack against it. There are many symptoms of lupus, depending on which part of the body is mistaken for being foreign. If the immune system targets tissues of the brain, or the muscles, blood vessels, or nerves near the head, these areas will become inflamed, and headache may result. More commonly, though, headache is one of lupus's many general symptoms; it can be a warning sign of an upcoming "flare" or be one of several flulike symptoms. It's estimated that up to 20 percent of people with systemic lupus suffer from chronic headaches, and up to 10 percent have migrainelike symptoms.[1]

Meningitis

Meningitis is caused by a bacterial or viral infection, which in turn causes inflammation of the *meninges,* or membranes surrounding the brain. Accompanying symptoms include a stiff neck, fever, and *photophobia* (sensitivity to light).

Temporal Arteritis

Temporal arteritis usually occurs only in people fifty years of age or older and is caused by inflammation of the large arteries, usually of the temporal, occipital, or ophthalmic arteries. The main symptom is a jabbing, throbbing, or burning pain felt around the ear, especially while chewing. The headache can be nonspecific, or accompanied by muscle aches, fatigue, and blurred vision.

Danger Signals: When to Call Your Doctor

The National Institute of Neurologic Disorders and Stroke recommends that you see a doctor if you have any of the following types of headache:

- Accompanied by confusion, unconsciousness, or convulsions
- Involving pain in the eye or ear
- Accompanied by fever or nausea
- Occurring after a blow to the head
- Accompanied by slurred speech, blurred vision, numbness, memory loss, or trouble walking
- Gets worse, lasts longer than usual, or changes
- Recurrent (especially in children)
- Persistent in someone normally free of headaches
- Interferes with normal life

While it is consoling at first to discover that your headache isn't life-threatening, this sense of relief is often quickly replaced by a sense of helplessness and frustration: What, then, is the cause of the headache? In the search for an answer, it's been estimated that people with migraine, for example, suffer up to eight years before finding an accurate diagnosis! Since there are no biological markers or tests for benign causes of headache, doctors rely on a patient history and reports of symptoms to reach a diagnosis. What follows in the next pages is a review of the major categories of headache.

MIGRAINE

Migraine has been part of recorded medical history for more than five thousand years. Though the word *migraine* is a French term, it traces back to the Greek *hemicrania* to describe one of migraine's distinguishing features: pain on one side (*hemi*) of the head (*cranium*). But anyone who has had migraines knows that head pain is just one of several symptoms that occur before or along with the headache and migraine pain is not always one-sided.

Migraine is most often a *syndrome* including one or more symptoms that either coexist or build progressively over time. For example many, but not all, people are warned of an impending headache by neurological (brain-related) disturbances called *auras*. Headache experts divide the migraine population into two major groups: those who have migraine with aura (once called *classic migraine*), and those who have migraine without aura (formerly *common migraine*). Only about 10 to 20 percent of migraine sufferers have auras.

Who Gets Migraine?

Migraine afflicts about twenty-three million Americans. Migraine is not selective based on wealth, fame, or intelligence. It has been known to plague such historical luminaries as Alexander Graham Bell, Julius Caesar, Virginia Woolf, Peter Tchaikovsky, and Queen Mary Tudor of

England. But migraine is gender-biased: Although men do get migraines, the vast majority (75%) of sufferers are women.

Migraine can begin as early as infancy. But symptoms in young children are often very *nonspecific*—expressing as nausea, vomiting or colic, or general malaise. Many very young children do not have headaches at all but exhibit other migraine symptoms (see Chapter 5). Mostly migraine and head pain start in young adulthood, with the first episode striking during the teenage years, peaking between twenty and thirty-five years of age and declining thereafter.

As mentioned, there are several types of migraine, the two major ones being migraine with aura and migraine without aura. The *aura* is a preheadache symptom characterized by visual or other sensory disturbances (see page 32).

Researchers believe that migraine sufferers inherit a genetic susceptibility to the disease: More than half of migraineurs have a family member with migraine. A gene for one rare form of migraine, *familial hemiplegic migraine,* has been found.

Migraine Without Aura (Common Migraine)

Migraine headache can be divided into three phases: the warning phase (known in medical parlance as *premonitory* or *prodromal* phase), the headache phase, and the resolution phase. Note: You may not have all of the symptoms described below.

Symptoms of Warning (Premonitory/Prodromal) Phase

It should be emphasized that many people don't have *prodromal symptoms*. But even if you don't experience a warning phase, you could still have migraine. Hours or days before the onset of a migraine you may have one or more of the following symptoms:

- Neck stiffness
- Shoulder tightness
- Drowsiness/yawning
- Speech problems
- Head congestion (teary eyes, stuffy and/or runny nose)

- Changes in appetite (less hungry; cravings for sweets)
- Mood changes and mood swings (irritated, anxious, depressed, elated)
- Sensitivity to light and sound
- Vague, undefinable feeling that a migraine is coming on

Headache Phase

LOCATION OF HEAD PAIN

- Usually located on one side of the head; but the side can change from attack to attack
- Pain may begin on one side of the head, then spread to the entire head

QUALITY OF HEAD PAIN

- Throbbing, pulsating
- Moderate-to-severe and often incapacitating
- Made worse by physical activity, light, noise, or odors

DURATION OF PAIN

- Lasts between four and seventy-two hours (untreated), but can last longer
- May last less than four hours in children

OTHER CHARACTERISTICS
Other symptoms seen in many people include one or several of the following:

- Nausea
- Vomiting
- Diarrhea
- Feeling of being cold

- High sensitivity to light and sound—the tendency is to lie down in a dark, quiet room

Some people may also experience one or more of these symptoms during the headache phase of a migraine:

- Dizziness
- Pallor
- Faintness
- Palpitations (rapid heartbeat)
- Sweating

Resolution Phase
The following symptoms often occur after the headache subsides:

- Feeling "washed out"
- Changes in mood and/or appetite
- Soreness of the scalp
- Fatigue
- Depression
- Sense of well-being

Pattern of Pain
Many people with migraines feel headache symptoms first thing in the morning. When the headache occurs at night or in the very early morning, it can be severe enough to wake you up from a deep sleep.

For some people migraines are brought on with regularity due to hormonal changes (PMS, birth control pills, menopause), exposure to certain foods or environmental factors, or emotional stress (see "Common Migraine Triggers," page 36). For others migraines have their own mysterious schedules, without any known trigger.

Migraine with Aura (Classic Migraine)

With the exception of the aura, the symptoms of the headache and resolution phases are the same as those just described. The aura occurs between the warning and headache phases of the migraine—ten minutes to an hour before the onset of headache. If it lasts longer or occurs for the first time, a physician must be consulted; it might indicate a stroke or other serious condition.

Aura is thought to be a neurological phenomenon, which means that it has to do with the nervous system. Though auras are more likely to build progressively, they are also known to come on all at once. The term *aura* (which means "wind") is used to describe visual disturbances and disturbances of other sensory faculties.

Visual Disturbances

The visual disturbances, which comprise 75 percent of auras, can assume a variety of forms:

- Flashing lights
- Sparkles, spots, or stars
- Zigzag patterns that "break up" the images in your visual field
- Distortion of object size or shape
- Blind spots

Sensory Disturbances

Other disturbances, in addition to visual disturbances or on their own, can also occur:

- Weakness or numbness on one side of the body
- Confusion
- Dizziness
- Difficulty speaking

Causes of Migraine—Nature or Nurture?

Conventional Western medicine considers migraine a distinct disease, with its own set of physical causes. But the medical community cannot agree on the nature of these causes.

We do know that migraines often run in families. If you get migraines, the chances are 50 to 75 percent that someone in your family has had them as well. But people don't inherit migraine in the same way they inherit hemophilia or sickle-cell anemia, for example. With the latter diseases there's a specific genetic link—and there are genetic and laboratory tests to confirm a family pattern. With migraine there are no laboratory tests, and symptoms are not all that specific, making it difficult to trace generation-to-generation migraine patterns. Also a migraine "gene" has yet to be definitely identified, except for the rare form of *familial hemiplegic migraine*. What seems to operate genetically with migraine is the tendency to pass down a physical *susceptibility,* perhaps a combination of genetic factors.

Lacking the discovery of a migraine gene, the question arises whether this susceptibility is nature or nurture. It's possible that some people inherit migraine as a physical response to emotionally stressful situations, in the same way that we take on our family's mannerisms, habits, or ways of coping with tension.

Whether migraine is genetically inherited or socially acquired (or both), the question remains, How does migraine happen in the body? Why do some people suffer from migraine even without a family history? Currently several theories hold sway, and are described below. Some alternative medical disciplines and healing practices uphold these theories; others, such as traditional Oriental medicine, macrobiotic approaches, and Ayurvedic medicine espouse different views, which are touched on in Chapter 1, and discussed further in Part II.

Vascular (*Blood Vessel*) Theories

The idea that migraine is caused by changes in blood vessel activity dates back to the 1600s and is still considered valid today. The theory contends that the aura results from spasm of blood vessels in the *occipital* lobe of the brain, located at the back of the brain, near the base of the skull. This constriction causes visual disturbances because these blood vessels carry blood to the visual cortex, located in the occipital lobe.

After the aura-causing spasm (which doesn't happen in all people with migraine), there is a period of *dilation*—an opening and swelling—of the blood vessels around the scalp and face. Pain results from nerve irritation due to swelling of the blood vessels and inflammation around the vessels; the throbbing nature of migraine pain is attributed to the flow of blood through the sensitized blood vessels.

The Serotonin Theory

Platelets are disk-shaped cells responsible mainly for clotting blood. These cells store *serotonin*. As a *neurotransmitter,* a natural chemical that sends messages to the brain and nervous system, serotonin helps regulate pain messages and causes blood vessels to constrict.

Serotonin is stored in platelets and is released by platelet *aggregation* (gathering, or clumping). Some studies show that the platelets of people with migraines have a greater tendency to clump, and in this way release higher-than-normal amounts of serotonin. After being released from platelets, serotonin finds its way to *receptors*—the ultimate destination for serotonin-carried information. At this point we know that serotonin receptors are found in three different places:

- Blood vessels in the brain.
- Nerve cells in certain parts of the brain and throughout the body.
- Nerve endings that surround the blood vessels at the base of the brain (the *trigeminovascular system*). The trigeminal nerves, as we will see below, transmit pain messages in the head and face to the brain.

Proponents of the serotonin theory, which is related to the vascular theory, believe that the release of serotonin is responsible for the vasoconstriction that occurs during the aura phase of migraine.

People with migraine are twice as likely to also have a condition known as *mitral valve prolapse*—a malfunction of the mitral valve in the heart—which is thought to increase platelet aggregation and damage.

The Neural (or Neurogenic) Theory

Neurogenic means "originating from the nerves." This theory maintains that blood vessels *inside* the brain become stimulated by the *trigeminovascular system,* which includes two *trigeminal* nerves at the brain stem. These nerves transmit a sensation of pain from the head and face to the brain. Irritation of the nerves or blood vessels of the head or face triggers a release of chemicals (substance P, a peptide that aids in transmitting pain signals, is an important player) that cause inflammation of the blood vessels, irritation of the trigeminal nerves, and pain.

The Unifying Theory

As its name implies, the unifying theory brings the preceding concepts together to explain the symptoms of migraine.

The belief here is that the migraine syndrome begins with electrical changes in the brain that affect the trigeminovascular system. The electrical changes happen after a repeated onslaught of stressing factors— emotional or physical. When the body can't take the stress anymore, these electrical changes trigger a cascade of biochemical events—platelet clumping, serotonin release, and contraction of the blood vessels— leading to inflammation of the vessels and a lowering of blood flow to the brain. The body reacts by opening blood vessels and releasing pain mediators.

Some researchers also think that there's a part of the population with a problem metabolizing serotonin, which is responsible for the release of chemicals that contribute to vascular and nerve inflammation. These same people are prone not only to migraine but to other serotonin-related disorders, such as depression and irritable bowel syndrome (IBS).

Magnesium Depletion

Recent studies indicate that *magnesium depletion*—that is, having lower-than-normal levels of the mineral magnesium—can influence serotonin and nitric oxide release, blood vessel size, and inflammation. Indeed it might be the common denominator for all theories. In our studies, we estimated that 50 percent of people with migraine are magnesium-deficient. It's also thought that people with mitral valve prolapse have lower-than-normal levels of magnesium.

Several studies have shown that magnesium depletion plays a critical role in blood vessel size. It seems not only to cause blood vessel constriction but to make blood vessels *more* sensitive to other chemicals that cause constriction and *less* sensitive to substances that cause blood vessels to dilate.

Studies have also shown that magnesium depletion seems to help release serotonin from its storage sites. It also helps make blood vessels in the brain more receptive to serotonin and thus clears the way for serotonin to cause constriction of blood vessels.

As we will see in Chapters 3 and 6, based on some of my studies and studies by other scientists, replacing magnesium has been shown to have a very positive effect on migraine symptoms in some people.

Common Migraine Triggers

If migraine is inherited, why don't all people experience symptoms most of the time like people with other inherited diseases, such as sickle-cell anemia? Part of the answer may be that a susceptibility to migraine leaves the body vulnerable to stresses that trigger a migraine attack. Another answer may be that headache is the physical expression of reaction to dietary or environmental factors. Some allergists, environmental doctors, and holistic practitioners believe that up to 90 percent of all migraine headaches are caused by allergies or multiple sensitivities to food products or other substances. We'll explore these in more depth in Chapter 3, but for now, see the table below for a brief review of headache triggers.

Keep in mind that your headache may be triggered by one or more of the following substances—but probably not all of them!

HORMONAL FACTORS (ALSO SEE CHAPTER 5)

PMS
Ovulation
Menstruation
Pregnancy (first trimester)
Birth control pills (estrogen)
Menopause (decreases in estrogen, use of estrogen replacement therapy) either naturally, or due to surgery

DIETARY FACTORS (ALSO SEE CHAPTER 3)

Alcohol (especially darker beverages, such as red wine, beer, or scotch versus white wine or vodka)
Foods containing tyramine (aged cheeses, red wine, pickled foods, figs, yogurt, freshly baked bread, bananas)
Food allergies
Sugar
Aspartame (artificial sweetener found in NutraSweet)
Food additives (e.g., nitrites, amines, benzoic acid tartrazine, and MSG)
Tobacco
Caffeine
Chocolate
Yeast
Spices
Corn
Brewer's yeast (also found in some vitamins)
High doses of vitamins, particularly vitamin A
Fasting or skipping meals

ENVIRONMENTAL FACTORS (ALSO SEE CHAPTER 4)

Environmental allergies (sick building syndrome, pollutants)
Carbon dioxide and other pollutants
Toxins in building materials (such as formaldehyde in wood treatments)
Changes in weather, time zone, sleeping patterns
Bright, flickering fluorescent lights
Certain odors (e.g., specific perfumes)
Noise
Emotional and physical stress
Cigarette smoke

Other Types of Migraine

There is also a category known as migraine equivalents (in medical-ese, *acephalgic migraine*) with many symptoms of migraine, but without headache. Other migraine types include:

- Hemiplegic migraine (difficulty moving one side of the body)
- Ophthalmoplegic migraine (double vision, inability to fully move eyes)
- Retinal migraine (periodic vision loss or darkening of the visual field)
- Basilar migraine (double vision, vertigo, faintness and incoordination)

Diagnosis of Migraine

Because there is no specific test for migraine, the diagnosis of this syndrome is based on a history of your symptoms, family history, and general physical examination. Since the symptoms are often nonspecific, it's very important to be as clear as possible when describing your symptoms to avoid misdiagnosis.

Headache and the Brain

The brain plays a central role in the Western view of migraine. Here are some brain basics to help you better understand how some headaches happen.

The brain resides within the protective cavity of the *cranium,* or skull. The spinal cord connects to the brain and is contained in the *vertebrae*—the backbones along the spine—through an opening at the base of the brain. The skull is made of bone, is covered with layers of muscle and skin, and is richly endowed with a web of blood vessels and nerves. These nerves give the muscles surrounding the skull the ability to feel sensations—pain, touch, and temperature.

The brain itself is made up of billions of cells called *neurons,* which exchange electrical signals in the brain. Many of the cells are programmed to serve specific functions. Neurotransmitters are messengers between cells that initiate electrical currents. Serotonin, nitric oxide, and other amines—ammonia-based, naturally occurring substances—are among the most crucial neurotransmitters.

Motor cells transmit messages for movement, *sensory cells* control physical feelings, and so on. These and other important cells are often grouped together in the brain to facilitate their functions. These functions are either spurred on or slowed down by other cells—they're engaged in a complex and continuous *feedback* system throughout the brain and the rest of the body.

Within the skull are two halves of the brain—the left and the right cerebral hemispheres. Both sit on a short pipe of brain tissue known as the *brain stem.* The brain stem is control-central for the body's automatic life functions such as breathing, heartbeat, and blood pressure, as well as hearing and eyesight and general consciousness. This is why, in trauma accidents, damage to the brain stem is often the cause of coma.

Cranial nerves from the head travel through the brain stem upward to the brain. These cranial nerves transmit motor and sensory information to the head, face, eye, and mouth muscles in the head.

Leading downward from the brain stem is the spinal cord, which extends down the back and is protected by the bones of the vertebrae; it is further encased by tissues called the *meninges,* as well as muscles and ligaments. Nerves that exit and enter the spinal cord are called *peripheral* nerves, which connect up with nerves throughout the body.

The nerves that are especially important to headache include:

- *Trigeminal nerves,* which are a pair of cranial nerves. They are mostly sensory nerves that transmit feelings from parts of the face and scalp, and from the meninges of the brain.
- *Cervical nerves,* or nerves of the neck. They carry feelings

from the neck and back of the head to the spinal cord and into the brain.

Under certain, not very well understood, conditions, pain felt in one part of the head can originate from the neck and other parts of the head. This phenomenon, known as *referred* pain, helps explain the pain in the head associated with dental problems or with muscle tension in the neck and shoulders.

The spaces, or cavities, in the head can also be the source of pain. The sinus cavities can cause head pain when they are inflamed or infected and filled with fluid. Similarly the spaces inside and between the cerebral hemispheres, known as the *ventricles,* house cerebrospinal fluid, which helps nourish and protect brain tissue—so changes in the amount or composition of fluid circulating around the brain can also cause head pain, as is sometimes the case with vitamin A overdose.

TENSION-TYPE HEADACHE

Tension-type headache is also known as "muscle contraction" headache, or simply, tension headache. Other names include "psychogenic" headache and "stress" headache. The current name came from new theories about the causes of tension-type headaches.

As the name implies, tension-type headache is thought to be brought on by muscular or emotional tension. But recent studies show that abnormalities in the brain's biochemistry may also play a part, as they do with migraine. Also the symptoms of tension-type headache and those of migraine often overlap. We'll examine these factors in more detail in the following sections.

There are two main categories of tension-type headache: *chronic* and *episodic.* Chronic headache symptoms are very disruptive and happen persistently, almost every day for weeks or years. Episodic headache symptoms are not as prolonged as they are in chronic headache.

Who Gets Tension-Type Headaches?

Tension-type headache is the most common of headache varieties. Some people have bouts of both migraine and tension headaches. People who take pain-relieving drugs on a regular basis are prone to a *rebound* effect—a syndrome whereby the pain becomes greater when the painkillers wear off. The rebound effect is implicated strongly as the cause of some chronic daily headaches. Tension-type headaches, just like migraines, can be a part of PMS.

Symptoms of Tension-Type Headache

LOCATION OF PAIN

- Both sides of the head at once
- Band of pain or pressure around forehead, scalp, back of head, or neck
- Pain, knotting, and/or stiffness in neck, shoulders, and/or upper back

QUALITY OF PAIN

- Tightness or intense "viselike" pressure
- Steady, dull ache (versus throbbing or stabbing)

OTHER CHARACTERISTICS

- *Not* aggravated by physical activity, light, or sound
- *Not* often accompanied by nausea and never vomiting
- *Never* preceded by aura
- Headache may begin as tension-type and turn into a migraine
- Some patients with chronic headache also suffer from depression

PATTERN OF PAIN

- *Chronic:* headaches every day or every other day
- *Episodic:* lasts a few hours, does not occur very often

Causes of Tension-Type Headache

The cause of tension-type headaches is under debate among Western medical doctors. Some argue that tension-type headache reflects biochemical changes in the brain that are caused by, or result in, muscle tension—and that the same mechanisms that cause migraine also cause tension-type headaches (see "Causes of Migraine," page 32). In short they believe that migraine and tension-type headache are two ends of a continuum of symptoms that emerge from the same underlying cause.

Others assert that tension-type headache is a distinctly unique disorder. Based on the name, conventional wisdom would have it that tension-type headache is due to tension of the muscles and underlying soft tissue around the head and neck and that it's a common result of emotional and physical tension. Emotional tension can cause a physical response—tensing of muscles. There appears to be much truth to this intuitive thought. People who have stressful jobs, who are under emotional pressure, or who have anxious dispositions seem to be more prone to tension-type headaches. In recent years chronic stress has been implicated in a wide range of chronic diseases, including headache.

Muscle tension could also be posture-related, or associated with underlying structural problems such as arthritis or spine injury. There is much evidence to support this concept (for details, see "The Mind-Body Connection," page 43). Indeed in studies of people with tension-type headache, muscular tension is often present but, confoundingly, not always at the time of the headache itself, suggesting that muscular tension sets off reactions that cause headache symptoms after the muscles relax. Many people with migraine have as much muscle tension as those with tension-type headache.

Common Triggers of Tension-Type Headache

Whether or not the mechanisms of tension-type headache are related to those of migraine is up for debate; what we do know, though, is that they share many of the same triggers. See pages 36–37 for a list of headache triggers.

The Mind-Body Connection

An understanding of how muscle contraction and soft-tissue damage lead to headache lays the theoretical groundwork for understanding many of the physical methods described in Chapter 7 as well as the mind-body methods in Chapter 8.

The body is composed of interconnected parts that influence one another. In health these parts are in balance, a condition known in medical parlance as *homeostasis*. Under stress the body can respond to such a degree that the balance is thrown off. In some people this imbalance can lead to pain and disease.

To illustrate this effect, think of the way you felt the last time something frightened you. You might have felt your stomach tense up, your muscles contract, your heart pound, and your mouth become dry. These are real physiological responses to stress, coined as the "fight-or-flight" response by Harvard physiologist Walter B. Cannon in the 1930s. The fight-or-flight response prepares the body for quick action.

This defensive mechanism can serve an important, immediate purpose: Without it we might not be able to react quickly when facing threatening situations such as oncoming cars. The fight-or-flight response was particularly useful when human beings faced many physical threats, such as wild animals. Today's "wild animals" take a different form: financial worries, job frustrations, relationship problems—the chronic emotional and psychological stressors that we face every day. Recent research has demonstrated a strong link between chronic stress and physical tension (and disease).

The body, it seems, was not made to endure chronic stress. Under normal situations the fight-or-flight response will give way to homeostasis once the threat is removed. But if the stress is ongoing, even at low levels, it can lead to negative changes in the body, such as muscle tension and blood vessel constriction. Headaches, high blood pressure, changes in blood sugar, and ulcers are just some of the negative responses to these effects.

There is another, and related, proposed mechanism for the mind-body stress connection. The early twentieth-century psychiatrist Wilhelm Reich, a protégé of Sigmund Freud, asserted that the physical body holds and reflects emotions—often hidden from the conscious mind—and that in psychotherapy working on the body is just as important to releasing pent-up emotions. Reich's findings have played a seminal role in the development of many bodywork methods (see Chapter 7).

THE PHYSICAL CAUSES AND EFFECTS

Chronic muscle tension can also alter the body structure, creating a self-perpetuating cycle of tension and pain that persists long after the stressful cause of tension has been resolved.

Chronic muscle tension can be caused by bad postural habits—standing or walking in ways that put unnecessary stress on the body, or work habits such as cradling a telephone between the shoulder and ear or hunching over a computer keyboard—or by underlying structural problems.

It can also result from prior physical trauma; if you hurt your shoulder, for example, the body's tendency is to protect it by tensing muscles around the area of pain, or to overcompensate by straining other muscles. This phenomenon is known as *splinting;* just as we apply a splint to a broken bone, the body may naturally develop a splint for an injured part of the body. After the injury has healed, the muscles and soft tissues have become habituated to the new structural situation and continue tensing when there is no need.

Biochemically when muscles become tense, they become starved of blood and oxygen. After prolonged periods of oxygen deprivation the muscles begin to "choke," resulting in an effect medically known as *ischemia*. Ischemia triggers the release of hormonelike chemicals such as *arachidonic acid* and *prostaglandin,* which make nerve endings more sensitive to pain signals—and sound the alarm for the body to take some action to relieve the pain.

Often we are not aware of how we contract these muscles because the actions have long become part of our habit or posture. Continued muscle tension can lead to ongoing irritation of the nerves that lead to the head, and to chronic headache. Body-education methods such as the Alexander Technique and the Feldenkrais Method aim to make students consciously aware of these habitual patterns, and offer new movement options to replace them (see Chapter 7).

The five groups of muscles that are closely linked with headache include

- Temporalis
- Frontalis
- Occipitalis
- Rectus capitis
- Trapezius

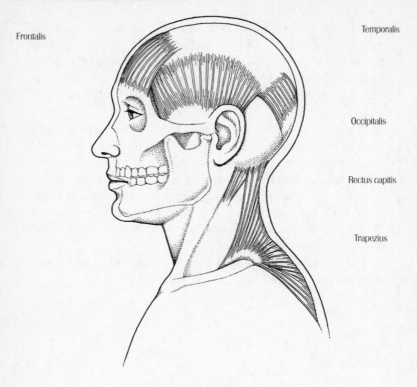

Frontalis

Temporalis

Occipitalis

Rectus capitis

Trapezius

Head and Shoulder Muscles

TEMPORALIS MUSCLE

Clench your teeth and trace your fingers from the side of your eyebrow back to the temple. This is your temporalis muscle. Now think of how often you might clench this muscle, when you're angry or under stress. Many people also activate the temporalis by grinding their teeth at night.

FRONTALIS AND OCCIPITALIS MUSCLES

Frown or squint. These expressions are controlled by the frontalis muscle, which extends from your eyebrow up to your forehead. Deep concentration, anger, or bad eyesight can contribute to chronic tensing of the frontalis, and resulting tension in the occipitalis.

RECTUS CAPITIS MUSCLES

With your body upright, look down as though reading a book in your lap—or crane your neck forward. The rectus capitis muscles at the nape of your neck allow you to do this. For many people these positions are postural bad habits that lead to strain of the occipitalis muscles. It was recently discovered that there is also a set of connective tissues at the base of the skull, behind the rectus capitis, that form a bridge between the deep neck muscles and the *dura mater,* the sheath of highly sensitive tissues that surround the brain and spinal cord. This muscle, called the rectus capitis posterior minor, has been directly linked to tension headaches.[2]

TRAPEZIUS MUSCLES

Raise your shoulders up to your ears, now lower them. This simple exercise exaggerates the way many people hold their trapezius muscles in tension, by hunching their shoulders or carrying heavy bags or by cradling telephones between their ears and shoulders. By the way, if your trapezius muscles are chronically tensed, this exercise might also give you a sense of relief and relaxation.

THE ROLE OF CONNECTIVE TISSUE

Connective tissue is any type of tissue in the body that serves a connecting function. The *fascia* is a connective tissue, like a stretchy cloth, that surrounds and permeates muscles, bones, organs, and blood vessels. The *dura mater* is a highly sensitive subtype of fascia that surrounds the brain and spinal cord.

When healthy, the fascia is flexible and slippery, giving the encased muscles and organs enough freedom of movement to perform their natural functions. But the influences of gravity, aging, accidents, or other stresses cause it to contract in certain areas and become rigid, putting pressure on the muscles, organs, and other internal body systems. Chronic structural imbalance contributes to rigid fascia. In addition distortion of the fascia in one area of the body may cause a tightening of this internal sheath in another.

By manipulating the fascia, the goal of osteopathic physicians, craniosacral therapists, massage therapists, and Rolfers, these practitioners aim to restore its flexibility, which in turn restores structural balance, freedom of movement, and functioning to the body's organs and other systems. A possible result of this manipulation is headache relief.

CLUSTER HEADACHE

It's been called the suicide headache and the demon of headaches. These monikers give you a sense of the intensity and severity of cluster headaches, which can indeed cause such ravaging pain that people have been driven to suicide.

Doctors have also described it as Horton's neuralgia, and Harris's neuralgia, for the physicians who first described the syndrome. In Europe it may be referred to as episodic migrainous neuralgia. Like migraine, cluster headache is a type of vascular headache. However, the mechanisms for cluster headache appear to be different from those of migraine.

Cluster headaches are so-called because the bouts often come on once a year and last for one to three months. During the cluster patients experience one to three attacks a day, lasting from fifteen minutes to two hours, followed by a period of pain-free remission. This pattern may continue daily for weeks or months with such regularity that people can virtually set their clocks by the attacks. However, a small percentage of people experience *chronic cluster headache,* and with this type there are no lasting periods of relief.

Who Gets Cluster Headache?

Unlike the situation with migraine, 85 percent of sufferers are men between the ages of twenty and forty, though rare cases have been reported in children. Many are smokers. Depression and sleep disturbances are also part of the cluster-headache profile. Sufferers may have a rugged complexion, tend to be taller than average, have blue or hazel eyes, and may have thicker blood (a high hemoglobin level).

Symptoms of Cluster Headache

In a report from the Fifth International Headache Congress, many of the two million Americans with cluster headaches are misdiagnosed as having sinus headache and undergo unnecessary surgery or treatment for allergies.[3] Needless to say, accurate diagnosis based on a thorough understanding of your symptoms is critical! What follows is a list of typical symptoms of classic cluster headache:

LOCATION OF PAIN

- Begins on one side of the upper face or head, typically near the temple, forehead, or one eye, as discomfort and aching
- Pain spreads over the same side of the face and/or neck (rarely, may alternate to the other side in a different episode)

QUALITY OF PAIN

- Begins as mild discomfort, but within minutes reaches high intensity
- Extremely painful, and almost unendurable. Differs for each individual; but it may be boring, throbbing, piercing, or burning

OTHER PHYSICAL CHARACTERISTICS

- Nose becomes stuffy or runny, often only on one side of the head
- Eye may tear, droop, become bloodshot, and the pupil may dilate

- Face may perspire
- The afflicted side of the face may feel warmer
- People become agitated, pace, and may even hit their heads against the wall due to the intense pain (unlike migraine pain, which worsens with movement)

PATTERN OF PAIN

- Daily attacks (one or more) lasting fifteen minutes to two hours, often at the exact same time every day
- Often occurs during sleep, awakening sufferers with excruciating pain
- After intense pain subsides, individuals might feel a dull ache for several hours
- Episodes may continue daily for weeks or months, followed by a remission lasting anywhere between six months and two years

Causes of Cluster Headache

From a conventional Western medical point of view, cluster headaches are a type of vascular headache—that is, they are caused in part by *dilation* (widening) of the blood vessels. Migraine headache is also thought to be a vascular headache. But the exact mechanisms of cluster headache are still an enigma.

Through study, researchers know that heredity does *not* play a major role in cluster headaches. However, many agree that the *hypothalamus*—the brain's home base for body rhythms and hormone regulation—is a key player in the development of cluster headaches. Studies have shown that blood flow to the brain increases during a cluster attack, which gives credibility to the vascular role. Others have noted a change in testosterone (male sex hormone) levels, which substantiates the body-rhythm-regulating hypothalamus as a possible participant—and helps explain why clusters occur with such regularity, and primarily in men.

Another theory about clusters involves *chemoreceptors,* which are located in the carotid (neck) arteries and which regulate the amount of oxygen and carbon dioxide in the blood. During a cluster attack, oxygen levels have been found to decrease.

As with migraine, we have found in our studies that some individuals with cluster headache have been found to be deficient in magnesium.

Much more research is needed to understand how these factors contribute to the unbearable pain of cluster headache.

Common Triggers of Cluster Headache

The following are the most common triggers for cluster headache, but other factors may also incite an attack. It's important to note that these factors bring on headache only during a cluster period—it's very rare for these triggers to initiate a cluster headache during remissions between cluster periods.

- Alcohol, even in small amounts, is the most common trigger
- Other vasodilating substances, such as foods that contain nitrates (hot dogs, bacon, etc.—see Chapter 3) and medications that contain vasodilators (nitroglycerine—see Chapter 3)
- Dramatic changes in temperature
- Exercise
- Stress

Other Types of Cluster Headache

The preceding pages describe the classic cluster headache. As mentioned, some people suffer from *chronic cluster headaches* that continue to occur one or more times a day without any pain-free periods of remission. *Chronic paroxysmal hemicrania* is a rare form of cluster headache, characterized by intense bouts that are shorter in duration (two to five minutes), but happen more often during the day (up to twenty or more times). Unlike classic cluster, women are more prone to chronic paroxysmal hemicrania. Also alternative methods usually do not work for these people—though there are some reports with certain modalities, such as inhalation through a mask of pure oxygen (which works for cluster, not other types) and certain herbal treatments. The anti-inflammatory drug, indomethacin, is highly effective for chronic paroxysmal hemicrania. Another rare type of cluster headache is *cluster-migraine syndrome,* which combines features of both cluster and migraine headache.

Diagnosis of Cluster Headache

Diagnosis is made on the basis of a medical history, with a focus on symptoms. But the symptoms are often misleading, resulting in long periods of painful misdiagnosis. The intensity of pain may raise false suspicions of brain tumors, head trauma, migraine, trigeminal neuralgia, or even dental problems. The nasal symptoms could seem to indicate sinus problems. Allergies may be suspected due to eye redness and tearing. It's important to communicate to your doctor or practitioner as precisely as possible the combination of your symptoms, with emphasis on the distinctive "cluster" pattern.

LESS COMMON HEADACHES

Sinus Headache

"Sinus" headache sufferers beware: TV ads tempt us to attribute headaches to sinus problems, but in the vast majority of cases, they're not. This doesn't mean that sinus headaches don't exist—it's just important to accurately diagnose true sinus headache to make sure you get the proper treatment.

True sinus headaches are usually caused by *sinusitis*—or inflammation of the sinus cavities. There are two categories of sinusitis: acute and chronic.

Acute sinusitis is a potentially serious condition that warrants immediate attention. In acute sinusitis the inflammation is due to infection of the sinus cavities. **Since the infection can travel to the brain, it's vital that you contact a doctor immediately if you have these following symptoms: headache, fever, tenderness over the sinus area, and a**

green-yellow discharge from the nose or back of the throat. Some people also experience nausea and dizziness.

Chronic sinusitis is caused by inflammation, not necessarily infection, of one or more of the sinus cavities. You might feel a sense of fullness in your head rather than outright pain, which is made worse by moving your head. The pain centers on the sinus cavities, with symptoms that are similar to, but less severe than, acute sinusitis. Usually people with chronic sinusitis *do not have a fever.*

In children chronic sinusitus can be difficult to diagnose and is often misdiagnosed as tension or migraine headache.

Temporomandibular Joint Headache

The temporomandibular joint (TMJ) is located in front of the ear, at the juncture of the jawbone and the skull. This headache is caused by spasm of the muscles around the joint. It is one of the most overdiagnosed conditions, leading to the unnecessary pain and expense of corrective appliances and surgery. In addition to pain—headache, ear, or jaw pain—true symptoms of TMJ syndrome include pain caused or aggravated by chewing, inability to open the mouth fully, and tenderness of the TMJ. Some people also hear clicks or pops in their jaw, but this symptom is also seen in people without headaches or TMJ syndrome. Tenderness of the joint is often due to prolonged clenching and grinding of teeth (caused by stress).

Eyestrain Headache

Eyestrain headache is felt around the eyes and front of the head. Reading in poor lighting and astigmatism are common causes of eyestrain headache. Similar but more severe symptoms might be indicative of *glaucoma,* which is caused by increased pressure in the eye. Symptoms of glaucoma include redness of the eye, bad night vision, or halos around lights at night. Since glaucoma can lead to blindness, it's important that you seek out the professional help of an ophthalmologist (the medical professional who diagnoses and treats disorders of the eye).

Sex-Related Headache

Not the same as the ''not-tonight-honey'' headache, sex-related headache is a condition that more often afflicts men. The medical term is *benign orgasmic cephalalgia.* This translates as harmless headache related to orgasm, which is a misnomer because sex-related headaches are not always benign, nor do they always occur with orgasm. The pain is intense and throbbing—like a migraine. Indeed some experts believe that the physiological effects of sexual excitement, such as dilation of blood vessels, sets in action the same biochemical mechanisms responsible for migraine. The pain can last minutes, or endure for several hours.

Though the tendency is to dismiss sex-related headaches as harmless, occasionally, they can be related to stroke (bleeding from a blood vessel in the brain). A small but significant percentage of strokes occur after sexual activity. On the other hand the release of endorphins during orgasm may relieve a migraine or tension headache.

Hormonal Headache

A significant number of women experience headaches that correlate with hormonal changes—due to PMS, menstruation, use of birth control pills, pregnancy, and estrogen depletion (related to menopause or surgical removal of the ovaries). These factors are discussed in Chapter 5.

Psychological Aspects of Headache

We express feelings in many ways—through words, actions, and sometimes through our bodies. When we feel joyful, we feel a clarity and springiness in our step. People notice, and may comment on, how well we look. We have more energy and strength. These physical feelings are very real, and very socially acceptable.

But when we feel anxious or depressed, our bodies also reflect it, sometimes with symptoms of illness. The medical world refers to this response as *somatization*—the conversion of feelings into physical symptoms that otherwise have no discernible physical cause. As a group, symptoms that arise from psychological sources (rather than direct physical injury or disease) are called *psychogenic*.

Lest you think that this explanation somehow diminishes the importance of these headaches, or dismisses them, allow me to reassure you: The pain is very real, and these headaches should be approached with the same seriousness and consideration as any other type of headache.

Conventional Western medicine has documented the effects of psychological stress on the body. Earlier in this chapter we looked at some of the muscular symptoms associated with stress. We also know that under stress the body prepares for action.

Internally the body responds to stress in several ways:

- Release of biochemicals
- Increased heart rate
- Increased blood pressure
- Muscle tension (including spasm of stomach)
- Constriction of the blood vessels
- Coldness of hands and feet as blood moves toward the area of injury

This response works very well in helping people react quickly and efficiently to the rare threatening situation. But the body is not well equipped to cope with chronic stress or pressure. When the pressure is ongoing, these physiological responses can cause chronic illness.

By reviewing the mechanisms of migraine, cluster, and tension-type headache, it's not difficult to see how stress can play a central role in triggering an attack—or predispose you to head pain. An acceptance of emotional or psychological stress as a critical part of the pathogenesis of headache, with measurable physiological consequences, underlies many of the mind-body therapies (to be discussed in Chapter 8)— particularly psychotherapy, biofeedback, hypnosis, imagery, meditation, relaxation, and prayer. Indeed honoring the relatedness of the mind to the body is one of the distinguishing features of most complementary approaches.

Depression appears to be closely related to chronic headache (migraine and tension-type) in several ways. First, several large population studies indicate that people with depression are three times more likely to suffer from migraines. Studies also show that people with migraines are three times more likely to develop depression. However, one condition does not cause the other; rather they probably share a similar mechanism. Indeed there's some evidence that both share an underlying serotonin disorder. Lower levels of serotonin are well documented in studies of people with clinical depression and are the basis for the development of new antidepressant drugs.

Exertional Headache

Some people experience headaches when they exert themselves physically. This doesn't mean that the exertion has to be strenuous. In fact exertional headaches are also known as the *cough headache* and the *laughter headache,* as well as the *lifting headache.* Symptoms are a throbbing, sharp pain that can last for minutes or hours. These headaches can sometimes be prevented by taking anti-inflammatory drugs (such as aspirin) or herbs (see Chapter 9) before engaging in physical activity. Since the sudden onset of any headache symptom could signal a dangerous underlying cause, it's important to seek medical advice if the headache persists.

Hangover Headache

The cause of a hangover headache is rarely a mystery to the individual who suffers from the throbbing head, nausea, and fatigue after overindulging in alcohol. There's some evidence that the alcohol itself is not the cause of the hangover, but rather other ingredients in the liquor.

Low Blood Sugar Headache

Abnormally low blood sugar, or *hypoglycemia,* can cause a variety of symptoms, including headache. While missing a meal or two will lower blood sugar, and induce headache symptoms, this temporary condition shouldn't be confused with hypoglycemia. True hypoglycemia is a potentially serious disease—often a precursor of diabetes—characterized by headache, light-headedness or dizziness, sweating, and trembling.

Constipation Headache

Headache is thought to result from constipation, either because of the resorption of toxic substances into the bloodstream or due to the inflation of the blocked intestines themselves. The resulting toxins can cause headache symptoms.

Travel Headache

Many people find that being a passenger in a moving vehicle—plane, automobile, train—can trigger the onset of headache, perhaps due to the visual stimulation or changes in atmospheric pressure. Missing meals, emotional tension, and hormonal imbalances due to changing time zones can all contribute to stress and headache.

Chronic Fatigue Syndrome Headache

Chronic fatigue syndrome is thought to be caused by the Epstein-Barr virus (EBV). The symptoms are varied, nonspecific, and flulike. Fatigue is the main symptom, but headache is often present as well. Because of the general symptoms, EBV is hard to diagnose, but it's estimated that tens of thousands of Americans have the virus, either with or without symptoms. Highly contagious, EBV is spread by close contact. Upon contracting EBV, the body forms antibodies, which can be measured but are not diagnostic. There is no vaccine or cure. Some researchers suspect *Candida albicans,* or yeast infection, as a potential instigator; 60 percent of EBV sufferers have candida infections. Some suspected contributing factors include low blood pressure due to too-low salt intake, chronic mercury poisoning from fillings, anemia, hypoglycemia, hypothyroidism, and sleep disorders.

CHAPTER 3

Diet, Drugs, and Headache

What is food to one is to others bitter poison.
—LUCRETIUS, On the Nature of Things

━━━━━━━

We are what we eat, so the saying goes—and many headache experts take the adage very seriously. But few of us have managed to avoid the experience of eating a type or quantity of food that leaves us feeling sick, or have failed to notice how changes in our diet affect our sense of well-being or physical appearance. In spite of these messages from our bodies, eating is often a less-than-mindful activity.

All of us, but especially people with headaches, could benefit from being more aware of what we feed our bodies. There's striking evidence that certain foods (and other ingested substances, such as drugs) can trigger headaches, either immediately or within a day. For example, an estimated 25 percent of people with migraine can trace its source to foods that contain tyramines (see page 62).[1] And that's just one food type, for just one type of headache. People with cluster[2] and tension-type headache[3]—and even sinus headache[4]—have also linked foods with their head pain.

Certain people are more predisposed to food reactions than others. Individuals with chronic headache seem to be especially vulnerable, for a variety of possible reasons, possibly linked to the same factors that cause headaches. For example, migraine- and cluster-headache sufferers might be particularly susceptible to certain *vasoactive* foods (foods that exert activity on the blood vessels) because of certain ingredients or components. As discussed in Chapter 2, these imbalances could be aggravated by other factors as well, such as stress, lack of exercise, changes in climate. In other words it seems that outside factors conspire with constitutional vulnerabilities to create conditions for headache.

Many holistic disciplines—Ayurveda, traditional Oriental medicine, and macrobiotics, for example—believe that our capacity for certain foods is influenced by our individual constitution, climate, and lifestyle. Ingesting an amount beyond that capacity might create an imbalance and a physical reaction. On the other hand you can raise your tolerance for specific foods by bolstering your strength in other areas of your life, as we'll see in Part II.

COMMON DIETARY TRIGGERS OF HEADACHE

Though many studies have been conducted to identify the food sources of headache, much of the information is *anecdotal*—that is, doctors know what they know because of what their patients tell them. The lists that follow come from a combination of studies and reports from headache sufferers to their doctors.

Keep in mind that no single person reacts to all of the foods, beverages, additives, and pharmacological agents listed below. Researchers generally agree that, with a few exceptions, headaches are brought on by a combination of substances, during a time of particular vulnerability. You might react to caffeine one day, for example, and have no reaction another.

Alcohol

Alcohol is a potent headache trigger—a fact well known even by people who otherwise never get headaches.

But the mechanism of a hangover headache is different from that of a migraine- or cluster-headache trigger. In hangover the headache is attributed mainly to impurities in the liquor. There are a few other ways that alcoholic drinks precipitate a headache attack as well. First, alcohol is a potent vasodilator. Flushed cheeks and red eyes are vivid outward signs of dilated blood vessels. In people with tension-type headaches, small amounts of alcohol might actually help relieve pain. But as you remember, part of the mechanism of headache is not just the dilation of blood vessels but spasm—opening and closing. One theory holds that migraines begin with constriction (causing aura) and progress to dilation (causing blood to rush forth, producing a pounding sensation). So when alcohol opens and stretches blood vessels, it could set in motion the mechanisms of headache.

In addition, though alcohol first opens blood vessels, the body reacts to this influence by closing them off. In effect alcohol acts ultimately as a vasoconstrictor.

Second, many types of alcohol contain additives or preservatives that precipitate headache. Red wines, for example, contain sulfites and tyramine, both prime headache-causing candidates. In general, the darker-colored alcoholic drinks—red wine, beer, scotch, etc.—are more likely to trigger headache.

People with cluster headaches are especially sensitive to alcohol, even in small quantities.

Caffeine

For headache sufferers caffeine is a double-edged sword. On the one hand small amounts of caffeine constrict blood vessels—which makes it useful in controlling migraine. In fact caffeine is an active ingredient in several migraine drugs. But too much caffeine (more than 240 mg, or two or three cups a day) consumed on a daily basis can make a headache worse.[5]

Caffeine is also a stimulant and can interfere with sleep patterns. People with chronic headaches are especially sensitive to changes in their environment and lifestyle. Interrupted or inadequate sleep increases stress, which we know can set the stage for headache.

The caffeine-withdrawal headache, common on weekends, is caused by sudden reduction or elimination of caffeine from the diet. If you're used to drinking two to three or more cups a day, you might have developed a dependency on caffeine, and cutting down or quitting can cause a caffeine-withdrawal headache.[6]

Foods and Drugs That Contain Caffeine

Cocoa
Chocolate (including milk chocolate)
Coffee
Drugs such as

- Anacin
- Cafergot
- Darvon Compound-65
- Dexatrim
- Esgic
- Excedrin
- Fioricet
- Fiorinal
- Midol
- No-Doz
- Norgesic
- Norgesic Forte
- Synalgos-DC
- Vanquish
- Vivarin tablets

Soft drinks such as:

- Coca-Cola (including diet)
- Pepsi-Cola (including diet)
- Dr Pepper
- Mountain Dew
- Tab
- Sunkist orange soda

Tea, including some teas that are often considered "herbal":*

- Chinese green tea
- Earl Grey
- Mint tea (not all)
- Oolong tea

*Herbal teas are generally caffeine-free, but it's important to read the label carefully, or ask before ordering or purchasing them.

Amines

Amines are amino acids found in many foods and are naturally occurring throughout the body. *Tyramine, tryptamine,* and *dopamine* are common amines found in foods. It's thought that amines trigger headaches either directly by constricting blood vessels or indirectly by activating certain biochemicals in the body that initiate a headache attack. Some studies have found that certain people with migraines have lower-than-normal levels of a digestive enzyme that breaks down dietary amines (see "Food Sensitivity, Intolerance, and Allergy," page 75).

Phenylethyl-amines are naturally occurring amino acids that work to improve memory and produce the mood-elevating neurotransmitter norepinephrine. They're also found in feel-good foods such as chocolate and aspartame (the artificial sweetener, see page 67). So while the phenylethyl-amines might be mood-elevators, they also carry the danger of triggering headaches.

It should be noted that people who take drugs known as *MAO inhibitors* may be even more sensitive to tyramines. These drugs include phenelzine (Nardil), and tranylcypromine (Parnate).

Some Amine-Containing Foods

Some alcoholic beverages (beer and wine)
Avocados

Bananas
Bean pods and broad beans (including soybeans)
Bread that is freshly baked
Cabbage
Cake that is freshly baked
Cheese (especially hard, aged cheeses)
Chocolate
Chicken liver and other livers
Citrus fruits
Cream and sour cream
Eggplant
Fermented foods
Figs
Fish that is pickled or preserved, including caviar
Meat that is aged or cured, organ meats, game meats, and pork
Nuts (including peanut butter and other nut butters)
Onions
Peas
Pickled foods
Pineapple
Raisins
Spinach
Tomato
Vinegar and foods that contain vinegar (e.g., catsup, relishes, mayonnaise, salad dressings, Worcestershire sauce, steak sauces, Tabasco sauce, horseradish, prepared mustards)
Yeast-extract-containing foods (e.g., bouillons, prepared soups)
Yogurt

Food Additives and Substitutes

Nitrites and *monosodium glutamate* (MSG) are food additives. Nitrites and nitrates are preservatives for meats, such as hot dogs and bacon, giving them a red color. They also add flavor and help prevent food poisoning. Nitrites are sometimes sprayed on fruits and vegetables in grocery stores and salad bars. Nitrites and nitrates are potent vasodi-

connection with headache. In animal studies they
ause cancer, but this link in humans has not been
satisfaction of the U.S. Department of Agriculture.

or enhancer most famous as an ingredient in Chinese
so added to many other prepared foods. An estimated
10 to 25 percent of the population is sensitive to MSG although the
FDA deems it completely safe.[7] It's also a vasoconstrictor. The symptoms—headache, sweating, dizziness, and a burning sensation—come
on about thirty minutes after eating the offending food.

Some Foods Containing Nitrites/Nitrates

Bacon
Bologna
Bratwurst
Beef jerky
Corn dogs
Corned beef
Food coloring agent FD&C yellow #5
Fruits and vegetables in some grocery stores (sprayed with nitrate-
containing preservatives)
Ham
Prepackaged lunch meats
Liverwurst
Meat tenderizers
Pastrami
Pepperoni
Pork and beans
Salad fixings at some open salad bars
Salami
Sauerkraut
Sausage
Seasonings and flavorings (read the label)
Smoked fish
Soy sauce

Spam
Vegetables packed in brine

Some Foods Containing MSG

Bacon bits
Baking mixes
Barbecue sauces
Bouillon cubes
Bread stuffing
Breaded foods
Canned meats
Cheese dips
Clam chowder
Corn chips
Croutons
Dry roasted nuts
Frozen foods
Gelatins
Oriental food
Potato chips
Processed meats
Relishes
Salad dressings
Salt substitutes
Seasonings
Soups, canned and dry
Soy sauce

Unmasking MSG in Prepared Foods*

MSG is most often used in prepared, packaged foods. But it's not always clearly labeled. It can be a hidden component of other products,

---

* Reprinted with permission from *Conquering Headache,* by Alan Rapoport, M.D., and Fred Sheftell, M.D., © 1995. Hamilton, Canada: Empowering Press.

or labeled as "natural flavoring." Here are some of the common "masks" for MSG:

Hydrolyzed protein
Sodium caseinate
Yeast extract
Yeast nutrient
Autolyzed yeast
Texturized protein
Calcium caseinate
Yeast food
Hydrolyzed oat flour

Chocolate

Chocolate can be triple trouble for the headache sufferer. First, it contains chemicals that constrict blood vessels. Second, it contains caffeine. Finally, it is high in sugar—and dramatic changes in blood sugar can trigger headache in sensitive individuals (see "Other Diet-Relataed Factors," page 79). People with migraine need to be particularly careful about chocolate because many find themselves craving it during the prodromal period, before an attack.

Other Potential Headache Triggers

The following list includes foods that contain vasoactive and other headache-causing substances:

Aspartame (NutraSweet and Equal)
Caramel candy
Corn
Corn syrup
Dairy products
Licorice
Olives
Mangos
Kiwi

Strawberries
Papayas
Shellfish
Wheat products

Artificial Sweeteners

The FDA has received many complaints about adverse effects associated with aspartame, the generic name for the artificial sweeteners NutraSweet and Equal—though it has not been proved in clinical study. In addition to headache, sensitivity reactions include dizziness, malaise, nausea, and visual disturbances. Many people add the sweetner found in NutraSweet directly to their food or beverages—but it should be known that it is found in many products, from multivitamins and breath mints to cereals and yogurt. Check the label of all diet products for aspartame.

THE STOMACH-HEAD CONNECTION

While it's clear that certain vasoactive substances can trigger headaches, scientists are at odds over why others might cause headaches. There are several possible explanations—some of which may overlap or aggravate the others. These include the following:

- *Digestive disorders,* which may manifest as improper or untimely digestion, disturbances of the natural bacterial flora in the digestive tract, and/or buildup of toxic substances
- *Nutritional deficiency,* which causes a host of problems that could lead to head pain
- *Food sensitivity,* which is a heightened physical awareness to a particular food but is neither an intolerance nor a true allergy
- *Food intolerance,* which is distinct from allergy, and is caused by digestive problems or a deficiency in the digestive enzymes
- *Food allergy,* which is due to immunological problems and can

either be genetically based or originate from nutritional deficiencies

- *Stress,* the ubiquitous troublemaker in headache, which can aggravate or cause any of the foregoing

Before entering this foray of conflicting theories, it helps to understand a little about the digestive system—the basics of how whole foods become micronutrients or toxins.

The Digestive System

The digestive process begins almost as soon as the fork leaves your mouth. Chewing food calls forth digestive enzymes in the saliva to make food softer and easier to swallow. The food then makes its nine- to ten-inch trek down the esophagus to the stomach.

In the stomach, digestive enzymes break food down even more. Protective antibacterial secretions help prevent food poisoning and regulate the healthy balance of good bacteria.

After three to four hours foods leave the stomach for the small intestine. Fats tend to linger longer, whereas carbohydrates beat a faster retreat. Chemicals in the small intestine break food down into its micronutrients and macronutrients. These constituents are then absorbed into the bloodstream—with the exceptions of alcohol, which is absorbed in the stomach, and oxygen (technically a nutrient), which is absorbed in the lungs. From the bloodstream, nutrients make their way to the liver and are then distributed to tissue cells throughout the body.

In health the body is very selective and efficient about what it takes in and what it eliminates. In cells nutrients are metabolized and made available to serve their life-maintaining or repairing purposes. Substances that are potentially toxic are excreted through the bowels and urinary tract.

When Good Foods Do Bad Things

Even healthy foods can cause unhealthy results when the digestive system isn't working optimally. Here are a few ways the digestive system can get into trouble and cause headaches:

Stress

Emotions can greatly affect digestion. Anger and hostility tend to speed up digestion, whereas fear and depression can slow or even stop it in its tracks, contributing to constipation or bacterial overgrowth, and possibly headache.

Undigested Foods

Due to stress, constipation, and/or other underlying physical problems, foods can sit in the large intestine partially undigested, resulting in absorption of toxins. The liver, in an attempt to carry out the waste product, becomes overloaded and cannot adequately process the toxic substance. Headache could be one of the symptoms of this toxic overload.

A relatively new and somewhat controversial finding is that food and bacteria can also pass across the intestinal wall—a phenomenon known as leaky gut. When the gut is weakened, either by disease such as *celiac sprue* (intestinal malabsorption) or by drinking alcohol or other factors (possibly genetic) these substances can circulate into the bloodstream. Over time the liver may become overloaded by toxic substances. The result: sensitivity to toxic substances circulating in the bloodstream or immunological dysfunction such as potential allergic reactions. We'll discuss the immune system and food allergy later in this chapter.

Imbalance of Bacterial Flora

Where there is life there are bacteria—and many foods carry these microorganisms. Most often, bacteria are not present in enough force to threaten the body, so the immune system can keep bacterial levels from flourishing out of control into infection.

The digestive tract is armed with a natural balance of bacteria, called the natural bacterial flora. Overuse of antibiotics can disturb the normal bacterial flora, resulting in possible overgrowth of specific bacteria such as *Candida albicans*—a yeastlike fungus found naturally in the healthy body. But when *candida* grows unchecked, *candidiasis* can occur.

Candidiasis manifests in many ways, including sore throat, vaginal yeast infections, irritable bowel syndrome (stomach pains, diarrhea, and constipation), and headache. There's some evidence that candida is linked with Epstein-Barr syndrome, in which headache is part of the constellation of symptoms. In addition candida infection is also known to impair the immune system, which is the underlying cause of food allergies, and possibly headache-related symptoms. Yeast-containing foods, such as breads, cakes, and crackers, can spur on candida growth. Other candida promoters include sweets and wheat. These foods are all on the headache sufferers' checklist of possible triggers.

Enzyme Deficiency

A genetic lack or deficiency in digestive enzymes, which are responsible for breaking foods down into nutrients, can result in food intolerance (see page 75).

Nutritional Imbalances

Researchers today know that there's a strong relationship between nutrients and the development and cure of diseases. A deficiency in nutrients can have many different effects on the body, depending on how much and how long one is deprived. Vitamin C deficiency, for example, is now known to contribute to immune system impairment and increase the risk of some types of cancer. Overconsumption of certain nutrients can also have ill effects—too much fat in the diet can lead to heart disease. Research also confirms that an imbalance of certain nutrients can contribute to headache. Here are some of the recent findings:

Magnesium Deficiency

Magnesium is a dietary mineral that helps regulate blood vessel size, serotonin function, and nerve activity in the brain, among other functions. From our research, we estimate that up to 50 percent of people with migraine (or more than ten million Americans) are deficient in this mineral.[8] Magnesium deficiency is thought to be at least one important factor in migraine attacks, among other conditions. There's also evidence that lower-than-normal magnesium levels contribute to a small percentage of patients with tension-type[9] headaches and up to 40 percent of patients with cluster[10] headaches.

Many studies suggest that magnesium might be a common denominator in both the vascular and the neural theories of migraine. In support of the vascular theory, magnesium deficiency results in blood vessel constriction[11]—and adding magnesium to the diet leads to the opening (*dilation*) of blood vessels. In support of the neural theory, magnesium deficiency has been linked with the production and release of substance P[12]—a biochemical that contributes to the inflammation of nerves and headache pain. (We'll discuss the role of magnesium as a treatment option in Chapter 6.)

Magnesium deficiency is commonly caused by a lack of this mineral in the diet. In addition magnesium can become depleted by the other factors:

• Stress
• Digestive disorders, such as irritable bowel syndrome
• Drinking water that is "soft" (that is, with few minerals)
• Long-term use of diuretics, a common blood pressure medication
• Alcoholism
• Malnutrition

How do you know whether you're deficient in magnesium? Magnesium depletion most severely affects the heart, muscles, nerves, and kidney tissues. Headache may be the only outward sign of magnesium deficiency. Others include

• PMS
• Leg muscle cramps
• Weakness
• Anorexia (appetite and weight loss)
• Nausea

- Digestive disorders
- Lack of coordination
- Confusion

High-fat Diets

A high-fat diet may be worse for you than you think. Though research is still in its early stages, there is mounting evidence that diets high in fat can mean a higher risk of migraine. According to a recent study and review of the medical literature, high fat intake is associated with many potential causes of headache, including: increased fatty acids, increased platelet clumping, damage to blood vessel walls, and higher serotonin levels.[13]

Copper Deficiency

Copper is a trace mineral that helps form bone, hemoglobin, and red blood cells. It works with zinc and vitamin C to create elastin and is important for healthy nerves. Recent research suggests that copper deficiency could contribute to high blood cholesterol and anemia, particularly in people with high-sugar diets. Along with zinc deficiency, copper's also associated with high blood pressure. Copper deficiency is also implicated in immunodeficiency.

The role of copper in migraines is not confirmed, but evidence strongly suggests that changes in copper metabolism can have a dual effect. First, it could have a direct effect on the functioning of blood vessels in the brain. Metabolic changes in copper cause the blood vessels to dilate or constrict, triggering migraine.[14]

Vitamin B Deficiency

Deficiencies in *niacin* (vitamin B$_3$) and *folic acid* are known to contribute to headaches. Niacin is needed for good circulation and a healthy nervous system. It also helps metabolize other nutrients (carbohydrates), certain drugs, and toxins. Folic acid, also known as folacin, is responsible for producing red blood cells and DNA synthesis. It aids in the metabolism of proteins and is vital for normal growth.

The role of these B vitamins in headache is not very well understood. Niacin helps increase blood flow to the brain, thus helping to prevent or reduce the vasoconstriction associated with chronic headache. Folic acid, as a key player in the production of red blood cells, keeps the body's supply of oxygen fresh. For these reasons it's thought that deficiencies in these vitamins could contribute to headache.[15]

Niacin deficiency, known as pellagra, can affect every cell of the body. The first symptoms include lassitude, weight loss, loss of appetite, and indigestion. In addition to headache, nervous-system symptoms include irritability, insomnia, emotional instability, and loss of memory. The skin may be rough, scaly, and uncommonly dark in areas that are exposed to sunlight. The digestive tract is afflicted in all areas, from the tongue, which becomes swollen and bright red, to the intestines, which may result in diarrhea. These symptoms are usually associated with other B-vitamin deficiencies as well.

Deficiencies of folic acid are among the most common, especially among pregnant women in the last trimester, and usually occur along with a deficiency in B_{12}. The symptoms include irritability, headache, weight loss, weakness, shortness of breath, palpitations, forgetfulness, emotional disturbances, and diarrhea.[16]

The causes of niacin and folic acid deficiencies are usually related to depletions in the diet. However, folic acid deficiency can also be caused by

- Intestinal problems
- Gastric surgery
- Certain medications, including aspirin and anticonvulsants

Vitamin A Excess

The health benefits of vitamin A are remarkably varied. It's important to good eyesight and prevents night blindness. It also promotes healthy skin. Vitamin A is an antioxidant and aids in immune function, helping to protect against pollution and cancer, colds, and flu. Beta-carotene is the food source of vitamin A.

Vitamin A overdose has been shown to trigger headache. Doses as low as 25,000 IU daily have been known to cause toxicity,[17] but the mechanism has not been well studied. Sometimes it's related to a side

effect called benign intracranial hypertension. It is caused by an inter-
ference of normal circulation and absorption of cerebrospinal fluids.
With vitamin A toxicity this frightening effect is usually transient—it
passes quickly.

In addition to headache, large doses of vitamin A are well known for
producing harmful effects, especially related to the eye. Children are
particularly susceptible to high doses. Other symptoms of overdose
include

- Yellowing of the skin
- Vomiting
- Weight and/or appetite loss
- Joint pain
- Abdominal pain
- Irritability
- Bone abnormalities
- Itching
- Dry, scaly, bleeding lips
- Stunted growth

Vitamin A overdose is not related to the beta-carotene received from
food; you probably need to be taking vitamin A supplements to reach a
point where you experience toxic effects.

Iron Deficiency

Iron is a mineral that helps oxygenate (give oxygen to) the blood and
form hemoglobin. It's vital to the production of many enzymes, as well
as disease resistance and growth in children.

The role of iron in headache is not well documented. But it's been
identified as an important factor in synthesizing neurotransmitters in
the brain. We know that the neurotransmitter serotonin is an important
regulator of headache. Iron deficiency occurs in the brain long before it
becomes apparent in the bloodstream. It's possible therefore that headache could result from lower-than-normal serotonin levels due to iron
deficiency.

Whatever the mechanism, headache can be a symptom of iron deficiency, as are tiredness, apathy, slower brain function, heart enlargement, and fingernails that are spoon-shaped and have lengthwise ridges.[18]

Iron deficiency is one of the most common deficiencies, particularly among women of childbearing age because high quantities of iron are lost monthly through menstruation. In fact any condition that causes blood loss can lead to iron deficiency, including chronic ulcers and hemorrhoids, blood donations, and surgery. Iron might also be less available in people with rheumatoid arthritis and cancer. Individuals with candidiasis and chronic herpes are more vulnerable to iron deficiency.

Food Sensitivity, Intolerance, and Allergy

There is a lot of confusion about the differences between food sensitivity, intolerance, and allergy. Though they are technically different conditions, there are researchers who believe that one or all can produce chronic headache.

Food Sensitivity

Sensitivity may be defined as a heightened, usually negative, response to a substance. In a way, it is a generic term that includes intolerance and allergy; it describes the *way* in which we react, not the reason why.

Chemical sensitivity, a specific subcategory of sensitivity, is a complex physiological process that produces allergylike symptoms but, unlike allergy, does not seem to involve the immune system. Its very existence as a clinical syndrome is disputed by most practitioners of conventional medicine. Chemical sensitivity is often dismissed as being a psychological problem. Through the efforts of people who suffer such sensitivities, several national organizations have formed to encourage basic research, national awareness, and information.

Briefly, chemically sensitive people appear to be highly sensitive to low levels of toxins (or other symptoms that most people consider benign) in foods and/or the environment. The latest research shows that chemical sensitivity is probably a combination of central nervous sys tem damage and enzyme deficiencies, which may be caused by genetics, chronic exposure to toxins, or both, according to the Chemical Injury Information Network.

According to people who study chemical sensitivity, the problem can be difficult to diagnose for several reasons. First of all, people who are chemically sensitive seem to react to very low levels of chemicals—levels that are generally considered safe for the general population. Thus the standard tests for chemical reactions—such as allergy tests or tests for blood levels of toxins—do not show up positive. This makes sense since chemical sensitivity does not seem to be an allergic response involving the immune system.

Second, the body's reactions to low levels of chemicals happen very slowly, causing minor but irreversible damage that progresses until the injury reaches a critical point.

Third, the mechanism of chemical sensitivity may be complex. According to the most recent theories, the body forms a sort of addiction to a chemical, so that if it fails to get the regular dose, the body goes into withdrawal. The withdrawal symptoms, such as headache, will mask the real problem, which is internal damage due to chemical exposure.

Fourth, once a person is sensitized to one chemical, the sensitivity can "spread" to include other, unrelated compounds. Once that happens, according to the Chemical Injury Information Network, chronic exposure will lower the body's tolerance level and make it all the more vulnerable to other chemical assaults.

Some substances in foods can cause chemical sensitivity, but more insidious are the hidden, and poorly regulated, toxins in the environment and commercial products. For more on chemical sensitivity, see Chapter 4.

Intolerance

Intolerance, according to the National Center for Nutrition and Dietetics, is defined as an adverse reaction to foods caused by

- Digestive problems and other physical conditions that can mimic food allergy symptoms

- Enzyme deficiency causing a physical inability to digest certain foods (such as lactose intolerance)
- Allergylike symptoms caused by ingestion of certain foods (wine, cheese) or exposure to certain substances

Clinical study has shown that some migraine sufferers lack an enzyme, *phenyl-sulfotransferase,* that helps in the digestion of certain foods, particularly foods that contain phenylethyl-amines. Chocolate and aspartame, the synthetic sweetener in NutraSweet, also contain phenylethyl-amines.

Allergy

Allergy is an abnormal response of the body's immune system to foods or ingredients. For some people, eating small amounts of an offending food can cause a life-threatening reaction. Less allergic people can tolerate small amounts. The National Center for Nutrition and Dietetics states that although 33 percent of people think they have a food allergy, true allergy exists in only 1 percent[19]—that is, conventional Western medical study has failed to find a clinical connection: Blood tests do not reveal signs of immune system dysfunction; there appear to be no family patterns; and skin tests are not always indicative of headache-related allergies.

There are two theories about why people who have toxic reactions to substances might not show positive blood tests. One is that headache represents a "delayed" allergic reaction that involves the immune system.[20] Another theory (as demonstrated in one study) is that the allergic response is significantly different in people with migraine.

The connection between sinusitis and allergy is better established; however, the allergens (see page 78) tend to be more environmental than food-related.

How Allergy Happens

An allergic reaction occurs when the immune system identifies certain substances as being harmful to the system. This can occur even when the substance is not present in threatening amounts.

The healthy immune system is on guard all the time for potential invaders, or antigens. *Antigen* is defined as any substance that does not rightly belong to the body (*anti* = "against"; *gen* = "type"). An antigen can even be foods and other nutrients that are in fact good for the body. When an antigen causes an allergic reaction, it's called an *allergen*. On exposure to an allergen, the immune system produces an antibody that recognizes only that specific allergen. One such antibody is known as IgE, which connects up with other substances in the blood and tissue. This IgE complex then snares the allergen, activating a series of events (including inflammation and dilation of blood vessels) aimed at protecting the body and ousting the intruder.

Once an antibody has formed, it is always there to fight off any repeat invasions—which is why people who are allergic to a certain substance remain so.

Most often, allergic reactions occur with amazing swiftness, within minutes of exposure. But allergies can occur over time, after repeated exposures, when the body becomes "overloaded"—that is, when the amount of substance has surpassed the person's natural level of tolerance. To further complicate the issue, ingesting certain substances can prime the body to react to others. And many different types of foods can be involved. These characteristics of delayed allergy make it much more difficult for the allergy sufferer to identify the offending substance. Making matters worse, victims of delayed allergy often crave the very foods that cause headaches.

Other Diet-Related Factors

Many people report headaches after skipping meals. Some research-ers relate this to hypoglycemia, or low blood sugar. While missing meals might in fact contribute to headache, there's little evidence link-ing this pattern with true hypoglycemia. Hypoglycemia is a very spe-cific clinical condition that may be an early sign of diabetes. Short periods of low blood sugar do not constitute true hypoglycemia; rather, this is defined as *functional hypoglycemia*. Symptoms of true hypogly-cemia—which often occur after carbohydrate-rich meals are con-sumed—include headache, dizziness, light-headedness, trembling, and possibly nausea. If you have more than one of these symptoms, contact your doctor for an evaluation of your blood sugar. In the nonhypo-glycemic headache sufferer, the physiological stress of missing a meal is a more likely headache trigger than low blood sugar.

DRUGS AND HEADACHE

We've already looked at some drugs—prescription and over-the-counter—which contain ingredients that could trigger headaches. Virtu-ally any drug taken incorrectly or at higher-than-recommended doses may cause headache as a side effect. But there are some that may cause headache even at regular doses.

Vasodilators

The most obvious culprits are vasodilators, which are often used to treat high blood pressure or angina—or even headaches. These include, but are not limited to, the following:

- Captopril
- Diltiazem
- Hydralazine
- Isosorbide dinitrate
- Minoxidil

- Nicardipine
- Nifedipine
- Nitroglycerin (oral drug and skin patch)
- Propranolol
- Reserpine
- Verapamil

Vasoconstrictors

Certain vasoconstrictive drugs can contribute to *rebound headaches;* upon stopping them the body responds with dilation of the blood vessels and, potentially, headache symptoms. Vasoconstrictive drugs that may cause rebound headaches include the following:

- Ergotamine
- Amphetamines
- Caffeine

Drugs That Result in Intracranial Pressure

Certain substances can cause pressure inside the cranium and produce headache:

- Vitamin A overdose (more than 25,000 IU daily)
- Tetracycline
- Lithium

Drugs That Contribute to Noninfectious Meningitis

Unlike bacterial meningitis, which can be life-threatening, inflammation of the meninges due to aseptic or noninfectious meningitis requires medical attention, though it is not as dangerous. Drugs that contribute to this effect include the following:

- Ibuprofen
- Sulindac
- Tolmetin

Estrogen Replacement Therapy

As you'll see in Chapter 5, changes in blood levels of estrogen—the "female hormone"—can create bodywide effects that cause headache. The birth control pill and estrogen replacement therapy (such as Premarin) are drug forms of estrogen.

Cigarette Smoking and Illicit Drugs

The following substances have been shown to trigger headache or cause rebound headache upon withdrawal:

- Cigarette smoke
- "Secondhand" smoke
- Benzodiazepines
- Cocaine
- Inhaled glue

Withdrawal from virtually any addictive drug can produce headache; withdrawal from alcohol, cocaine, and opiates should be monitored carefully to avoid severe, potentially life-threatening reactions.

CHAPTER 4

The Headache Environment

The air bites shrewdly.
—*WILLIAM SHAKESPEARE*, Julius Caesar

———

Just as the foods we eat can set the stage for headache, toxic substances and/or allergens in the air we breathe can also bring head pain. Other environmental factors such as the weather, noises, and light can also trigger a headache attack.

The question arises (as it did in Chapter 3), Are these triggers direct causes of chronic headache, or do they switch on other mechanisms that are lying in wait? With certain headache types, such as eyestrain headache or sinus headache, there is an organic cause. But for chronic tension-type, migraine, and cluster headache, the mechanisms are under dispute. The same theories apply for environmental toxicity as for dietary toxicity (see Chapter 3, "Food Sensitivity, Intolerance, and Allergy," page 75). Briefly, reactions to substances in the environment may result from

- *Intolerance*—due to a functional problem in breaking the substance down or eliminating it
- *Allergy*—an immunological problem whereby the body mounts an immune response against an offending substance

- *Chemical sensitivity*—a nonimmunological syndrome, probably a combination of central nervous system damage and enzyme deficiencies, which may be caused by chronic exposure to toxins, or genetics, or both

Removing the sensitivity-causing substance might relieve the headache for the time being. But in its unbalanced state the body remains poised for reactions to other substances. So while identifying and eliminating toxic causes of headache is obviously important, it's also important to explore whether other, deeper factors are at play.

THE AIR WE BREATHE INDOORS

By now most of us know that air pollution is bad for our health, but it may be surprising for many of you to learn that *indoor pollution* can incur health consequences that are as grave, or even more serious, than those caused by outdoor pollution. Here are some startling facts:

The National Academy of Sciences estimates that indoor pollution contributes up to $100 billion annually in health care costs. The Occupational Safety and Health Administration (OSHA) estimates that more than twenty million Americans work with chemicals known to cause nervous system damage, even when used in small amounts. And according to the National Research Council, complete toxicity information is available for only 2 percent of the seventy thousand chemicals in daily use.[1]

Poor Ventilation

The energy crisis in the 1970s can be blamed for many ills, not the least of which is setting the stage for environmental illness. To conserve energy, the government encouraged weatherization and energy-efficient construction. The upside was savings on energy bills; the downside was poor ventilation in new buildings. As a result all of the new materials and products that contain petrochemicals, formaldehyde, and other toxins (and they are ubiquitous) become trapped in our superinsulated environments.

Offices or homes built in the fall or winter in colder regions are particularly prone to causing indoor environmental problems. These new building materials are often treated with substances that, without the chance to escape through ventilation, will give off gasses and "percolate" in an enclosed space. Environmental toxins that normally would have a chance to escape by opening a window in spring or summer are, in the winter, trapped and accumulate—resulting in higher-than-normal levels of toxins and a higher potential for causing toxic reactions.

Hidden Headache Hazards

Some of the biggest headache-causing suspects on the home front are humidity, dust mites, molds, yeast, and algae. But other factors to consider include chemicals that emit from cleaning solutions, personal-care products, dry cleaning, wood preserving, and other sources to be discussed on the following pages.

Humidity

I know of one headache sufferer who can predict humid weather more accurately than any weather reporter. But she is not alone. Many headache sufferers know when it's going to rain and can presage drops in barometric pressure. These individuals seem to be more prone to headache during air travel or while climbing to high elevations.

There are a few possible explanations for her talent: Perhaps her body is reacting to a change in the weather, or maybe it's reacting to factors that thrive under humid conditions, such as dust mites, molds, yeast, and algae.

Dust mites are microscopic insects that flourish under conditions that are common in today's American household. It should be noted that the dust mite itself is not the offender but its droppings. The more dust mites you have, the more droppings. Yeast, algae, and molds coexist and proliferate under similar conditions.

The Kitchen

We've already discussed how the foods you cook on your stove can trigger headache, but what about the stove itself? Gas stoves can be particularly hazardous due to the emission of *nitrogen dioxide, benzene,* and *carbon monoxide.* Cleaning solutions might also contain ingredients that trigger headaches. Moist areas, for example under the sink, can be breeding grounds for dust mites, yeast, algae, molds, and fungi. Cookware made of aluminum, or dishes made of plastic, might be the source of sensitivities.

The Bathroom

As mentioned above, moist areas are perfect for the growth of common household allergens. The shower stall creates an ideal habitat for the proliferation of molds. Again, cleaning solutions should be suspected as possible headache-producing sources.

The volatile molecules in *highly scented personal products* (such as shaving lotions, soaps, moisturizers, shampoos, etc.) also can quickly assault the nervous system and bring on a headache.

Housewide Considerations

Dry cleaning, treated woods, and insulation materials often emit *formaldehyde.* Polyurethane, a clear plastic sealant often used in finishing woods and other materials, can be toxic for several months after its application. Other products used in the process of pressure-treating woods may incite headache attacks as well. *Carbon monoxide* from home heating systems is a potentially dangerous source of headache, an early symptom of possible poisoning.

The rapid changes in temperature in heating/cooling ventilation systems are good breeding grounds for molds and fungi, which then become distributed throughout the building.

Insecticides often contain vasoactive agents that could trigger a headache. Consider also your *water supply,* which can harbor chemicals leached from nearby factories or farms. In one study headaches plaguing a western Illinois community were traced to water pollution with trichloroethylene (TCE). Even if water testing fails to uncover toxic levels of chemicals, many headache sufferers are highly sensitive to even low levels of toxins—levels that may be considered safe for the general population.

Hidden Ingredients That Can Cause Headache

According to the Environmental Protection Agency, the following ingredients—found in common personal-care and cleansing products—have been found to cause headache.[2]

	Benzyl Alcohol	Ethyl Acetate	Alpha-Terpineol	Methylene Chloride
Aftershave		•	•	
Air freshener	•		•	
Cologne	•	•	•	•
Deodorants	•		•	
Dishwashing liquid		•		
Fabric softener		•	•	
Hairspray			•	
Laundry bleach	•		•	
Laundry detergent			•	
Nail polish		•		
Nail-polish remover	•	•		
Paint				•
Perfume	•	•	•	
Shampoo	•	•		•
Soap	•		•	
Varnish remover				•
Vaseline lotion	•		•	

Headache on the Job

Office politics aside, lurking within the carpeting and walls of your office building could be toxic substances that bring on chronic headache. Factory workers may be exposed to noxious inhalants or chemicals absorbed through the skin that may cause headache (see "Chemicals," below). Consider the following environmental factors in your place of work:

Chemicals

What types of chemicals are commonly used? If you work in a dynamite factory, for example, suspect *nitroglycerine*. A potent vasodilator, nitroglycerine is a common headache-triggering factor. In fact any chemical-factory work should raise a red flag. People who work with welding, mining, metalizing, metal grinding or finishing, paint (that contains lead), or any sort of combustion might be exposed to headache-causing inhalants. Farmers and farm workers should consider pesticide exposure. People who work in printing or art might not be aware that the fixatives and markers they use daily are noxious, especially for the sensitive headache sufferer. Individuals who work in building and construction might want to explore whether they're exposed to chemicals used for treating woods—both in the woods themselves (formaldehyde and others) and in their sealing (polyurethane and others). Also, many offices have regular pest-control schedules; consider whether your headaches coincide with fumigation.

Fumes and Noxious Odors

People with chronic headache might also be highly sensitive to odors, such as fumes from the above-mentioned sources, perfumes, automobile exhaust, and cigarette smoke.

Lighting and Computers

As mentioned, those of you who suffer from migraine with or without aura can be especially sensitive to changes in light. Bright or flashing lights can precipitate a migraine attack. Infrared lights (from welding and other operations) can also precipitate headache. Fluorescent lights, which tend to flicker—sometimes almost imperceptibly—can also bring on headaches. Reading, poor lighting, or astigmatism are common causes of eyestrain headache.

Job Activities

Sudden exertion can bring on a headache, as may bad postural habits. See Chapter 7 for more information.

Travel

Many factors that occur during travel can, either alone or in combination, bring on a headache attack. For example, when hiking to altitudes above ten thousand feet, people who are not susceptible to headaches may experience them. Changing time zones can throw off your internal biological clock, resulting in stress and hormonal changes that may set the stage for headache. Travel-related factors that may cause headache include

- Atmospheric changes (page 89)
- Changes in time zones
- Constant motion
- Altitude
- Enclosed environment (particularly during air travel, see "Poor Ventilation," page 83)
- Skipping meals (see Chapter 3)

Is Your Office Making You Sick?

Complete the following questionnaire. If you answer yes to any of the questions, investigate the sources as possible headache triggers.

Yes   No

/ /   / /   I am exposed to chemicals in my workplace.

If yes, please list (e.g., glues and fixatives, aerosol sprays, sealants, pesticides):

_____

_____

_____

_____

_____

/ /   / /   The windows in my office building cannot be opened.

/ /   / /   The heating system uses gas or oil for fuel.

/ /   / /   I use a computer much of the day.

/ /   / /   My job requires a lot of air travel.

/ /   / /   The lighting source is fluorescent lights.

/ /   / /   My work requires physical exertion.

/ /   / /   My job environment is noisy.

/ /   / /   My coworkers smoke.

/ /   / /   I am exposed to perfumes, sprays, or other fumes on the job.

Weather Changes

It's hay-fever season, and while everyone else is sneezing and wheezing, you're getting headaches. Is there a connection? Some headache experts might attribute it to allergies, while others point to changes in the weather. Many headache sufferers seem to be exquisitely sensitive to barometric and/or humidity changes. As we discussed on page 84, humidity is a common headache trigger, possibly due to the proliferation of allergens. Other researchers attribute this weather reaction to ionic changes—positive and negative charges in the air—during changes in atmospheric pressure.

We'll explore ways of detecting and reducing environmental headache hazards in Chapter 6.

CHAPTER 5

Special Populations: Women, Children, and Teens

I am, being woman, hard beset.
—ELINOR HOYT WYLIE, "Let No Charitable Hope"

Throughout this book we've emphasized that each person with headache is unique. You may share some characteristics with other headache sufferers, such as a sensitivity to particular foods or environmental toxins, but certain populations deserve special attention because their patterns of head pain are often quite distinct. These groups include women, children, and teens.

Until puberty the incidence of headaches is evenly distributed between males and females. But at puberty hormonal changes set in, and set the stage for headaches—in girls.

Before going any farther, it may help to understand the role of hormones in headache.

THE HORMONE-HEADACHE CONNECTION

Hormones help the body keep a healthy biochemical balance by informing it of outside stimuli and regulating its responses. Essentially they are messengers that are produced mostly by *endocrine* glands, distributed throughout the body, and that travel through the blood to activate necessary changes in the body. Some of these changes contribute to headache.

The Endocrine System

Adrenal Glands

Located above the kidneys, the two adrenal glands produce two different types of chemicals: *catecholamines* and *steroids*.

The catecholamines include hormones that activate the fight-or-flight response to stress. The greater the stress, the higher the output of hormones such as adrenaline.

There are three categories of steroid hormones: *mineralocorticoids,* which regulate the balance of fluid in the body; *glucocorticoids,* which perform several functions, including the control of blood pressure; and *sex hormones,* estrogens (female hormones) and androgens (male hormones). We'll look more closely at estrogens and their role in headache later on in this chapter.

Pancreas

The pancreas is an organ located behind the stomach that produces insulin and other hormones that regulate blood sugar levels—the energy of the body. In Chapter 3 we talked about how skipping meals can cause headaches due to low blood sugar levels.

Pituitary Gland

Found in the head, the pituitary gland is control-central for the hormone system. The pituitary is connected to the *hypothalamus,* which teams up with the pituitary to help it control hormonal functions. For example the pituitary produces hormones that control other hormone-producing systems. The pituitary produces *gonadotropins,* which are vital in the female reproductive cycle, including follicle-stimulating hormone (FSH) and luteinizing hormone (LH).

The pituitary glands also make *prolactin,* which is responsible for producing breast milk in pregnant women. Prolactin levels are also known to jump during periods of stress and might be part of why headache sufferers respond to stress triggers.

Thymus

The thymus is a gland located behind the breastbone and seems to play an important role in the immune system.

Thyroid

The thyroid is a gland that sits in the hollow in the front of your neck. It secretes hormones that help control metabolism. Higher-than-normal thyroid levels (known as *hyperthyroidism*) speed up the body's metabolism and produce symptoms such as headache, nervousness, palpitations, fatigue, and loss of weight. Lower-than-normal thyroid levels (known as *hypothyroidism*) slow the body down, creating symptoms such as headache, accumulation of fluids in the body (*edema*), dry hair and skin, weight gain, a slow heart rate, and others.

THE HEADACHE CYCLE IN WOMEN

We mentioned earlier that in women the adrenals produce estrogens and that the pituitary gland produces gonadotropic hormones, LH and FSH. From puberty through menopause, women are ceaselessly influenced by fluctuations in these hormones due to the repeated cycles of menstruation and sometimes pregnancy. In some women precipitous drops in estrogen are thought to be responsible for premenstrual headaches.

The Menstrual Cycle

Next we'll look at how hormone levels change during the menstrual cycle and how these changes can contribute to headache. Keep in mind that while twenty-eight days is the average length of a menstrual cycle, most women have shorter or longer periods.

Days 1–5: Menstruation

The first day of menstruation marks the first day of the cycle. At this time progesterone levels have dropped and the uterus contracts, causing painful cramps in some women, to help release the lining of the uterus—menstrual bleeding. The following are some of the possible factors contributing to headaches:

- *Migraine:* Before menstruation estrogen levels drop quickly. It's thought that this sudden fall triggers migraine. The premenstrual phase sets the stage for a migraine during menstruation.
- *Tension-type headache:* Stress and pain combine during menstruation to create ideal conditions for a tension-type headache.

Days 5–9: Postmenstruation

With the exception of FSH, hormone levels are now low. FSH levels are increasing to stimulate the ovaries to ripen an egg within the follicle (a kind of nest that forms on the ovary), which in turn puts estrogen production in faster motion. During this time women are feeling what one woman I know calls her midcycle high—as a result, headaches are generally at an all-cycle low.

Days 9–14: Proliferative Phase

This is when the egg starts to mature. FSH levels decrease, estrogen levels increase, and luteinizing hormone begins to accumulate. Again the slow, steady rise in estrogen does not cause many headache-related problems during this time.

Days 14–28: Premenstrual Phase

The oocyte, or egg, has matured and is expelled from the ovary to the fimbrae, where it makes its way down the fallopian tube and ultimately to the uterus. During this time estrogen and LH levels fall dramatically; LH first, then estrogen. The ovaries produce progesterone to nurture the developing egg in case it has been fertilized by sperm.

The vasculature of the uterus is now growing, producing more blood. If the egg is not fertilized, the uterine lining will shed during the process of menstruation.

Now the abrupt fall in estrogen and progesterone levels sets the stage for migraine. Simultaneously prostaglandin, a hormone that increases sensitivity to pain, also increases as a result of these hormonal swings. The result is not only conditions for migraine but a greater sensitivity to pain.

Magnesium

There is also evidence that magnesium levels are reduced during the premenstrual phase. As mentioned in Chapter 3, magnesium deficiency has been linked with blood vessel constriction[1] and with the release of substance P,[2] the biochemical that sets in motion pain-causing inflammation. In my studies about 50 percent of people with a migraine attack appear to be magnesium-deficient, and this deficiency strikes women with migraines more often than men.[3] Low magnesium levels seem to also be responsible for other PMS symptoms.[4]

Birth Control Pills

We've just seen how monthly hormonal changes, particularly in the levels of natural estrogen, can lay the groundwork for headaches in women. Hormonal changes also occur due to other biological events in a woman's life, including pregnancy and menopause. Estrogen-containing drugs, such as the birth control pill and estrogen replacement therapy (such as Premarin), which is used to ease the symptoms of menopause, can also affect estrogen levels, and a woman's vulnerability to headache.[5]

Migraine is one of the most common side effects of oral contraceptives, commonly known as the Pill.[6] It can set off a migraine, worsen its severity, or increase its frequency. Though migraine is most common among women who are prone to headache, for some women, taking the Pill triggers their first attack.

The Pill helps prevent pregnancy by raising estrogen levels; it's the increase in estrogen that produces headache-causing changes in blood vessels. Estrogen can increase platelet aggregation, which increases the risk of headache-triggering events.

Certainly the Pill does not cause migraine in all women, nor does it trigger migraine in all women who are vulnerable to it. In fact some women notice a reduction in the severity and frequency of their headaches when taking the Pill. This effect may be more common among women who normally experience great fluctuations in estrogen and who, by taking the Pill, find that their estrogen levels are more stabilized.

Menopause and Hormone Therapy

Menopause is defined as the cessation of menstrual periods. But with the exception of women who undergo surgical removal of their ovaries, menopause is a process—a natural series of biological events that result in the end of menstruation. It takes an average of four years for a women's menstrual periods to come to a complete halt. During these years before menopause (*premenopause*), women slowly start to experience hormonal changes that can cause headaches. The length of periods may change and the cycle between periods can get longer or shorter. This cyclic instability is caused by changes in hormone levels. The key word here is *instability;* estrogen levels (and levels of other hormones, such as progesterone) tend to rise and fall even more sharply during this time. The decline in estrogen will often result in dilation of blood vessels—a setup for headache, as well as hot flashes.

Women who undergo surgical menopause due to removal of the ovaries (*oophorectomy*) or removal of the ovaries and uterus (*total hysterectomy*) are more likely to have a more intense reaction because of the abrupt decline in estrogen.

For many women who suffer from migraines, menopause often heralds a new headache-free era. But a great many women experience other disruptive effects, such as hot flashes, vaginal dryness, heart palpitations, joint pain, and possibly headache. These effects are directly linked to the loss of ovarian estrogen and progesterone.

Other long-term effects of menopause include osteoporosis (bone loss) and an increased risk of heart attack. For these reasons many women take estrogen therapy, or hormone therapy, which combines estrogen and progesterone. Hormone therapy takes the form of a pill, creams, and skin patches.

Clinical studies have shown that hormone therapy can help prevent osteoporosis and ease the physical discomfort of menopause; but it could also aggravate headache. In much the same way as the Pill, estrogen therapy in any form (pill, cream, or skin patch) can set in motion the biochemical events that lead to headache—platelet aggregation, serotonin release, substance P release, inflammation of nerve endings, and vasospasm (see Chapter 2 for more on the mechanisms of headache).

Any change can bring stress. And "the change of life" can be a substantial stressor for women. As anyone who has experienced a hot flash knows, the physical symptoms alone can be a source of emotional stress. Loss of sleep due to nighttime hot flashes (also known as night sweats) disrupts the body's biorhythms, setting the stage for stress and headache. Also, laden with negative social symbolism, menopause may be seen by some women as an adverse change, causing a decline in self-image. Today menopause is no longer as veiled a subject as it once was, and there are many articles, books, and magazines devoted to helping women gain an understanding of menopause—which hopefully will help change some of the negative stereotypes surrounding this natural process (see "Resources" for more information).

Pregnancy

Hormonal changes are highly charged during the first three months of pregnancy. The fluctuations in estrogen can be great enough to bring on the first migraine attack in some women—or heighten the pain for those who already suffer. After the third month, however, as hormone levels fluctuate less severely, most women experience relief.

After pregnancy, when estrogen and progesterone resume their normal fluctuation, headaches might recur, or come on again after several headache-free years.

HEADACHES AND CHILDREN

We often think of headaches as an adult disorder, so we may become particularly alarmed when a child complains of chronic head pain. While any sudden pain should be taken seriously in children since it may signal a serious underlying problem such as brain tumor or meningitis or encephalitis, the vast majority of headaches in children are benign. (See page 27 for the warning signs of potentially dangerous headaches.)

But chronic benign headache is surprisingly common among children. It can occur in children of any age, from infancy through teenage years. Unlike adults, headaches strike young people with less gender bias than adults: Males and females are almost equally afflicted.

Headache Sources in Children

Children are prone to the same types of headaches as adults (except of course hormone-related headaches), and a lower incidence of cluster though they may be more vulnerable to headaches related to trauma due to falling down or bumping their heads. They may also be more sensitive to infections, reporting headache symptoms that are really caused by an ear infection, cold, or sinus infection. With teenagers, particularly young women, the relatively sudden escalation of hormones could be a powerful headache trigger, often potentiating the first headache attack.

As with adults, headaches can be brought on by stress, improper posture, dietary factors, environmental assaults (bright lights, odors, etc.), or emotional distress. Indeed the child may be more sensitive to the toxins in the environment, and is not yet well armed to cope with food allergies.

Migraine in Children: Variations on a Theme

Migraine is not uncommon among children; more than half of migraineurs have their first migraine attack before the age of twenty.

Very young children may not be able to express the source of their discomfort. They may appear restless and irritable, pale and "fragile."

If they have a severe headache, they may seek out a quiet, dark room—just as adults would. Most migraine symptoms mimic those experienced by adults (see Chapter 2); children are more likely, however, to have pain on both sides of their head, whereas adults usually have pain only on one side. In addition to the migraine described for adults, migraine in children may take other forms:

- *Abdominal migraine.* Expressed as nausea and/or vomiting, with or without headache, lasting for hours or days. Children may be more prone to motion sickness. Clearly it is important to rule out other potential causes for abdominal pain before marking it as a migraine.
- *Basilar migraine.* A prodrome to head pain, or along with head pain, experienced as weakness or numbness of the limbs, unsteadiness, dizziness, or loss of consciousness. Some children also experience an *acute confusional state,* which can occur separately from the headache, where they become drowsy and/or listless and irritable. They may see changing shapes, or smell odors that do not exist. These symptoms usually disappear within an hour. This type of migraine may continue into adulthood.
- *Hemiplegic migraine.* Numbness and/or weakness of an arm or leg on one side of the body, along with head pain. May also persist into adulthood.
- *Ophthalmoplegic migraine.* Weakness of the eye muscles causing double vision, usually accompanying headache. Again, it is important to rule out other possible causes before settling on a diagnosis of migraine. May also persist into adulthood.

Tension-type Headache in Children

Children are subject to the same responses to stress as adults. Bodily stresses caused by improper posture might be a source of headache-causing muscle tension—which is more easily corrected at a young age. Also, as with adults, the source of tension-type headache can often be traced to emotional issues. Symptoms of tension-type headache in children are similar to those in adults.

Emotional Factors of Children's Headache

Children are often exquisitely sensitive to emotionally charged issues at home, with friends, and at school. In their book *Headache Free* Roger Cady, M.D., and Kathleen Farmer, Psy.D., describe the sick child as "an emotional barometer for the climate at home." Just as headache may be a symptom of an underlying physical disorder, it may also be the clearest signal of deeper emotional problems—depression, anxiety, frustration, or hopelessness. How is the child doing at school? Is she experiencing great pressure from friends or schoolwork demands? Does he have fears or insecurities about his role in the family? Rather than view the child's chronic headache as a mere play for attention, parents may be well advised to see it as a real call for help.

Evaluating the Child's Headache

Even the most articulate and self-aware adult can spend several frustrating years before finding a doctor who can diagnose the cause of his or her headache. Children are at an even greater disadvantage. How do you distinguish between a headache that is potentially severe and life-threatening and one that is benign? Cady and Farmer suggest asking the child the following questions:

- Where does it hurt?
- When did the hurt begin?
- How did the hurt begin?
- Does it hurt as bad as skinning your knee?

If the headache continues to recur, Cady and Farmer suggest looking into emotional issues relating to school, friends, and other concerns.[7]

Headache Alternatives for Children

An understanding of the sources of your child's headache is your best guide to the solution. Pay special attention to the timing of your child's headache: Did it occur after eating a particular food? Does it always happen after going to a certain friend's house? There may be a food or environmental sensitivity at school. You'll find pointers for detecting these sensitivities—and solutions for averting them—in Chapter 6.

Opening discussions about emotional issues with your child can help defuse anxieties. Children are especially responsive to relaxation and biofeedback techniques, described in Chapter 8.

Postural problems can be detected, and reversed, in several ways—see Chapter 7.

In short, holistic alternatives described in the next half of this book may be particularly appealing to the parents who want to avoid chronic drug therapy for their children with headache.

PART II

The Alternatives

Medicus curat, natura sanat—Medicine treats, nature heals.

———

There are hundreds of alternative routes that motivated self-healers can take to relieving their headache. How do you find the one that is right for you, or for your child? Here are my recommendations:

• *Start with your instincts.*   Can something as unscientific as instinct be the right way to select a health method? In fact there is some scientific basis for following instincts in this matter. First, there is mounting evidence that the mind has a powerful effect on the health of the body. If you understand and want a treatment to work, it is more likely to be successful. The power of the placebo effect is evidence of this success. As we will see in Chapter 8, the mind can control much more than we have been generally taught to believe.

Second, scientific study shows that commitment, or as doctors like to say, *compliance,* is a key predictor of success—even with drug therapy. A significant percentage of drug therapies fail because people fail to take them correctly, or for long enough. Your commitment to many of the complementary approaches we review in Chapters 6–10 will need to be substantial. Expect no overnight miracle cures. Expect instead to spend time—brewing teas or visiting therapists, following exercise programs or sorting out your nutritional needs, practicing postures or meditating. In short expect to become actively and intimately involved in the fate of your own health. The upside of this committed work may very well be a greater chance of success—with any method you select.

That being the case, you might as well start by finding a treatment approach for which you have a *natural affinity*. For example, if you love to exercise and work on your body, explore the physical approaches first. If you are introspective, you might start with the mind-body approaches. If you are an avid gardener, you may enjoy growing and brewing your own herbs. You can mix different techniques as well. Children respond particularly well to interactive approaches, such as biofeedback, guided imagery, and progressive relaxation.

We have organized the complementary methods roughly by category. There are some spillovers. Some of the physical approaches, such as yoga, clearly cross over into the mind-body realm. And while the underlying theories of homeopathy differ greatly from herbal therapy, it does often employ botanical substances.

Finally, you will not find chapters devoted exclusively to macrobiotics, naturopathic approaches, traditional Oriental medicine, or Ayurvedic medicine. For overviews of these healing philosophies, see Chapter 1. Specific practices from these disciplines are interwoven throughout the book, as they apply to different categories of healing. More information can be found in the "Resources" section at the end of this book.

• *Evaluate your response and your progress.*   Generally we rely on doctors to photograph and prod our bodies, process the information, then feed it back to us. With many complementary therapies, you will be taking the lead. It will be up to you to keep in touch with your body's responses and to gauge your own progress. Self-knowledge techniques are new skills for many of us—but well worth cultivating. It is very helpful to keep a diary of your headaches, their duration, and their severity. The diary should also contain possible triggers, such as stress, foods, and weather changes.

How long before you give up on a technique? Many treatments take much longer to do their work than drugs; as a rule of thumb, if an approach does not yield some positive change within one or two months, you should move on to a different practice. There are exceptions. For example, riboflavin may need to be taken for more than two months before results begin to appear, according to one study.

• *Find a reliable partner in health.* While we encourage you to take responsibility for your health, we recommend that you find a reliable partner to help you get started at first. If your regular doctor is open to complementary approaches, he or she should be your first choice. If not, we have compiled a list of organizations (see ''Resources'') to guide you toward practitioners in different areas of complementary medicine.

This book must not be used in place of a physician or qualified health care practitioner. Most of the complementary approaches we describe in the following pages have not undergone the rigors of clinical study. Many are not considered therapeutic and have not been investigated or approved by any government or regulatory medical agency in this country. In some cases the practitioners themselves do not make therapeutic claims. We urge you to exercise caution when evaluating a practitioner or an approach.

In presenting the information on the following pages our aim is to educate you, to the best of our ability, to the many *options* available to you. We neither recommend nor suggest their use, and disclaim any responsibility for harm that might result from this information. Only you and your health care professional are qualified to make decisions regarding your health. We strongly recommend that you consult your doctor or health care professional before engaging in any medical treatment plan, particularly if you are pregnant or have an underlying health condition.

CHAPTER 6

Nutritional and Environmental Approaches

Tell me what you eat, and I will tell you what you are.
—A*NTHELME* B*RILLAT* -S*AVARIN*

▬▬▬

After reading Chapters 3 and 4, you might feel daunted by the task of (a) discovering *whether* foods or environmental factors are contributing to your headaches; (b) identifying *which* factors are at play; and (c) figuring out *how* to cope with them. We'll try to give you some guidance here. In this chapter you'll get the basics of a healthy diet according to several schools of thought. We'll also offer a method for identifying which, if any, substances are triggering your headache. And we'll recommend some ways to help you remove headache-causing toxins from your body, boost your immune system, and lessen your sensitivity or allergy to substances.

CREATING YOUR HEADACHE-FREE DIET

How do you know whether your headaches stem from the foods you eat? It's possible that in reading the lists of headache-causing foods, one type of food jumped out at you and triggered the thought "Yes, that's it! Whenever I eat chocolate (for example), I get a headache!" I would recommend that you follow your intuition and avoid chocolate to see if it helps. But few of us are that lucky. In the absence of a striking revelation, we offer here several approaches you can take.

Start with a Healthy Diet

A balanced diet is the foundation of good health. As adaptable as it is, the human body requires nourishment to function properly. This statement might seem too obvious for words, but it bears real consideration. We know that the lack of nutrients is a significant stressor on its own: Our immune system fails to function properly, we lack energy, our organs fail to do the work they should. We become more vulnerable to headache and other physical ailments. In this weakened state we are less able to cope with the emotional and psychological stresses that can also trigger headache, or set off other disease processes.

Even if you discover that you're sensitive to certain types of foods and get headaches as a result, you need to replace the offending foods with others or supplements that provide similar nutrients. So, before trying to isolate food allergies or sensitivities, first evaluate your basic diet.

What, then, constitutes a good diet? There are several theories.

Conventional Western Medicine

Nutritional guidance in the United States was first devoted to ways of preventing nutritional deficiencies and of promoting consumption of agricultural products. Over the past few years public-health policy has taken aim at lowering the risk of diseases caused by overconsumption. The shift reflects changes in the U.S. food supply over the past century—from one of lack to one of abundance. The current consensus of federal nutritional policy makers—including the United States Department of Agriculture and the Food and Nutrition Board of the National Academy of Sciences—is expressed as the Food Guide Pyramid.

The Food Pyramid was designed to give the general public information on how to adjust the proportions of common foods so that the diet includes the Recommended Daily Allowance (RDA) of nutrients while reducing the risks of nutrition-related diseases. The diet is high in fiber, low in fat, and balanced nutritionally. There are no exotic foods or supplements recommended. It's also important to keep in mind that these foods and their proportions are recommended for the general healthy population—a broad-sweeping generalization that doesn't take into account special populations (e.g., pregnant women, children, and people with specific disease conditions) or lifestyles (e.g., very physically active).

However, dieters beware. Too much emphasis is being placed on low-fat diets. Too little fat combined with too much carbohydrates is also proving to be unhealthy—and counterproductive to weight loss. The ideal diet should be balanced.

FOOD PYRAMID GUIDE

Fats, Oils, and Sweets Use Sparingly	
Milk, Yogurt, and Cheese Group 2–3 servings	Meat, poultry, fish dry beans, eggs, and nuts 2–3 servings
Vegetable Group 3–5 servings	Fruit Group 2–4 servings
Bread, Cereal, Rice, and Pasta Group 8–11 servings	

Source: U.S. Department of Agriculture and U.S. Department of Health and Human Services, 1990.

The Food Pyramid Guide, as we mentioned, is based on the RDA. According to nutritional experts, some people might need higher dosages of certain vitamins and minerals, including those who are

- Physically active
- Pregnant or lactating mothers
- Under stress

- Mentally or physically ill
- Taking other medications
- Recovering from surgery
- Smokers
- Alcoholics

In Chapter 3 we identified some vitamin and mineral deficiencies that could contribute to headache. Check the chart below for natural ways to supplement your diet with these nutrients. Briefly they include the following:

Vitamins/Minerals That Could Contribute to Headache

Too Little	**Too Much**
Magnesium	Vitamin A
Niacin	Fatty food
Folic acid	
Iron	

Nutrients and Dosages for Maintaining Good Health

What follows are the Recommended Daily Allowances put forth by the National Research Council in 1989. Keep in mind that these are average doses, for the healthy, average-weight adult male. Some nutritional levels should be slightly lower for females (except for vitamin D, calcium, and phosphorus) and somewhat higher for pregnant and lactating mothers. Levels are often significantly lower for infants and young children. And they may be very different for people with underlying diseases. Consult a registered dietitian, nutritionist, or other expert for dietary recommendations that are right for you.

Vitamins	**RDA**	**Food Sources**
Vitamin A	4,000–5,000 IU	Chicken and turkey, dark green leafy vegetables, root vegetables, yellow fruits
Vitamin B_1 (thiamine)	1.5 mg	Dried beans, brown rice, egg yolks, fish, peas, pork, poultry, wheat germ
Vitamin B_2 (riboflavin)	1.7 mg	Beans, cheese, eggs, fish, meat, poultry, spinach, yogurt
Vitamin B_3 (niacin, niacinamide)	16–20 mg	Beef, broccoli, carrots, cheese, corn, flour, eggs, fish, milk, potatoes, tomatoes, whole wheat
Vitamin B_5	4–7 mg	Beans, beef, eggs, saltwater fish, pork, fresh vegetables, whole wheat
Vitamin B_6 (pyridoxine)	2–2.5 mcg	Brewer's yeast, carrots, chicken, eggs, fish, meat, peas, spinach, sunflower seeds, walnuts, wheat germ
Vitamin B_{12} (cyanocobalamin)	3–4 mcg	Beef, shellfish, eggs, salmon, yogurt
Vitamin D	400 IU	Fish liver oils, fatty saltwater fish, fortified dairy and eggs, sunlight, alfalfa, butter, cod liver oil, egg yolk, milk, oatmeal, salmon, sardines, sweet potatoes, tuna, vegetable oil

Vitamins	**RDA**	**Food Sources**
Vitamin E	12–15 IU	Cold-pressed vegetable oils, whole grains, dark green leafy vegetables, nuts and seeds, legumes
Vitamin K	65 mcg	Alfalfa, broccoli, dark green leafy vegetables
Vitamin C with mineral ascorbates	60 mg	Green vegetables, berries, citrus fruits
Folic acid	400 mcg	Barley, beans, beef, bran, brewer's yeast, brown rice, cheese, chicken, dates, dark green leafy vegetables, lamb, lentils, liver, milk, oranges

Minerals	**Daily Dosages**	**Food Sources**
Calcium (chelate)	800–1200 mg	Dairy, salmon (with bones), sardines, seafood, dark green leafy vegetables
Chromium*	50–200 mg	Meat, whole grains, broccoli, brewer's yeast, fortified cereals
Copper*	2–3 mg	Shellfish, beans, nuts, seeds, organ meats, whole grains, potatoes
Fluoride*	1.5–4 mg	Fluoridated water, marine fish
Iodine	150 mcg	Iodized salts, seafood, saltwater fish, kelp
	175 mcg during pregnancy	

Minerals	Daily Dosages	Food Sources
Iron*	10 mg 30 mg during pregnancy	Eggs, liver, fish, meat, poultry, dark green leafy vegetables, whole grains, enriched breads and cereals
Magnesium	280 mg, men 350 mg, women	Wheat bran, whole grains, dark green leafy vegetables, meat, nuts, beans, milk, bananas
Manganese*	2.5–5 mg	Whole grains, nuts, vegetables, fruits, tea, beans
Molybdenum*	75–250 mg	Whole grains, liver, beans, dark green leafy vegetables
Phosphorus	1,200 mg 2,300 mg during pregnancy 800 mg over age 25	Plentiful in almost all foods
Potassium*	1,600–2,000	Oranges, bananas, potatoes with skin, dried fruits, yogurt, meat, poultry, milk
Selenium	55 mcg, women 70 mcg, men 65 mcg, pregnancy	Fish, shellfish, red meat, grains, eggs, chicken, garlic, organ meats
Sodium*	2,400 mg maximum	Salt
Zinc	12 mg, women 15 mg, men, women during pregnancy	Seafood, liver, eggs, brewer's yeast

Other Nutrients*	Daily Dosages**	Food Sources
Biotin	300 mcg	Cooked egg yolk, saltwater fish, meat, milk, poultry, soybeans, whole grains, yeast

Choline	100 mg	Egg yolks, legumes, meat, milk, whole-grain cereals
Inositol	100 mg	Fruits, vegetables, whole grains, milk, meats
PABA (para-aminobenzoic acid)	25 mg	Kidney, liver, molasses, whole grains
EFA (Vitamin F) (essential fatty acids)	25 mg	Apricots, cherries, grapefruit, grapes, lemons, oranges, prunes, rose hips
Coenzyme Q_{10}	30 mg	Mackerel, salmon, sardines
Garlic	60 mg	Garlic, kyolic supplements
L-carnitine	100 mg	Food supplements
L-cysteine	50 mg	Food supplements
L-lysine	50 mg	Food supplements
L-methionine	50 mg	Food supplements
L-tyrosine	100 mg	Food supplements
Lecithin	200–500 mg	Soybeans, eggs, brewer's yeast, grains, legumes, fish, wheat germ
Pectin	50 mg	Apples, carrots, beets, cabbage, citrus fruits, dried peas, okra
RNA-DNA	100 mg	Food supplements

*No RDA established; ranges of Estimated Safe and Adequate Daily Dietary Intake from the National Academy of Sciences.

**No RDA established; ranges from *Prescription for Nutritional Healing.*

Sources for chart: National Research Council, American Dietetic Association; *Prescription for Nutritional Healing* (Avery Publishing Group, Inc.) with permission; *University of California Wellness Letter* vol. 8, no. 11, August 1992.

Some Vitamin Pointers

• Women should get the RDA for folic acid (400 mcg) to reduce the risk of neural tube birth defects.

• If iron levels exceed the RDA, there may be increased risk of heart disease.

• Very high doses of zinc (above 50 mg/day) may compromise immune function.

• Magnesium and calcium must be taken either in a slow-release form or in several daily doses.

VITAMIN SOURCES: SUPPLEMENTS VERSUS FOOD

As you can see from the preceding chart, constructing a healthy diet can be a complicated and time-consuming matter. Wouldn't it be *easier* to just take supplements? Easier, yes. Healthier? Not necessarily.

Most experts would recommend that you get nutrients from your diet rather than vitamin/mineral supplements. I generally agree. The nutrients in foods are more easily taken in by the body and often confer other beneficial qualities that are important to health, such as dietary fiber. Also it is very difficult to overdose on vitamins or minerals from food. Finally, taking dietary supplements provides no greater guarantee that your body will "utilize" the nutrients you take. Many factors can influence whether your body is actually using these nutrients properly—your age, exercise level, underlying diseases, and so on.

With all of this said, there are some cases where vitamin/mineral supplements are of value. For instance people on food-restricted diets, due to allergy or other conditions, might need to take vitamin supplements. In addition it is difficult to get the RDA of certain nutrients from a healthy diet alone. For example studies show that at doses of 100 to 400 IU daily, vitamin E is a powerful antioxidant, helping to reduce the incidence of heart attack and cancer. But to get this amount in food, you might need to consume a lot of fats (vegetable oils), which can have negative health effects.

Similarly people with calcium deficiencies—especially vulnerable are women of menopausal age—often must turn to supplements to help stave off osteoporosis. In addition the elderly (over the age of seventy) often do not eat enough to get the nutrients they need such as magnesium and the B vitamins. Our caloric needs might decrease with age, but our need for nutrients doesn't.

If you think you need vitamin supplements, here are some guidelines to help you select brands that meet your needs:

- Look for expiration dates. If they aren't obvious, ask the pharmacist to help you.
- Store in a dark, cool, dry place to optimize shelf life.
- Choose multivitamins that provide 100 percent of RDA.
- Generally, time-release and sustained-release supplements are not only more expensive but unnecessary. An exception: time-release iron for pregnant women.
- In large doses vitamins and minerals can be toxic. In 1991 U.S. poison control centers received fifty-six thousand calls about supplement-related vitamin/mineral toxicity. Getting your nutrients from foods avoids this problem.
- In large doses (more than 300% of the RDA), vitamins and minerals can cause a deficiency of other nutrients. (For example, taking too much copper or iron could result in a zinc deficiency.)
- In large doses nutrients may suppress your own natural immune system.
- Avoid high doses (more than 1,500 mg daily) of sustained-release niacin, to minimize toxicity.
- Higher doses of iron may be harmful, especially for men.

NATUROPATHY

Nutrition is the mainstay of naturopathy, which often relies on foods and herbs as therapeutic approaches in and of themselves. Naturopathy espouses the healing power of nature. An eclectic system, naturopathic doctrine advocates a variety of holistic approaches to help individuals maintain or regain a state of vital, dynamic health. The naturopathic diet emphasizes natural and unprocessed foods—particularly plants (fruits, vegetables, grains, beans, seeds, and nuts), with very little refined food (honey, fruit juices, dried fruit, sugar, and white flour). It may be seen as a more natural version of the diet devised by modern Western science—and one that focuses on cleansing the body.

VEGETARIAN DIETS

Vegetarians will be happy to hear that plant- and dairy-based diets have been shown to be healthier than those relying on meat as the main course. In general they are more plentiful in foods that help lower the risk of nutrition-related diseases, such as grains, fruits, and vegetables. Even with this said, vegetarians must be just as mindful of their menus as carnivores to make sure that they get adequate nutrition. The *Harvard Women's Health Watch* (January 1996), a health journal published by Harvard Medical School Publications Group, recommends that vegetarians pay particularly close attention to the following nutrients, which are easy to miss in many vegetarian diets:

- Folic acid or folate—leafy green vegetables such as kale are high in folate
- Vitamin D—found in dairy products or derived from exposure to sunlight; needed for calcium absorption; vegans should consider supplements
- Calcium—citrus fruits increase calcium absorption, whereas spinach can inhibit it
- Iron—citrus fruits enhance iron absorption from other foods, whereas legumes, beets, grains, and fortified flour can deplete it
- Vitamin B_{12}—found in dairy products; vegans should consider vitamin supplements
- Protein—soy products are excellent sources of protein, equal to meat

The risk of nutritional deficiency is especially high among people who follow *vegan* diets, which omit all meat and dairy products such as cheese, eggs, yogurt, and milk. These diets should not be fed to children under the age of five because they may be more vulnerable to developmental problems due to anemia (iron deficiency) and B_{12} deficiency. The Vegetarian Food Pyramid, below, shows how you can build a nutritionally sound diet from vegetarian or vegan sources.

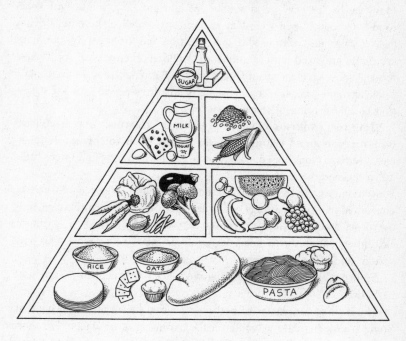

Vegetarian Food Pyramid

ORTHOMOLECULAR MEDICINE (MEGADOSE NUTRITIONAL SUPPLEMENTS)

Linus Pauling, winner of the Nobel Prize in 1968, coined the term *orthomolecular* to describe an approach to medicine that recognizes illness as a deficiency in nutrients—and the use of nutrient supplements to reestablish health. Orthomolecular physicians use nutritional therapy as their primary means of treating disease, often supplemented by vitamins in doses that far exceed the RDA range.

HERBALISM

Many herbs are very good sources of nutrients and, along with other foods, are considered excellent therapies by medical herbalists. They have traditionally been used to aid digestion and for flavoring, but many are richly endowed with vitamins and minerals themselves. As "whole foods" they have an advantage over supplements; they often contain vital nutrients *plus* the complementary qualities needed for the digestion and absorption of these nutrients.

However, while many herbs are rich in vitamins, some herbalists do not recommend taking them on a daily basis to correct deficiencies. Herbs, as mentioned, often contain other nutrients that might build up in the body over time.

Remember, herbs are not by definition safe. While some can be consumed in high quantities or for long periods of time without causing overdose, others should be prepared very carefully and taken sparingly; still others should be avoided during pregnancy or by people who have certain underlying illnesses.

Before taking any herbal preparation, it's best to consult a qualified herbalist.

The healing properties of herbs go beyond their nutritional content. Some are medicinally valuable for the treatment of headache. For more about herbal remedies for headache and their preparation, see Chapter 9.

MACROBIOTICS

Macrobiotic teachings assert that as warm-blooded beings, humans are constitutionally yang (see Chapter 1 for definition of *yang* and *ying*). To balance our yang tendencies, we generally need yin foods—our complementary opposite—to maintain good health. Yin foods include vegetables that are harvested during spring or summer and generally grow above ground (lettuces, peas, beans, herbs, cucumbers, etc.), as well as *some* fish, especially whitefish and shellfish.

Yang foods include plants that are harvested later in the year and generally grow below ground (roots, such as carrots, beets, and parsnips; winter squashes; etc.), as well as most meats.

Brown rice is regarded as the most balanced of foods. However, dietary requirements differ depending on several factors. For example men require more yang foods than women.

Common sense confirms what macrobiotic thought tells us, which is that the climate and season of the year affect our food requirements. For example, those living in a very cold, yin climate generally need to balance out with foods that are very yang, such as animal meat. On the other hand, those living in hot tropical, yang regions require the complementary opposite—yin foods (more fruits and vegetables)—to maintain a balance. This is why practitioners of macrobiotics often espouse foods that are natural to one's own region.

Our lifestyle and physical makeup also play important roles in our food needs, and vice versa. Each person has his or her own capacity for yin and yang foods, and an intake beyond that capacity might create an imbalance and a physical reaction. For example, consuming small amounts of chocolate every day might not bother you until, one day, you've reached your limit and react with chronic headaches—without ever really understanding the cause because you've become so used to eating chocolate. However, if you were to balance that intake with physical activity, you might never experience a reaction.

The way macrobiotic meals are prepared and eaten is almost as important as the meals themselves. The attitude of the cook, the cookware used, the cleanliness of the kitchen and utensils, and the manner in which foods are eaten all influence the overall healthfulness of the food, and ultimately the health of the person consuming it. (See "Resources" for books on macrobiotic diets.)

AYURVEDA

Ayurvedic medicine also relies on a variety of healing tools to prevent illness and maintain health—but good nutrition is central. Poor nutrition is viewed as being an almost surefire way to cause illness.

As you might remember from Chapter 1, the Ayurvedic belief is that all living things, foods included, embody different proportions of the five fundamental energies of the universe—ether, air, fire, water, and earth. Human beings are regarded constitutionally as three predominant types of bio-energies, or *doshas: vata* (ether and air), *pitta* (fire and water), and *kapha* (earth and water). Similarly foods have different energies that have different effects on each individual.

The Ayurvedic diet is highly individualized, with foods matched to counterbalance disturbances in an individual's bio-energy. For people with an overabundance of kapha characteristics, a kapha-balancing diet will be recommended, and so on. Similarly you can be of a kapha dosha and have illness that results from disturbances in vata or pitta, which might require an anti-vata or anti-pitta diet.

Just as emotions can influence the way we digest (or don't digest) foods, foods can also influence emotions, according to Ayurvedic thought. Certain foods are known to expand consciousness. These foods are whole foods of wheat, rice, milk, sugar, green vegetables, fruits, and nuts. Others are known as passionate foods, and include spicy foods, alcoholic and caffeinated drinks, fried foods, and others. Canned and frozen foods, strong alcoholic beverages, and others induce greed, pessimism, and laziness. These are just a few examples.

Based on your bio-type (see Chapter 1), you can get a *general* idea of the types of foods that are best suited for you. However, keep in mind that your age, climate, digestive process, and general health will all influence the type of diet that is best for you.

To Balance Vata

- Most recommended: grains (wheat, oats, rice); most vegetables; most fruits; most nuts and seeds; sesame oil; most spices; dairy products; natural (unrefined) sugars
- To be avoided: dry grains (cereals and soybeans); raw onions; pork and lard; refined sugar and chocolate.

To Balance Pitta

- Most recommended: grains (wheat, mung beans); raw vegetables; most fruits; unfermented milk products; mild spices; unrefined sweets
- To be avoided: raw onions; peanuts; peanut oil; pork, lamb, beef, and shellfish; salt and very hot spices (peppers, garlic, mustard); refined sugar

To Balance Kapha

- Most recommended: some cooked vegetables (especially celery, broccoli, cabbage, and carrots); hard fruits (apples and pears); hot spices
- To be avoided: white rice and wheat; bananas; peanuts; peanut and olive oils; pork, beef, and lamb; refined salt; molasses, refined sugar, raw sugar, and maple syrup

When and how you eat is almost as important as what you eat, according to Ayurvedic tradition. The timing (ideally, between ten A.M. and one P.M. for the main meal, when digestion is heightened), atmosphere (calm for adequate digestion), and spacing (allow eight hours for full digestion) of meals should all be considered.

It cannot be overemphasized that the Ayurvedic approach is very individualized. We offer these *general* guidelines to give you an idea of the Ayurvedic view of nutrition, but they cannot replace your own study of the subject or the advice of an Ayurvedic practitioner (see "Resources" at the end of this book).

TRADITIONAL ORIENTAL MEDICINE

As with Ayurveda and macrobiotics, traditional Oriental medicine puts great emphasis on diet. Air, physical health, and diet are the three main ways that we generate a healthy flow of qi (see Chapter 1 for more on the principle of traditional Oriental medicine). We have more control over our diet than we do any other health-influencing factor.

As Bob Flaws explains in *Migraine and Traditional Chinese Medicine,* the digestive process is one of heating and processing foods in the "Fire" of the Stomach; it is distilled by the Spleen; then the "Pure" essence of the food is sent to the Heart and Lungs to be transformed into Blood and qi. At the same time, the "Turbid" residue is eliminated by the body. (Remember, in traditional Chinese medicine, the Stomach, Spleen, Heart, and Lungs refer not only to the organs themselves but to the meridian channels that cross them—the biosystem connected to them.)

Chinese medicine teaches that cooking foods gives the digestive process a head start. Similarly drinks should be taken only sparingly with meals—and they should never be cold. The liquid weakens the digestive process, and the coldness works against the important heating process of digesting foods.

During digestion, if the Pure and the Turbid are not separated, the foods undergo negative changes that can disrupt the flow of qi. For optimal digestion the stomach should be half full of food, one-quarter full of liquid, and one-quarter empty.

In traditional thought, foods are characterized by many different qualities—yin and yang are at the foundation. Food temperature, or "nature," is also important. This refers not only to the food's temperature but to other intrinsic characteristics as well. Foods should be warm or room temperature when eaten. And they should be Warm or Neutral in quality. Spices and alcohol are, by nature, Hot or Warm. So, small quantities can be helpful in digestion. But, if they are taken in excess, they create too much Heat.

The important food qualities include the following:

- Taste (salty, sour, bitter, sweet, pungent, and neutral)
- Direction (ascending, descending, floating, sinking)
- Meridian route
- Yin/Yang balance
- Five Elements (based on temperature and Taste)
- Contraindications (powerful adverse qualities)

Taken together, these qualities help determine the place of a certain food in an individual's diet. As with Ayurvedic medicine, diet can become a powerful therapy. Chinese dietary medicine is not only individualized but complex. Interested readers are urged to explore books mentioned in the "Resources" section.

IDENTIFY FOODS THAT TRIGGER YOUR HEADACHE

There are several excellent books devoted exclusively to the dietary causes of headache. You can either follow these prescribed diets, which may mean making drastic changes, or you can try to identify the food(s) that trigger your headaches and make corresponding adjustments to your diet (see "Resources"). Both approaches require some commitment and effort. But the second approach, which we'll describe here, may actually help you overcome your food sensitivity, and ultimately enable you to reintroduce that food into your diet.

As we've mentioned in Chapter 3, there is evidence that certain foods and drugs produce biochemical effects that can set headaches in motion. But the link between diet and headache is controversial. The "allergy" theory is not widely accepted by conventional Western medicine. Indeed most mainstream experts believe that only 10 to 30 percent of headaches stem from food sensitivities and that only 1 percent are due to allergy.[1]

On the other hand, others believe that most chronic migraines, tension-type headaches, and cluster headaches are caused by food allergy or sensitivity and that removing intolerance- or allergy-inducing foods helps control headaches. In one study eighty-two out of eighty-eight children with chronic, severe migraine were identified as having food allergies—most commonly milk, eggs, chocolate, oranges, and wheat. And when the children were free of their food allergies, they also had higher tolerance for other headache-triggering factors, such as exercise, bright lights, noise, emotional stress, and perfume.[2]

Finally, many environmental physicians believe that food intolerance may stem from a combination of factors resulting in *chemical sensitiv-*

ity—which is different from allergy (which is not based in the immune system).

Whatever the mechanism, many clinical studies have confirmed that detecting and removing foods that cause headaches can either eliminate or reduce symptoms. In a review of five different studies of people with migraine, for example, food offered some relief for 30 to 93 percent of them.[3]

There are several ways you can go about identifying, and cleansing your body of, headache-inducing foods. An allergist may administer one of several different kinds of skin tests, whereby allergens are injected into the body, and if the skin reacts with an immune response such as redness, the test is positive for that allergen. Other allergists believe that this type of test might not be a good way to diagnose headache-related allergies because the immune system, overstressed by the onslaught of allergens, is unable to respond adequately to show up in the skin test. One of the tests, the lymphocyte test, which measures the immune system's white blood cell response to an antigen, is considered to give a more accurate reading of allergy. But many allergic people, according to some experts, even fail this test.

There are other ways to determine your food allergy or intolerance, which involves eliminating foods. There are two ways you can do this. You can follow all of the steps below, or simply try an *elimination diet,* followed by *sensitivity testing.* We'll go into more detail about each step on the following pages. Here's a quick overview of the long process, as outlined by several nutritional experts, including James F. Balch, M.D., and Phyllis A. Balch, C.N.C., in their book *Prescription for Nutritional Healing*:

1. *Identify the foods you eat most often.*   Look back at the past month. Which foods do you eat more than four times a week? This phase is simply to identify how often you normally eat certain foods.

2. *Keep a food diary.*   Look at your food record. Eliminate all foods you eat or drink more than four times a week. Do this for thirty days. The idea is that when you eat certain foods habitually, your body starts to become intolerant to them and you are more likely to have an allergic

reaction. By omitting these "habit foods" for thirty days, you're giving your body time to cleanse itself and rebuild your immune system.

3. *Take the food-sensitivity pulse test.* Now that you've given your body a rest from all the foods you eat on a regular basis, try each "habit food" again. Each time you do, take the sensitivity test. If your body reacts to the food, omit it from your diet for another thirty days.

4. *Cleanse your body.* After you've eliminated the offending foods from your diet, give your body a thorough cleansing. There are several options, depending on your preference and overall health, including fasting and enemas. For most people, fasting is recommended. (We'll address other cleansing methods at the end of the chapter.) If you fast for more than two days, be sure you are under a doctor's supervision.

5. *Reintroduce foods.* Start with very simple foods, then slowly add foods that you eliminated, one at a time, back into your diet. Be conscious of whether these foods cause a reaction.

6. *Rotate your diet.* Follow a specific diet for one week, changing it every day, including only foods that agree with you.

Step 1: Identify the Foods You Eat Most Often

Fill out this form. Each week list the foods you eat in the different categories. Then mark down how many times you eat that specific type of food.

Type of Food Beverages	Week 1	Week 2	Week 3	Week 4
[list beverages here]	[list how many times you drink them each week]			
_____	_____	_____	_____	_____
_____	_____	_____	_____	_____
_____	_____	_____	_____	_____
_____	_____	_____	_____	_____
_____	_____	_____	_____	_____
_____	_____	_____	_____	_____
_____	_____	_____	_____	_____

Type of Food	Week 1	Week 2	Week 3	Week 4

Breads and starches

[list breads/starches here]   [list how many times you eat them each week]

_____   _____ _____ _____ _____
_____   _____ _____ _____ _____
_____   _____ _____ _____ _____
_____   _____ _____ _____ _____
_____   _____ _____ _____ _____
_____   _____ _____ _____ _____
_____   _____ _____ _____ _____
_____   _____ _____ _____ _____
_____   _____ _____ _____ _____

Condiments and spices

[list condiments here]   [list how many times you use them each week]

_____   _____ _____ _____ _____
_____   _____ _____ _____ _____
_____   _____ _____ _____ _____
_____   _____ _____ _____ _____
_____   _____ _____ _____ _____
_____   _____ _____ _____ _____
_____   _____ _____ _____ _____
_____   _____ _____ _____ _____

Dairy products

[list dairy products here]   [list how many times you eat them each week]

_____   _____ _____ _____ _____
_____   _____ _____ _____ _____
_____   _____ _____ _____ _____
_____   _____ _____ _____ _____
_____   _____ _____ _____ _____
_____   _____ _____ _____ _____
_____   _____ _____ _____ _____

Type of Food	**Week 1**	**Week 2**	**Week 3**	**Week 4**

Fruits and juices

[list fruits/juices here]   [list how many times you eat/drink them each week]

_____	_____	_____	_____	_____
_____	_____	_____	_____	_____
_____	_____	_____	_____	_____
_____	_____	_____	_____	_____
_____	_____	_____	_____	_____
_____	_____	_____	_____	_____
_____	_____	_____	_____	_____
_____	_____	_____	_____	_____
_____	_____	_____	_____	_____
_____	_____	_____	_____	_____
_____	_____	_____	_____	_____
_____	_____	_____	_____	_____

Grains

[list grains here]   [list how many times you eat them each week]

_____	_____	_____	_____	_____
_____	_____	_____	_____	_____
_____	_____	_____	_____	_____
_____	_____	_____	_____	_____
_____	_____	_____	_____	_____
_____	_____	_____	_____	_____
_____	_____	_____	_____	_____
_____	_____	_____	_____	_____
_____	_____	_____	_____	_____
_____	_____	_____	_____	_____

Type of Food	Week 1	Week 2	Week 3	Week 4

Meats, poultry, fish

[list meats, etc., here]   [list how many times you eat them each week]

_____   _____ _____ _____ _____
_____   _____ _____ _____ _____
_____   _____ _____ _____ _____
_____   _____ _____ _____ _____
_____   _____ _____ _____ _____
_____   _____ _____ _____ _____
_____   _____ _____ _____ _____
_____   _____ _____ _____ _____
_____   _____ _____ _____ _____
_____   _____ _____ _____ _____

Nuts and seeds

[list nuts/seeds here]   [list how many times you eat them each week]

_____   _____ _____ _____ _____
_____   _____ _____ _____ _____
_____   _____ _____ _____ _____
_____   _____ _____ _____ _____
_____   _____ _____ _____ _____
_____   _____ _____ _____ _____
_____   _____ _____ _____ _____
_____   _____ _____ _____ _____

Oils

[list oils here]   [list how many times you use them each week]

_____   _____ _____ _____ _____
_____   _____ _____ _____ _____
_____   _____ _____ _____ _____
_____   _____ _____ _____ _____
_____   _____ _____ _____ _____

Type of Food
Spreads   Week 1   Week 2   Week 3   Week 4

[list spreads here]   [list how many times you eat them each week]

_____   _____   _____   _____   _____
_____   _____   _____   _____   _____
_____   _____   _____   _____   _____
_____   _____   _____   _____   _____
_____   _____   _____   _____   _____
_____   _____   _____   _____   _____

Sweeteners

[list sweeteners here]   [list how many times you use them each week]

_____   _____   _____   _____   _____
_____   _____   _____   _____   _____
_____   _____   _____   _____   _____
_____   _____   _____   _____   _____
_____   _____   _____   _____   _____
_____   _____   _____   _____   _____
_____   _____   _____   _____   _____

Vegetables

[list vegetables here]   [list how many times you eat them each week]

_____   _____   _____   _____   _____
_____   _____   _____   _____   _____
_____   _____   _____   _____   _____
_____   _____   _____   _____   _____
_____   _____   _____   _____   _____
_____   _____   _____   _____   _____
_____   _____   _____   _____   _____
_____   _____   _____   _____   _____
_____   _____   _____   _____   _____
_____   _____   _____   _____   _____

Type of Food Other food	Week 1	Week 2	Week 3	Week 4
[list junk foods, candy bars, chips, etc., here]	[list how many times you eat them each week]			
_____	_____	_____	_____	_____
_____	_____	_____	_____	_____
_____	_____	_____	_____	_____
_____	_____	_____	_____	_____
_____	_____	_____	_____	_____
_____	_____	_____	_____	_____
_____	_____	_____	_____	_____
_____	_____	_____	_____	_____
_____	_____	_____	_____	_____

From *Prescription for Nutritional Healing* by James Balch, M.D., and Phyllis Balch, C.N.C. © 1990. Published by Avery Publishing Group, Inc., Garden City Park, New York. Reprinted by permission.

Step 2: Keep a Food Diary

- Look at your list from last month. Make a list of your "habit foods"—what you ate or drank more than four times a week:

Habit Foods (foods/drinks I consume more than four times a week)

_____   _____
_____   _____
_____   _____
_____   _____
_____   _____
_____   _____

- For the next thirty days, eliminate all of the above foods.
- Keep a *daily* food diary of all the foods and drinks you consume.
- Describe in your diary the way you feel after you consume them. Your food diary should look something like this:

Date	Meal	Time	Foods/Drinks/ Medications	Symptoms
_____	Morning	_____	_____	_____
_____	Snack	_____	_____	_____
_____	Noon	_____	_____	_____
_____	Evening	_____	_____	_____
_____	Snack	_____	_____	_____
_____	Bedtime	_____	_____	_____

Step 3: Take the Food-Sensitivity Pulse Test

Now try your "habit foods" again—as well as any foods from your food diary that caused headaches. The food-sensitivity pulse test was developed by Arthur F. Coca, M.D. He and other allergists have found that the pulse rate increases after ingesting foods to which one is sensitive or allergic.

- You will need a watch with a second hand.
- Sit down and relax completely for five to ten minutes.
- Take your pulse by putting your index finger on your wrist.
- For one minute count the number of beats.
- Eat the food you think might be causing your headaches.
- Wait twenty minutes.
- Take your pulse again.
- If your pulse goes up more than ten beats per minute, stop eating that food for a month and then test it again.

From *Prescription for Nutritional Healing* by James Balch, M.D., and Phyllis Balch C.N.C. © 1990. Published by Avery Publishing Group, Inc., Garden City Park, New York. Adapted by permission.

Now that you've given your body a rest from all the foods you eat on a regular basis, try each "habit food" again. Each time you do, take the sensitivity test. If your body reacts to the food, omit it from your diet for another thirty days.

Step 4: Cleanse Your Body

Note: Do not fast if you are pregnant, anemic, under the age of sixteen or over seventy, diabetic or hypoglycemic, or think you might be, or have any medical condition. Everyone should consult a doctor or another health provider. Fasting for more than three days should be done only under qualified medical supervision.

Fasting can be very safe and effective if you follow certain guidelines, and if you are generally healthy. A fast does not mean you do not eat or drink anything. In fact it is vital that you take in nutrients during your fast. Vegetable and/or fruit juices are the mainstay of a fast. You should not chew anything, including gum. Here are some guidelines for a healthy, cleansing fast:

- Two days before the fast: Eat only raw fruits and/or vegetables
- During the fast:

DO drink distilled or spring water and/or fruit and/or vegetable *juices* at least three times a day. Green drinks, made of leafy vegetables, are a good choice, as are apple and grape juices.
DO NOT drink tomato, orange, or grapefruit juice.
DO NOT chew anything (even gum), as this will stimulate digestion.
DO take fiber such as bran (diluted in distilled water) or other natural fiber drinks.
DO drink freshly made vegetable broths.
DO NOT smoke cigarettes or drink coffee.
DO get plenty of rest, taking naps once or twice a day.
DO exercise gently—walk or stretch.
DO avoid chemicals from deodorants, soaps, cleansing agents, sprays.
DO take vitamin supplements if they are recommended by your health professional.

- After the fast: Eat only raw fruits and/or vegetables for two days.

To hasten the cleansing process, you might also consider taking enemas, using lukewarm distilled water or lukewarm chamomile tea.

Step 5: Reintroduce Foods

After fasting, and eating only fresh, raw fruits and vegetables for a few days, slowly start to expand your diet again.

- For two weeks follow a very simple regimen of fresh fruits, vegetables (raw, steamed, or broiled), chicken or turkey, fish, brown rice, herb teas, and unsweetened juices.
- Every day after that introduce other foods—only one new food per day. Pay attention to how you feel after eating each new food.
- If you have a reaction to a food, keep it out of your diet for two months. Then try it again. If it still causes a reaction, stop eating it entirely.
- Do not eat the same type of food every day. Skip four days between eating a specific type of food, such as bread.

Step 6: Rotate Your Diet

Because eating the same food every day increases your chances of becoming sensitive or allergic to it, you might want to try a rotation diet. This way you are ensured of maintaining variety, which helps avoid sensitivity reactions.

You can use the ''Vegetarian Food Pyramid'' (page 117) as a starting point to construct your own menus to get a good distribution of nutrients. Develop four days' worth of menus, making sure that you don't repeat any food types (for example, if you have bread one day, don't have it for the remaining three days).

This six-step program not only helps you identify foods that cause headaches but may help lessen or eliminate your sensitivity/allergy to them.

Abbreviated Allergy-Cleansing Process

You can bypass some of the preceding steps by following an elimination diet and using the food-sensitivity pulse test. Stop eating all foods except one or two (such as a ripe, seasonal fruit like melon or a vegetable like potatoes). Be sure to drink plenty of liquids. After one day or more, but no more than five days, note whether your headaches disappear. If headaches go away, suspect foods as a source. Then add one food at a time back into your diet. Each time you do, test your pulse using the food-sensitivity pulse test. The "allergic" foods can be reintroduced into your diet after six months to a year without symptoms.

NUTRITIONAL RECOMMENDATIONS FOR HEADACHE SUFFERERS

There is, as mentioned, considerable evidence that nutritional deficiencies, or excesses, can contribute to headache. Balancing these nutritional problems has been shown, in some cases, to prevent headaches—or even stop them in their tracks.

For Migraine Headaches

Magnesium

For many years researchers have suspected that magnesium deficiency contributes to headache. As mentioned in Chapter 3, magnesium plays a vital role in maintaining blood vessel health and serotonin function. In deficiency magnesium causes blood vessel contraction. This mechanism has been implicated in migraine in studies that I have conducted as well as in other studies. We estimate that 50 percent of migraine sufferers are deficient in magnesium.

In a recent study published in the medical journal *Clinical Science,* we reported an 85 percent success rate in treating migraine with an intravenous injection of magnesium.[4] In the study 85 percent of the magnesium-deficient men and women in the middle of a migraine attack experienced rapid and dramatic relief of symptoms when they received magnesium. Within minutes individuals felt relief of migraine pain. They also felt relief from nausea and from sensitivity to light and noise. Aside from a very few patients who had short-term light-headedness during the infusion, there were no side effects. In the study people who were not deficient in magnesium at the outset did not experience relief. This indicates that improvement was not due to a placebo effect.

The first double-blind study of the effect of magnesium supplementation on menstrual migraines was published in 1991.[5] In this study improvement in migraines correlated with an increase in intracellular magnesium levels.

Using slow-release magnesium we treated fourteen women who suffered from menstrual migraines and PMS symptoms.[6] In nine of these women, not only headaches improved but also symptoms of PMS.

In a 1996 study,[7] eighty-one men and women suffering from an average of three to four migraines a month received either 600 mg of magnesium or a placebo each day for 12 weeks. By the last 3 weeks of the study, the number of migraines was reduced by 42 percent among people taking magnesium, but only 15.8 percent among those taking a placebo. The difference between the two groups was statistically significant—which means the results are in fact true.

The results of these studies suggest that having adequate amounts of magnesium in your diet might help prevent migraines.

First, make sure you are getting the Recommended Daily Allowance of magnesium in your diet. See the chart beginning on page 110 for recommended foods. The most magnesium-rich foods include the following:

- Nuts
- Legumes
- Dark green leafy vegetables
- Wholegrain cereals
- Wholegrain breads
- Seafoods

Ironically several of these foods (nuts, legumes, breads) also appear on headache hit lists in Chapter 3. If you are sensitive to these foods, you might want to consider a supplement. It appears that when the magnesium supplement is *chelated,* or slow-release, absorption is better. Many magnesium supplements are poorly absorbed and some can cause diarrhea.

At RDA doses magnesium does not cause side effects. But at much higher-than-recommended doses it can cause drowsiness, weakness, and lethargy. Severe overdose may result in irregular heartbeat, paralysis, inability to breathe, and even death.

People with kidney disorders, including the elderly, who often have reduced kidney function, are especially vulnerable to toxic effects.

Riboflavin (B₂)

Megadoses of this vitamin, 400 mg daily (RDA for riboflavin is 1.7 mg), were shown to improve migraine headaches in a double-blind study performed by a respected research group in Belgium.[8] This was a relatively small study, but it was statistically significant. Improvement was observed after only two months of treatment. Of the fifty-four patients, only one developed a side effect, which was diarrhea.

Unsaturated Fatty Acids (EPA, Fish Oil Concentrate)

EPA is eicosapentaenoic acid—an unsaturated fatty acid that is one of several omega-3 fatty acids natural to the body. It is most famous for its proposed role in lowering cholesterol. But several small studies in the mid 1980s suggested that in some people the severity and frequency of headache can also be reduced by adding EPA to their diets. The research showed that EPA helps lower levels of prostaglandin (the biochemical in the blood that increases nerve sensitivity to pain and contributes to platelet clumping and constriction of blood vessels). It also reduces serotonin activity. In both these ways it is thought that omega-3 fatty acids such as EPA can help prevent headache.

Here are the results of three studies in which migraine sufferers received EPA supplementation (15–20 g per day):[9]

- Among eight people with frequent and severe migraine who took the supplement, the frequency and severity of headaches were cut by 50 percent.
- Among six people with chronic migraine, five experienced significant relief.
- In a slightly larger study of fifteen people, fish oil concentrate

reduced the number and severity of migraines in eight people, but four people became worse.

The government hasn't established a recommended daily allowance for EPA. Although the above-mentioned studies used extremely high doses of 15 grams of EPA daily to prevent headache, others more conservatively recommend 600 mg per day in three equally divided doses (I tend to agree with this lower dose).[10]

Foods richest in EPA are fish that inhabit cold, deep waters, such as salmon, tuna, mackerel, and herring. However, you would need to consume one-quarter pound of salmon to get 3 grams of EPA. Also, pollution of our waterways has made consumption of fish a somewhat risky matter, especially for people who eat a lot of it; toxins accumulate in the fatty tissues of fish. Essential fatty acids (EFA—also known as vitamin F) are related to EPA, and can be found in many vegetables and many unsaturated vegetable oils, such as safflower and olive oils. When these oils are heated, however, the EFA becomes inactivated. Evening primrose oil and black currant oil are also good sources of EFAs. Several EPA supplements are also available.

EPA should be taken with caution in people who are diabetic, and those who are at risk of stroke, nosebleeds, or bleeding disorders.

Other Nutrient Recommendations

Make sure your diet includes the RDA of the following nutrients:

- Niacin (B_3) increases blood flow
- Pantothenic acid (B_5) boosts the adrenal glands
- Vitamin B complex (B_1, B_6, and B_{12}) feeds the nervous system
- Pyridoxine (B_6) improves brain function, enhances immune function

As mentioned in Chapter 3, there's some evidence that low levels of copper in the diet might contribute to migraine, but the results are not conclusive. Copper is essential to the health of blood vessels and their normal dilation and contraction; it's possible that copper deficiency causes the blood vessels to react abnormally. The RDA for copper, and good food sources, appears in the chart beginning on page 110. **Warning: Do not exceed iron or copper RDA by more than 300 percent, as this may result in deficiencies of other nutrients, or cause toxicity.**

For Cluster Headaches

Choline (*Lecithin*)

Choline is a B vitamin that is found in lecithin—an essential fatty acid (see page 136) found in every cell. It helps keep cell walls soft and pliable; the meninges that surround and protect the brain are made up largely of lecithin. Lecithin helps break up and distribute hardened (saturated) fats in the body.

At least one study, reported in the *British Medical Journal,* has shown that choline levels are low in people with cluster headaches.[11] And increasing choline in the diet may help improve symptoms.

The recommended daily intake of lecithin is between 200 and 500 mg. Good food sources are soybeans, eggs, brewer's yeast, whole grains, legumes, fish, and wheat germ. Keep in mind that several of these foods might also trigger headaches (yeast and legumes, for example). Lecithin supplements, in granular and liquid forms, are available.

Magnesium

As with migraine, magnesium has been shown to help people with cluster headaches. In our study of twenty-two people, 40 percent experienced relief with magnesium lasting two days to several weeks to complete remission.[12]

To Reduce Stress-Related (Tension-Type) Headaches

The body is better able to handle stress of any kind when it is well nourished. The body under stress produces hormones that interfere with the immune system, which plays a role in food and environmental allergies. A good basic diet is the first line of action. To boost the body's defenses against stress, the following are recommended:

B Vitamins

The B vitamins, particularly vitamin B complex (100 mg daily) and B$_5$ (100 mg three times daily), are the most important antistress vitamins. B$_5$, also known as pantothenic acid, is abundant in beef, beans, eggs, fresh vegetables, and whole wheat. Though there have been no reports of problems with B$_5$ overdose, large doses of B complex can cause toxicities. Refer to the RDA guide beginning on page 110 and make sure not to exceed the dose by more than 200 percent.

Magnesium

Magnesium is depleted from the body during times of stress. And deficiencies can reduce tolerance to stressors. Guidelines for increasing dietary magnesium are listed on pages 134–136.

Vitamin C

Vitamin C has been extolled for many virtues. It is vital to the adrenal glands, which controls the stress response, as well as production of important hormones that play a role in headaches. Vitamin C may also help reduce high blood pressure, boost the immune system, and protect against platelet clotting (the latter sets in motion biochemical reactions that can lead to headache). A free radical scavenger, vitamin C is a potent antioxidant that lends protection against the onslaught of various environmental toxins (see below) that can contribute to headache. The best food sources of vitamin C include green vegetables, berries, and citrus fruits; but remember that citrus may potentiate headache. The daily amount shouldn't exceed 5,000 mg, especially in pregnant women. The optimal dosage appears to be 500 mg, twice a day.

CREATING A HEADACHE-FREE ENVIRONMENT

Like tracking down headache-causing foods, identifying headache hazards in your environment takes some detective work. Start with the "clues" offered in Chapter 4. For professional help, seek the aid of an allergist, particularly one who specializes in environmental medicine (see the end of this chapter). These specialists can not only help you identify the source of your problem, they can give you recommendations for correcting it. Clearly the best route to relief is to dodge the offending substance.

Humidity in the Home

Humidity, as you remember, breeds molds, dust mites, yeasts, and algae. Eliminating humidity—and reducing the population of headache-causing molds and mites—can be as simple as investing in a dehumidifier, or as complex as overhauling your home. Consider these room-specific tips for reducing humidity and allergens in the home recommended by William E. Walsh in his book *An Allergist's Approach to Treating Headache:*

Problem Area	Possible Solutions
In the basement	*To reduce humidity due to poor soil drainage:*
	• Install gutters and downspouts to direct rainfall away from house and prevent it from seeping into basement
	• Dig trenches to direct water away from house (whether from your own roof or from that of your neighbors)
	• Consult with a landscape architect to determine other ways of keeping water away from the home
	General guidelines:
	• Ventilate properly
	• Install a dehumidifier (keep humidity to 35%–50%)
	• Cover floor with plastic
	• Insulate ceiling and install vapor barrier
	• Remove all dust-mite-harboring objects (books, stuffed furniture, carpeting, boxes)
	• Add a paint-mold inhibitor to paint
In the bathroom	• Use an exhaust fan or open window to remove humidity after showering

- Wash shower curtain and all surfaces with mold-killing solutions
- Do not carpet
- Use only natural, hypoallergenic cleansing products, especially personal products

In the bedroom
- Use only synthetic, hypoallergenic bedding (mites love natural fibers and feathers) but avoid foam rubber
- Replace mattress every few years
- Encase box spring, mattress, and pillows in allergen-impermeable covers
- Wash all bedding—pillows, blankets, sheets, and mattress pad—in very hot water (130 degress) every two weeks
- Remove all carpeting or clean often with a tannic-acid solution to inactivate allergens
- Cover hot-air vents with filters, or close and use an electric radiator
- Avoid heavy curtains, or wash frequently
- Avoid overstuffed furniture
- Install an air cleaner
- Use a dehumidifier to keep humidity at 40%–50%
- When vacuuming, use a vacuum cleaner with high allergen containment, such as a multilayer dust bag and exhaust filter

In the kitchen
- Use an exhaust fan to remove humidity while cooking
- Clean refrigerator and garbage containers often to keep mold down
- Avoid plastic utensils and plates, which contain petrochemicals; use glass or ceramic instead

General Tips
- If refinishing floors, painting with oil-based paints, or laying new carpet, ensure proper ventilation for at least two months

- Replace cleansers with environmentally friendly solutions
- Eliminate aerosol sprays
- Avoid all products with a scent
- Avoid dry cleaning
- Use only scent-free, hypoallergenic soaps
- Wear only natural fabrics, never permanent press, which contains formaldehyde
- If you must fumigate, allow for proper ventilation (luckily fumigation is mostly needed during warm weather months)
- Each winter before installing storm windows, have your heating system and gas appliances inspected to reduce the chance of carbon monoxide toxicity
- Never leave your car idling in the garage
- Place a carbon monoxide detector in your home, make sure that it is labeled UL-approved

Water Contamination
- Have your water tested for environmental toxins
- If you suspect toxic chemicals, install a water filter

Where Carbon Monoxide Lurks in the House

Carbon monoxide is an odorless, invisible substance that commonly causes headache—it is also potentially deadly. Here are some common sources of carbon monoxide, and ways to reduce your risk of toxicity:

- Tobacco smoke
- Car exhaust—do not leave car idling in the garage
- Blocked or leaky chimney; clean on an annual basis
- Furnaces—have annual inspections
- Gas cooking ranges—have inspected periodically
- Fuel-burning heaters—have annual inspections
- Hibachis and grills—grill only outdoors

- Badly vented appliances—have them checked by service-repair person regularly
- Badly vented woodstoves and fireplaces—look for woodstoves that are EPA-approved and don't burn wood that has been chemically treated, and have regular clean-outs

Headaches at Work

If you have headaches during the work week, if your coworkers also complain of headaches or other vague symptoms (fatigue, difficulty breathing, dizziness, etc.), or if you work with known noxious chemicals (see Chapter 4), you might be suffering from an occupation-related headache.

Unfortunately it is often more difficult to control the workplace environment than it is your home. Here are some suggestions:

- *Gather evidence.*   See if your symptoms are shared by your coworkers. Try to identify the source. For example, if you're exposed to fumes or chemicals, find out whether they commonly cause toxic reactions (see Chapter 4 for starters). Noise, light, heat, and cold can contribute to headaches. In office buildings the headache hazards can range from inadequate ventilation to fluorescent lighting to exposure to computer screens. Contact the Human Ecology Action League (see "Resources") for ways of identifying work-related toxicities, and ways to reduce them in your workplace.
- *Find out your rights.*   Employers are required by law to provide a safe working environment. They should provide the means necessary to limit your exposure to occupational toxins, either through the manufacturing process or by offering protective clothing and/or masks. Ventilation should be adequate. Smoking in the workplace is prohibited in many cities. Noise and light (visible and infrared) may cause headache, and protective devices should be available for workers exposed to high levels. Unfortunately requirements and monitoring of businesses for environmental protection varies from state to state, and very small operations may be exempt from state laws entirely. To find out your rights, contact the National Organization of Legal Advocates for the Environmentally Injured or the Chemical Injury Information Network (see pp. 361, 362).

• *Address issues with management.*   If you are part of a union, you may get help from it. However, if you are not or are the only employee experiencing symptoms, or if your employer *is* following safety regulations, it may be difficult to garner the support of the union. You may be on your own. Speak with your supervisor or employer about your problem and try to develop creative solutions. You may not be able to convince your boss to change the air filtration system to cut down on molds, but you might be able to obtain some level of protection (such as a fan near your desk).

• *Take care of your health.*   In the end you are responsible for your own health. If your employer refuses to acknowledge a problem, find out what you can do to protect your health. It may involve keeping to a cleansing regimen that helps reduce the toxins in your body.

Clearing the Air with Plants

Air filtration and purification systems, ranging from buildingwide systems to room areas, can be installed to remove indoor pollutants in some environments. But this method might not be economically feasible, or impossible to effect in your workplace. According to recent findings from NASA's Skylab Project, indoor plants could offer a pleasant and effective alternative. Researchers have found that plants have a powerful ability to clean the air of certain toxins. And they need not be exotic species to be great cleansers. Common office and houseplants that often thrive in shady spots and sustain benign neglect are actually the best. For optimal cleansing, each hundred square feet requires three eight-inch pots.

Toxins	**Purifying Plants**
Formaldehyde	Spider plants, Boston ferns
Trichloroethylene	Peace lilies
Benzene	English ivy, chrysanthemums
Carbon dioxide	Orchids, bromeliads
Acetone	
Methyl alcohol	
Ethyl acetate	

Other air-cleansing plants include

African daisy
Aloe vera
Areca palm
Corn plant
Date palm
Diffenbachia (poisonous to animals)
Dracaena palm
Dragonplant
Ficus
Golden pothos
Philodendron
Poinsettia
Snake plant
Spathe flower

Adjust the Lights, Check Your Eyes

As we explained in Chapter 2, migraine can be triggered by flickering lights; eyestrain headaches can be caused by poor lighting. To help prevent headaches, consider these tips:

- Replace fluorescent lights (which may flicker, even imperceptibly) with incandescent bulbs.
- Always ensure adequate lighting when reading, sewing, typing, or similar activities.
- Get your eyes checked; eyestrain headaches may be the result of straining to compensate for bad vision.
- If you are working at a computer for long periods, be sure to look up and away from the screen periodically; better yet, take short breaks every half hour.
- Avoid watching television in a dark room for long periods of time.

KEEP YOUR BODY CLEANSED OF TOXINS

I know of one woman who suffered severe headaches for no known reason. Finally she traced it to recent renovation work in her house. She'd had her floors refinished in an art studio and, unwittingly, sustained progressive accumulation of toxins. She underwent a cleansing regimen to remove the toxins from her body, and her headaches disappeared.

Cleansing methods can offer you an extra measure of protection against headache-triggering substances from foods. As asserted by some allergists, environmental doctors, macrobiotic practitioners, and naturopathic physicians, the body reacts with illness when it has overloaded its toxic capacity. Headache is a common symptom. Here, then, are some options you might want to explore to cleanse your body:

General Dietary Guidelines

- Eat organic foods, with emphasis on fruits and vegetables.
- Drink at least eight cups of water daily, preferably distilled or purified water.
- Supplement your diet with choline (lecithin), vitamin C, and fiber.
- Make sure your diet covers the daily requirements of nutrients.

Fasting

Fasting has been considered a therapeutic modality for centuries. A well-controlled food fast, preferably under medical supervision, can jump-start the cleansing process. We described one method earlier in this chapter. For more information, see the "Resources" section.

Nutritional and Herbal Supplements

To cleanse the blood and remove toxins from the body, evaluate whether your diet includes enough of the following vitamins. Also consider choosing from herbal or other supplements. For best effects make sure your diet does not include processed, refined foods, sugar, and heated oils:

VITAMIN SUPPLEMENTS

Vitamin A (5,000 IU daily)
Vitamin C (500 mg twice a day)
Vitamin E (400 IU daily)

OTHER SUPPLEMENTS

Chlorophyll (from juiced greens or in supplements)
Alfalfa
L-lysine (an amino acid)
Garlic capsules
Coenzyme Q_{10}
Apple cider vinegar drink (warm water and one tablespoon apple cider vinegar)—helps cleanse the body and add potassium

Chelation Therapy

Chelation is a therapy that uses specific agents to bind with toxic metals in the bloodstream (such as lead) and help draw them out of the body. The chelating agents, as they are called, are taken orally or by injection. Intravenous chelation therapy should be performed only by a professional certified by the American Board of Chelation Therapy (see ''Resources'').

If you are exposed to metals, consider the following oral chelating agents to purify the blood:

Alfalfa
Coenzyme Q_{10}
Garlic tablets
L-lysine

Rutin
Vitamin C

Internal Cleansing of the Colon

The colon, or large intestine, functions not only to digest food but as the main route for removing undigested foods. It is a hollow organ that extends from the small intestine about five feet to the rectum. It is here that water and many minerals are absorbed into the body. Also here the body deposits wastes. As discussed in Chapter 3, improper digestion—due to stress, bad nutrition, or underlying disease—can cause constipation. This in turn can produce a buildup of toxins in the colon, which are reabsorbed into the blood—and produce illness. One symptom is headache.

Colon cleansing can take the form of *regular bowel movements, enemas,* which remove waste from the lower third of the colon, or full *colonic cleansing,* also known as colonic irrigation or colonic hydro-therapy.

Regular Bowel Movements

To promote regular bowel movements, follow these recommendations:

- Try to move bowels first thing in the morning, either before or after breakfast, whether or not you feel the urge. Allow plenty of time, breathe deeply, and relax. Get your body into the habit of regular elimination.
- Eat plenty of raw vegetables and fruits each day.
- Chew foods thoroughly.
- Drink at least two quarts (eight cups) of water a day, preferably distilled or purified.
- Avoid processed foods, refined sugars, coffee, nuts, fried foods, and pork.

Enemas

Used to bathe the lower third of the colon, therapeutic enemas date back to 1500 B.C. With the help of an enema bag two quarts of warm fluid are infused into the lower colon and either flushed back or retained for ten to fifteen minutes.

- Be sure to use purified or distilled water.
- To lubricate the anus, use natural vitamin E oil.
- Fennel tea, coffee, lemon juice, wheatgrass juice, or garlic juice can be used for nonretention enemas.
- After inserting the fluid, slowly roll side to side on your back.

Colonic Irrigation

Colonic irrigation, or hydrotherapy, is conducted by a professional (such as a naturopath, colon therapist, or natural hygienist) with the aid of a colon-irrigation machine. It involves use of warm, pure water to bathe the colon, along with gentle abdominal massage. The benefits of colonic irrigation include removal of impacted waste from the colon, massage of the colon, and stimulation of the colon to regenerate muscle activity.

The procedure often begins with a period of relaxation. A speculum is inserted into the anus. It is attached to a hose, which in turn is attached to a machine containing water. The machine can be adjusted for water volume, pressure, and temperature. The procedure averages forty-five minutes, during which time water is inserted and waste material removed several times to remove waste throughout the length of the colon. In severe cases several sessions may be required. If administered by a medical professional, the treatment is usually painless and completely safe. Some people experience abdominal discomfort after the procedure, which usually disappears within a day.

Before undergoing colonic irrigation, make sure that you consult with your doctor to rule out any reasons why it might be unsafe or unhealthy for you.

Skin Brushing

Like the colon, the skin is the repository of many of the body's toxins. When they are not removed, the toxins may reabsorb into the bloodstream. Macrobiotic practitioners endorse skin brushing, as do several traditional healing disciplines.

For best effects use brushes with natural vegetable bristles. The brushing is not done in the shower, but when you are dry. At first you may need to brush lightly until you get used to the feeling. Brush the skin over your entire body (except for your face). Do this for five minutes daily, working always toward your heart. This is believed to help remove toxins and improve blood circulation and skin appearance.

Ayurvedic Cleansing

In Ayurvedic medical belief internal cleansing is an important way of balancing the doshas and treating disease. Generally used as part of a complete regimen, *Antha-Shodoma,* or internal cleansing, can include one of several therapies: emesis (or vomiting), purging (stool elimination with therapeutic laxatives), nasal therapy (to remove mucus using oils and nasal massage), enemas (using special cleansing medications, either an oil or an herbal preparation, that is right for the individual), phlebotomy (blood removal). These procedures are often preceded by preparatory treatments. For example enemas are often preceded by sweat therapy or oil therapy (massage with oils). The cleansing of bodily toxins prepares the body for the final step, which is a rejuvenating or strengthening treatment.

The type of cleansing procedure you receive, and the accompanying herbal or oil therapies, depends on your individual constitution or *dosha,* your ailment (beyond the symptoms of headache), and other factors, such as your nutrition and lifestyle. It is strongly recommended that you seek a qualified Ayurvedic physician to guide you in these and other Ayurvedic practices.

GETTING HELP

For referrals to experts in the areas we've addressed in this chapter, contact the organizations listed in the "Resources" section at the end of this book.

CHAPTER 7

Physical Approaches

*The healer must be acquainted with many things
and assuredly with rubbing.*
—HIPPOCRATES

In recent years machines and drugs have largely become proxies for the sensitive tools that once served as the healer's primary means of diagnosis and treatment: the physician's hands. As patients we've become distanced from our healers, and out of touch with the healing ability of our own bodies. We, too, have come to rely on outside forces to fix our ailments, including headache.

Touch is probably the most basic form of healing known to humankind. Instinctively when we feel discomfort, our tendency is to massage or rub the area in pain. Think of how often your hands move naturally to your head whenever you feel a headache coming on. The healing effects of touch are innately understood by the infant, who finds comfort from contact with a caring person. Scientific studies of this natural phenomenon suggest that contact and touch help the body mobilize its own healing powers, for example, by reducing the production of stress hormones.

In a related way, movement is evidence of life—and in itself it can be an energy- and health-generating tool. The way we move our bodies (or don't) can create patterns of tension that contribute to headaches, and other illness.

These general healing concepts underlie many of the alternative therapies to prevent or treat headache that are discussed in this chapter. They range from mind-body methods that intimately engage the individual's self-awareness of movement patterns that contribute to headache, to those which make use of physical manipulations to correct structural or muscular problems, to those that vitalize and balance the body's own healing energies. In addition exposing parts of the body to heat or cold can open or close blood vessels to help regulate blood flow, or open sinus cavities, and in this way help relieve headache.

The name of this chapter may be misleading. We call it "Physical Approaches," which implies treatment of physical disorders. But most of these methods engage the whole person—physically, emotionally, mentally, and, if it is your intent, spiritually—not just symptoms or a specific part of the body. All of the physical approaches require some interaction of the body and mind. In some cases this communication occurs at first on an unconscious level. Pressing trigger points of sensitive muscles, for example, is thought to retrain the brain to release spasms that bring on headaches. In other cases most of the work is being done by the conscious mind. The Alexander Technique, for instance, is an educational method by which insidiously habitual patterns of movement are brought into the light of consciousness and, through this awareness, corrected.

Since the causes of headache extend beyond the limits of concrete physiology, it makes perfect sense that the methods for treating it may also reach beyond, or deeper into, the body.

With the exception of acupuncture, acupressure, and TENS, most of the methods described in this chapter have not been specifically studied for their effects on headache.

Indeed, effectiveness is often attributed to the placebo effect, and until reliable studies are conducted, I can neither support nor refute that claim. Many of the bodywork methods, for example, are *educational* processes that may, as a *by-product* of increased awareness of postural tension, help relieve headache. However, most practitioners make no claims for effectiveness in headache.

MASSAGE THERAPY

Many of the methods discussed in this chapter are based on some form of massage. Through the use of pressure, holding, or guiding, a practitioner manipulates the soft tissues to stimulate the body's own healing abilities. The American Massage Therapy Association defines seven types of massage:

• *Swedish massage*—Uses a system of long strokes, kneading, and friction techniques on the more superficial layers of the muscles, combined with active and passive movements of the joints. Used primarily for a full-body session, it helps promote relaxation, improve circulation and range of motion, and relieve muscle tension.

• *Deep-muscle/connective-tissue massage*—As the name implies, this type of massage uses deep finger pressure and slow strokes on contracted areas, either following or going against the grain of muscles, tendons, and fascia to release chronic patterns of tension in the body. Massage therapists, osteopathic physicians, Rolfers, and related disciplines use this approach.

• *Trigger-point therapy*—This method applies concentrated finger pressure to "trigger points"—painful irritated areas in muscles—in order to break the cycle of spasm and pain. It is often used to deal with pain. Bonnie Prudden Myotherapists and massage therapists employ this technique.

• *Shiatsu and acupressure*—These are Oriental-medicine-based systems of finger-pressure massage that target special points along acupuncture meridians—the invisible channels of energy (qi) flow in the body. Blocked energy along these meridians can cause physical discomforts, so the aim is to release the blocks and rebalance energy flow. Used by specialists in Oriental medicine, shiatsu (and related techniques), and massage therapists.

• *Reflexology* (*zone therapy*)—Uses principles similar to shiatsu and acupressure, except that the method is organized around a system of points on the hands, feet, head, and ears that are thought to correspond, or "reflex" to all areas of the body. Used by reflexologists and some massage therapists.

• *Hydrotherapy*—Traditionally used as an adjunct to massage and employed by some massage practitioners. It includes modalities such as hot packs and ice applications, along with saunas, steam baths, and whirlpools.

In this section we'll focus on Swedish massage, the most common form of massage in this country. The other massage approaches will be addressed later in the chapter.

Swedish Massage

History

Massage is one of the earliest forms of treatment, dating back at least to ancient China and continuing as a recommended treatment throughout history. In the United States massage took hold during the mid 1800s. Its popularity in the medical community waned in the mid 1900s in deference to more "advanced" medical technologies. In the 1970s massage experienced a renaissance. Today massage is recognized as a therapeutic practice, requiring certification in nineteen states. It is one of the most popular alternative therapies sought by Americans; an estimated twenty million have received massage.

How It Helps Relieve Headache

Massage in the United States is generally based on Swedish massage, which employs five basic techniques: effleurage (gliding strokes), petrissage (kneading), friction (rubbing), tapotement (percussion), and vibration. These techniques lightly manipulate the superficial muscle tissue so that blood flows toward the heart. In this way, massage proponents maintain, blood circulation is improved. And when blood circulation is improved, the body receives more oxygen and nutrients, and toxic wastes are more readily removed. Some massage researchers have found that massage stimulates the body's production of endorphins, which have painkilling and relaxing effects on the body.

Who Can Be Helped

People with headaches triggered by emotional stress or anxiety, postural problems, or muscle tension may benefit from massage therapy.

What to Expect

A reliable massage therapist will begin by asking questions about your reasons for getting a massage, your physical condition, medical history, lifestyle, and stress level—as well as areas of pain. You will be asked to undress in private and drape your body with a sheet, towel, or gown. You can leave your underwear on if you like. Lying down on a padded table, the therapist may apply some oils to facilitate the massage. Often your massage therapist will start with your feet or hands to help you get used to the feeling of being massaged. Using a variety of techniques (described on page 154), the therapist will work on all of the muscles of your body. You should feel free to communicate with the massage therapist if you feel discomfort or pain.

Effectiveness

The effectiveness of massage in some forms of headache has been documented. In one study of twenty-one patients suffering from chronic tension headache, general massage, as well as deep tissue massage of specific pain points, significantly reduced the frequency and severity of chronic pain by 50 percent—and these effects lasted for six months after treatment.[1] Cranial massage can be of particular benefit to headache sufferers (see page 240).

The effectiveness of massage may be explained in several ways. First, it has been shown to have an overall relaxing effect. By helping to keep tension in check, massage may help eliminate the trigger for tension-type headache and migraine.

Second, massage specifically helps relax tense muscles and tissues. As we explained in Chapter 2, muscle contraction is one of the accepted mechanisms of headache. Massage has been shown to help release restrictions of the fascia—the deep connective tissue that envelops and permeates bones, muscles, and organs.

Third, by helping to improve circulation, massage also helps maintain the health of blood vessels.

Finally, massage has been shown to stimulate the body's production of endorphins, which helps reduce pain.

Treatment Schedule

Periodic massages can be a helpful adjunct to other headache-controlling regimens. In the study mentioned on page 156, headache sufferers were massaged ten times over a two-and-a-half-week period, with long-lasting results. Unless massage has been prescribed by your physician for a specific number of sessions, you might consider getting one whenever you feel particularly anxious or tense, or are entering a time that you know will be tense, to help prevent headaches.

Side Effects

If performed by a trained and knowledgeable therapist, there should be no side effects from having a massage. Afterward some of your muscles might feel tender, as though you had been exercising.

Warnings

Let your massage therapist know of any illness. Massage should be avoided near areas of infectious, open wounds or bruises. Massage is not recommended for people with circulatory problems, especially phlebitis and thrombosis. In addition it isn't recommended for people with high fevers, infectious diseases, cancer (some types), cardiac problems, certain skin conditions, inflamed or infected injuries, areas of hemorrhage or heavy tissue damage, or recent fractures or sprains.

Finding a Reliable Massage Therapist

It should not be difficult to find a qualified massage therapist—there are over ten thousand in the United States. Word of mouth is your best starting point, or ask your physician or physical therapist. But since massage is not regulated in all states, look for a massage therapist who is licensed (some states have licensing requirements), and who received training from a school that's been accredited or approved by the American Massage Therapy Association (AMTA) Commission on Massage Training Accreditation/Approval. The AMTA and the Associated Bodywork & Massage Professionals provide referrals. Licensed massage therapists will carry the initials L.M.T. after their names, which stands for Licensed Massage Therapist. This means that they have received at least five hundred hours of instruction. The International Association of Infant-Massage Instructors offers short classes for laypeople to become certified in the massage of infants and young children. Organizations which require that members meet specific educational requirements and follow a strict code of professional conduct and ethics are listed in the ''Resources'' section.

Questions and Answers

• *Does massage hurt?*   If given by a qualified therapist, the massage should be a very pleasant experience. You may feel some tenderness of tense muscles after a massage. If you have any discomfort during the massage, let your therapist know and he or she will either work more lightly on that area or move to another spot.

• *I'm embarrassed about being naked. Is it absolutely necessary?*   Many people have this same concern before their first massage. A professional massage therapist will honor your ethics or sensitivities; if the therapist insists on your being nude, you should find another one. As you become more comfortable with the therapeutic aspects of massage, you may change your mind. But until you do, make certain that you feel comfortable.

• *Can massage be of benefit to children with headaches?*   I do not know of any studies regarding the effectiveness of massage and headache in children, although massage has been shown to reduce anxiety in children, which may be a trigger for headache. Massage of infants is a traditional practice in India and is becoming more common in the United States (see above); research shows that massage of premature babies helps improve weight gain and reduces hospital stay.

• *Can I be massaged if I am pregnant?*   Yes, a reliable massage therapist will have the knowledge and skill to help reduce stress, improve the flow of oxygen and blood to your tissues, and relieve swelling and edema as well as backaches. It is quite safe, however, be sure to speak with your doctor before starting a massage program.

• *Is massage covered by medical insurance?*   Massage may be covered by some insurance plans if it is prescribed by a physician. Ask your insurance carrier for details.

TRADITIONAL THERAPIES

Albert Einstein changed our view of the world when he developed the equation $e = mc^2$. What it means, in very simple terms, is that all physical matter is made up of formless energy. Energy that coalesces creates matter; matter dissipates into energy. Energy and matter are in a constant state of flux. In Eastern tradition this idea is not new. It is in fact the basis for a cosmology that guides a sophisticated system of medicine. In traditional Oriental medicine, *qi* (pronounced ''chee'') is an ancient expression of Einstein's recently rediscovered concept. Qi is the essential life force in all living things; it is the transformative energy that manifests as matter. In the traditional Indian medicinal system of Ayurveda this phenomenon is known as *prana,* also translated as breath.

Today researchers at esteemed institutions such as Stanford University and New York City's Mount Sinai Hospital are exploring this invisible phenomenon with scientific seriousness. And while research is still in its nascent stages, investigators are finding proof of what is now referred to in alternative-medicine circles as the *human bioelectric energy field,* or *bioenergetic medicine,* or simply energy medicine.

Traditional systems of medicine, such as Ayurveda and Chinese medicine, have a head start on Western bioenergetic-medicine pioneers. Over the past five thousand years physicians in these areas have developed formal therapeutic methods that harness (perhaps *access* is a better word) the power of this primary energy. Yoga and meridian therapies such as acupuncture, acupressure, and qigong (pronounced ''chee-kung'') are four common examples.

Meridian Therapies

After sustaining wounds at certain points in their bodies, warriors in ancient China noticed a paradoxical aftereffect: They experienced relief from diseases they'd suffered for long periods before. In exploring this effect, Chinese physicians discovered and began mapping *acupoints*— potent areas on the body that influence the health of vital organs and other body systems by regulating the flow of vital energy, or *qi*. This method of disease diagnosis, prevention, and treatment became an important part of the sophisticated medical system today known as traditional Oriental medicine.

Rooted in the ancient Taoist philosophy of yin and yang in China, the practices of meridian therapy have made their way over the past five thousand years to other Asian countries, notably Japan and Vietnam, and over the past two hundred years to Europe and the United States. In its cross-cultural transit, this basic language of healing has taken on the dialects of the societies that embraced it.

While it is useful to visualize qi as an energy that travels through hollow tubelike channels to nourish the body and the soul, its true meaning is more profound in traditional Chinese thought. Qi is the elemental force of life, found in all parts of all living things. It travels through the body via channels that are invisible but not random. These channels, also referred to as *meridians,* mark the natural patterns of qi flow.

The meridians are the body's qi superhighways—each relating to a specific organ or body system. In health qi flows freely along the meridians to vital organs, bones, tendons, muscles, and tissues—enabling different parts of the body to work as a unified whole. When the body is not in good health, there may be jam-ups or vacuums along the channels that inhibit the flow of qi. The stimulation of acupoints is believed to activate the body's own resources to remove blockages or fill the vacuum, thus reducing pain, restoring the balance of qi, and maintaining overall health.

According to traditional Chinese belief, we are all born with a certain amount of qi. Over the years, as we age and endure the physical and emotional challenges of everyday life, such as illness and stress, our storehouse of qi becomes depleted. There are also physical and meditative techniques (notably *qigong*) for accessing, renewing, and directing qi to bring about spiritual and physical health.

In the body, qi circulates primarily along twelve major meridians, which are connected to the twelve vital organs. There are also twenty-three channels circulating through the body, but we'll focus on the twelve main ones. Because they are bilateral—mirrored symmetrically on both sides of the body—there are actually twenty-four channels. Each also has a yin or a yang quality of its own. There are more than 2,000 acupoints on the skin that connect with the channels; conventionally 365 of them are the most commonly used.

Meridians of Chinese Medicine and Their Relation to Head Pain

Symptoms in This Part of the Head	Might Indicate Problems in These Pairs of Meridians
Back of head	Small intestine & Bladder
Side of head/temples	Gallbladder & Triple Burner
Front of head/forehead	Stomach & Large Intestine
Band around entire head	Lung & Spleen
Crown of head	Liver & Pericardium
Cheeks and teeth	Heart & Kidney

Remember that these are generalizations. Each individual is unique, and while the location of pain might point generally to a pair of channels, other factors come into play in the diagnosis of obstructed qi, such as the person's overall health, diet, and emotional state.

Western clinical study has confirmed the effectiveness of acupoint stimulation, describing its success in terms of its mechanisms of action, which are only partly understood. So far modern science has verified that stimulating acupoints also stimulates small nerve fibers in the muscle, which launches a three-pronged attack on pain. The spinal cord responds by activating chemical messengers—neurotransmitters called enkephalin and dynorphin—to block incoming pain messages. In this way the pain is blocked on a local level. But pain is also lessened by triggering the body's centralized pain-control processes, located in the brain. The neurotransmitters make their way to the brain to stop pain in two ways:

- In the midbrain, enkephalin mobilizes serotonin and norepinephrine, two other neurotransmitters, to block pain messages.
- In the hypothalamus-pituitary, endorphin is released into the blood and cerebrospinal fluid. As you might know, endorphins are the body's own painkilling chemicals.

In spite of these documented findings, and more than 150 generations of clinical practice in Asian countries, many Western doctors are skeptical about the healing effects of meridian therapies. As scientists we are trained to demand clinical proof in the form of rigorous study. Meeting this requirement is no small task.

The gold standard for clinical study is the double-blind placebo-controlled study design, where neither researcher nor patient knows whether the treatment has been given or the placebo. With this design it's impossible to compare drugs to acupuncture; "sham" acupuncture techniques, which serve as a placebo equivalent, have shown benefits, but there is much debate over the validity of these study designs. Single-blind studies are under way across the world, and continue to confirm the efficacy of acupuncture and acupressure. Yet it may just be that meridian therapies cannot yet be fully proven in Western terms. Our views of health and disease are framed through different lenses.

While one does not need to understand or endorse the Taoist beliefs that shape traditional Chinese medicine to benefit from any of the practices, an understanding of the concepts that govern this sophisticated medical system can help explain the integrated logic behind its effectiveness (see "Resources" for more information).

From a scientific point of view, the most compelling reason for considering acupuncture is clinical proof. Over the past fifteen years acupuncture has earned a solid scientific status through clinical studies. For people with tension or migraine headache, there are several studies—with positive results—but relatively few have been clinically studied. (For an explanation of clinical studies, see the Glossary.) But the consensus is that, for many people with migraine and tension-type headache, acupuncture reduces the number and severity of headaches.

Acupuncture

Though acupuncture originally derived from China, a growing number of physicians in the United States are beginning to learn the art and science of this time-proven method. An estimated ten million acupuncture treatments are performed each year in the United States. At the New York Headache Center, for example, I administer acupuncture frequently to help reduce my patients' head pain—and I am not alone in this practice. Many physicians and osteopaths are beginning to fuse alternative methods such as acupuncture with modern Western approaches.

History

A Chinese surgeon named Hua Tuo (A.D. 110–227, Han dynasty) is credited with being the first to use acupuncture for the treatment of headache. Acupuncture was introduced to U.S. physicians by Sir William Osler, one of the founders of modern medicine, who prescribed it one hundred years ago for back pain.

Effectiveness

In studies acupuncture has generally proved to be effective in 55 to 85 percent of people in reducing the number and severity of their headaches. But at least 15 percent of people don't respond to acupuncture at all.

The effectiveness varies depending on who administers the treatment and the duration of treatment. In one study conducted in the People's Republic of China, where proficiency would be expected to be quite high, 93 percent of migraineurs who failed to respond to Western medicine experienced relief with acupuncture.[2] In a study of people with tension-type headache, acupuncture significantly reduced the frequency and intensity of headaches, and the effects persisted for the duration of the study—up to twelve months after treatment.[3] Another large-scale study of people with tension headache and/or migraines showed acupuncture effective in reducing severity and frequency of pain.[4]

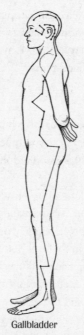

Gallbladder

For the prevention of migraine, hair-thin acupuncture needles are often inserted in the scalp, face, and hands for 20–30 minutes.

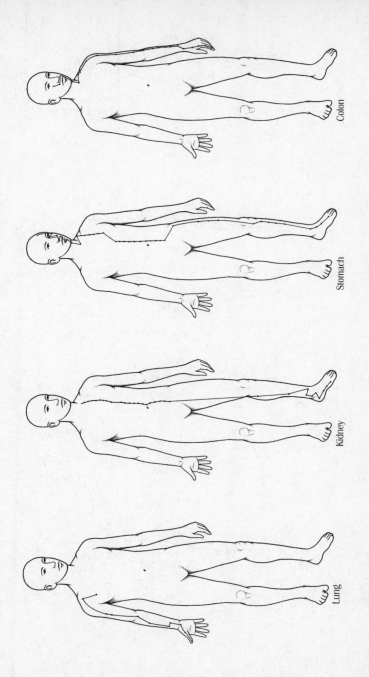

Lung

Kidney

Stomach

Colon

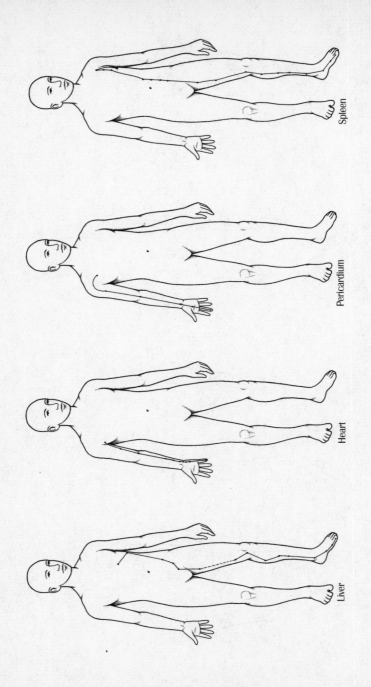

Spleen

Pericardium

Heart

Liver

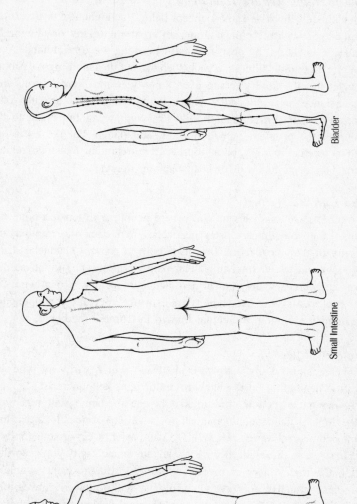

Three Heater

Small Intestine

Bladder

How It Helps Relieve Headache

As already discussed, the concept behind acupuncture is that there are key pain-control points along different meridians on the body. Headache is caused by obstructions in qi along these meridians. Acupuncture not only induces physical changes but according to proponents, it has the ability to tap deep emotional and mental levels that help balance an individual's entire being. Its effects are not only targeted to help correct specific physical symptoms, but reach to the source of the problem—the mind-body imbalance. For these reasons acupuncture can be applied as a preventive treatment for stress-related headaches, or as first aid for headaches in progress.

Who Can Be Helped

Acupuncture has been shown to help people with tension-type, migraine, and sometimes cluster headaches to reduce the number and severity of their headaches. It is used both to prevent headaches (prophylaxis) and to stop existing head pain (treatment). Though studies have not been as widely performed, acupuncture may prove beneficial for people with other headache types as well, especially if acupuncture is administered by an individual trained in Chinese medicine.

What to Expect

The session begins with an evaluation—which varies in type and duration depending on the background of your acupuncturist.

A person trained in traditional Chinese medicine will take your pulse, look at your tongue, and ask you a variety of questions that may seem odd or irrelevant, such as, "Do you prefer sweet or sour foods?" The answers to these questions help the clinician classify you according to the Chinese system of medicine, and help diagnose the source of your headache. By contrast a neurologist will follow a conventional headache "workup" consisting of a physical evaluation and medical history.

You will probably be asked to lie down on your back and relax. The practitioner will then apply hair-thin needles to specific acupoints. The needles are made of stainless steel and are usually disposable, so there is no risk of disease transmission. (Some practitioners sterilize and reuse their needles; *you should insist on disposable needles to eliminate any risk of infection.*)

The needles are usually inserted at various points on the scalp, face, and hands—depending on the type and location of your headache or facial pain—to a depth of one-half to one inch (shallower for children). Usually they are applied at the same points on both sides of the body. However, other points may also be used if your head pain is associated with other conditions. In traditional acupuncture the practitioner may also twirl the needles slightly or flick them lightly to provide additional stimulation.

The acupoints for prevention may be different from those used for first aid of headaches in progress. When applied for first aid, acupuncture may first make a headache feel worse—in a way, speeding up the course of symptoms—before it begins to dissipate.

After the slight initial discomfort of having the needles inserted, you may feel a variety of sensations—tingling, heat, or a feeling of pressure. These are good signs that the correct acupoints are being activated. You should have no discomfort from the needles after their insertion. This does not mean that you cannot move at all; the needles are very flexible and should not break even if bent.

You will then be asked to relax for twenty to thirty minutes with the needles in place. Since you will need to remain more or less motionless for the treatment, you may be offered a very light blanket to keep you warm.

You may then experience a deep sense of calm and even fall asleep. Again, this is a positive sign that the treatment is working—in traditional Chinese medicine it reflects the freeing of the flow of qi. After the allotted time your practitioner will remove the needles.

Some Variations on Acupuncture

Applying the same principle that stimulating acupuncture points will relieve pain, many doctors and practitioners employ similar methods.

Japanese acupuncturists, for example, use thinner needles and insert them less deeply.

Some schools of acupuncture limit application of needles to points in the hand, feet, or ears.

Some practitioners pass weak electrical currents through the needles to enhance their effect—a technique called *electroacupuncture.* Some also combine acupuncture with a traditional Chinese method called *moxibustion,* which is thought to predate acupuncture. With moxibustion a small cigar-shaped roll of dried herbs (*Artemesia vulgaris*) is placed a short distance from the acupoint and burned. When acupuncture and moxibustion are combined, a piece of dried herb is placed at the end of the needle away from the skin and burned. Another technique, *cupping,* uses a warmed glass to create a vacuum over acupoints. A few practitioners use *laser beams* instead of needles to stimulate acupuncture sites. Acupressure, the use of fingertip pressure to stimulate acupoints, is discussed on page 173.

Treatment Schedule

Typically the treatment course consists of weekly or twice-weekly sessions, which may continue for several weeks. Over time, if the treatments prove effective for you, their frequency can be reduced to once a week or every few weeks to maintain pain relief. Acupuncture can also be used for first aid of a headache in progress.

Side Effects

When done properly by an experienced practitioner, acupuncture is very safe. Some people experience minor redness and irritation at the acupuncture site, but this usually disappears within a few days. Others may feel anxious about the needles. Some people may even faint. (Practitioners have noticed that men are more likely to faint than women.) This is one of the reasons why people are asked to lie down for treatment.

There have also been rare reports of puncturing the lung and damage to the eye, which is why it's so important that you find a practitioner with experience.

Warnings

Let your doctor or practitioner know if you are pregnant, of any health conditions, or if you are taking medications.

While you can still safely receive acupuncture treatments during pregnancy, there are acupuncture sites that should be avoided, as they may cause miscarriage.

People taking prescribed blood-thinning agents such as warfarin (Coumadin) or heparin should not receive acupuncture, because it will increase the risk of bleeding. Taking over-the-counter drugs that may thin blood, such as aspirin, ibuprofen, or naproxen, will not generally increase your risk, but do let your practitioner know.

Finding a Reliable Practitioner

There are an estimated 6,500 acupuncturists in the United States. There are several routes you can take to find a qualified person to administer acupuncture. Word of mouth is a good start.

If you are looking purely for someone who is qualified in acupuncture (but not an M.D. nor a doctor of Chinese medicine), the National Commission for the Certification of Acupuncturists sets rigorous standards and can refer you to a licensed acupuncturist in your area (see below). The following states require that nondoctors meet or exceed the NCCA's standards in order to practice: Alaska, California, Colorado, Florida, Hawaii, Maine, Maryland, Massachusetts, Montana, Nevada, New Jersey, New Mexico, New York, Oregon, Pennsylvania, Rhode Island, Utah, Washington, Wisconsin, and the District of Columbia.

In addition there are more than forty schools and colleges of acupuncture and Oriental medicine in the United States. About half of them are approved with the National Accreditation Commission for Schools and Colleges of Acupuncture and Oriental Medicine, which also sets standards for educational achievement.

There are also more than three thousand conventional M.D.'s or D.O.'s who have become qualified in acupuncture through medical institutions. Many are licensed by the American Academy of Medical Acupuncture (AAMA), which sets standards for physicians (see "Resources"). The number of medical colleges that offer courses in acupuncture is growing all the time. There are two advantages to having an M.D./D.O. administer acupuncture: First, the physician can use acupuncture to complement other treatments; second, physician-applied acupuncture might increase the likelihood of receiving reimbursement by your insurance company.

To find a physician who is knowledgeable in all methods of Oriental medicine—acupoint therapy, herbology, nutrition, and meditation—contact the American Association of Acupuncture and Oriental Medicine. It is an umbrella organization for schools of acupuncture and Oriental medicine that meet basic requirements. More than twenty-eight schools are now members. They can refer you to a school in your area, which can in turn refer you to a local practitioner. Addresses are listed in the ''Resources'' section.

Questions and Answers

• *Does acupuncture hurt?*   Many people envision large, hypodermic-sized needles when they think of acupuncture. In fact acupuncture needles are so thin and light, most people barely feel their insertion. Others experience a distinct prick or tingling (like hitting the funny bone) at certain acupoints, which can be momentarily uncomfortable. Sensation is generally a good sign that the correct point has been stimulated. Some practitioners use ''needle guides'' to lessen the pain even further. As mentioned, traditional practitioners often twirl or flick the needle slightly to provide extra stimulation.

• *How long do the needles need to stay in?*   A typical treatment session lasts twenty to thirty minutes.

• *Can I "overdose" on acupuncture?*   No. There are no reports of adverse effects due to having too many acupuncture treatments.

• *What happens if the needle is inserted in the wrong place?*   Make sure that your practitioner is well qualified in acupuncture to ensure safety. But except in the case of pregnant women or underlying illness, there is very little risk.

• *Will I need other treatments besides acupuncture?*   The answer depends on your practitioner. If your acupuncturist is also a physician of Chinese or Oriental medicine, you might also receive herbs and/or recommendations for nutrition, meditation, and physical exercise. Some doctors of Chinese medicine may recommend *qigong* (see page 182). Some M.D.'s, osteopathic physicians (D.O.'s), and naturopaths are also skilled in acupuncture and may recommend complementary treatments for your headache.

• *I've heard of people keeping acupuncture needles in for a long time—will this happen for me with headache?*   Occasionally, for the treatment of addictions or weight reduction, tiny thumbtacklike needles are left in the ear for periods of days or weeks. Having a foreign body left in the ear carries a risk of infection. Few reports of a complication of this sort have appeared in the medical literature. Since the advantages of this method are not clear, it is best avoided.

• *Is acupuncture covered by health insurance?*   The answer depends on your health insurance. More than eighty private insurers and Medicare programs cover acupuncture. Many plans now accept acupuncture when it is either recommended or performed by a licensed medical doctor (M.D.). As complementary medicine becomes more accepted, and preventive approaches are seen as being economical, more insurance companies are beginning to offer coverage for alternative therapies, such as acupuncture.

• *Can children receive acupuncture?*   Yes. Even infants can safely receive acupuncture, except that it is important that they keep still. For this reason it is recommended that children not begin until they are old enough to stay motionless. In general the needles are smaller and thinner, inserted to a shallower depth, and left in for shorter periods of time (five to ten minutes, or just a few seconds).

Acupressure and Related Therapies

As with acupuncture, acupressure, shiatsu, and related Japanese techniques stimulate and direct the vital energy force (qi or ki). With these techniques, the same acupoints and meridians that are activated by acupuncture can be stimulated directly by the fingertips of a therapist—or self-applied.

History

Acupressure, which is said by some to predate acupuncture, is more than five thousand years old. It has undergone some transmutations over the years and is now a popular way to prevent and treat a number of chronic conditions.

Effectiveness

There are fewer clinical studies for acupressure than there are for acupuncture—possibly because it is considered less a medical technology than acupuncture is. However, the proof is in its endurance over thousands of years of use as a primary therapeutic tool.

How It Helps Relieve Headache

The same principles that guide acupuncture apply to traditional Oriental forms of acupressure. However unlike acupuncture, acupressure can be applied with or without a therapist.

Guidelines for Self-use

You can use acupressure techniques on yourself to prevent or treat a headache in progress. Because it takes only a few minutes, acupressure can be done virtually anywhere, though a regular preventive regimen performed at the same time every day is more likely to produce good results. Michael Reed Gach, Ph.D., acupressure expert and author of several books including *Acupressure's Potent Points,* offers the following guidelines and technique pointers:

- Do acupressure in a relaxing environment.
- Do not do acupressure one hour before or after eating a heavy meal.
- Pressure should produce a *twinge*—neither extremely painful nor overly soothing; it should "hurt good."
- Apply pressure gradually—don't push down too hard all at once.
- Pump pressure lightly, in a steady, rhythmic way, until you reach your "edge"—your twinge point.
- Breathe deeply to encourage energy flow and relieve tensions.

Acupressure Points for Relieving Headache

Like acupuncture, acupressure points are identified by their location along different meridians, or channels. There are about twenty different acupoints for the variety of chronic headaches we've discussed in this book—and the acupoints that are right for you depend on the type of headache you have. It is difficult to generalize, since headaches are outward symptoms of an underlying problem that relates to your general constitution, diet, and other lifestyle factors. But many experts in Oriental medicine agree that obstructions in qi along the gallbladder, stomach, and liver meridians are the most strongly implicated in vascular-related headaches, such as migraine. These meridians may also play a role in TMJ and tension-type headache. Eyestrain and sinus-related headache *may* be associated with qi obstructions in the bladder meridian, as may some anxiety-related headaches.

What follows are some recommended acupressure points. In addition we've included a sample of shiatsu exercises, described by Toru Namikoshi, author of *Shiatsu and Stretching,* (HarperCollins, 1985). This is just a sample of several points that *may* be of help for different types of headaches. For more recommendations specific to your headache syndrome, consult a qualified practitioner of acupressure or shiatsu.

Shiatsu Technique for Headaches
The following technique is helpful for migraines and headaches related to constriction or dilation of blood vessels near the head:

1. At the first sign of headache, apply medium pressure to the point of pain with your index, middle, and fourth finger for five seconds.
2. Apply pressure with your entire palms for ten seconds.
3. Repeat the above steps three times.
4. Apply pressure with both palms flat over your temples (right palm

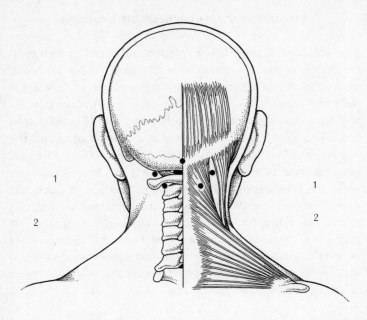

1. Migraine, eyestrain, neck pain and tension headache, and TMJ*
Located in the hollow between the neck muscles, just below the base of the skull. Tilt head back and use *thumbs* to press firmly for two to three minutes while breathing deeply. Relax for five minutes afterward.

2. Nervous tension, heaviness in the head, eyestrain, stiff neck*
Located on muscle one inch or so on either side of the spine, one finger width below the base of the skull. Hook *index, middle, and fourth fingers* on the muscles and press for three long breaths.

*Adapted with permission from *Shiatsu and Stretching,* by Toru Namikoshi, HarperCollins, 1985.

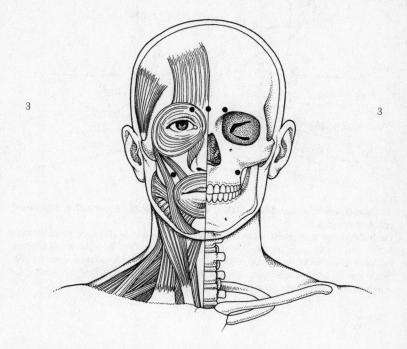

3. Sinus headache, eye pain, tension-related headaches*
Located on sides of nose, in the hollows between where the nose bridge meets the brow. Use *thumb and index finger* to press this point, hold and breathe deeply for a minute or two.

*Adapted with permission from *Shiatsu and Stretching,* by Toru Namikoshi, HarperCollins, 1985.

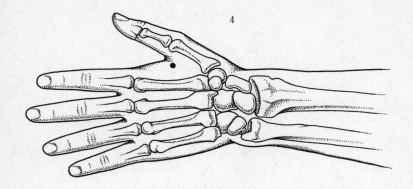

4

4. Constipation-related headache, sinus headache, toothache, tension-related headache*
Forbidden for pregnant women. *Located at the top of the mound that forms when you bring your thumb and index finger together.* Spread fingers apart. Squeeze point with *thumb* on back of hand, other fingers hooked under palm. Angle thumb toward the bone of index finger. Breathe deeply while pressing for one minute. Repeat on other hand.

*Adapted with permission from *Shiatsu and Stretching*, by Toru Namikoshi, HarperCollins, 1985.

for right temple, left palm for left temple) for ten seconds. Repeat three times.

5. Apply pressure with both palms over the top of your head for ten seconds. Repeat three times.

6. Place palms again over your temples (right hand over right temple; left hand over left temple). Applying pressure, rub the right hand up and down for five seconds. Move the left hand up and down for five seconds. Repeat, alternating hands, three times.

7. Now, with palms still over the temples, move the right hand forward and back for five seconds. Do the same thing with the left hand. Repeat, alternating hands, three times.

Variations on Acupressure

Shiatsu is a Japanese variation of acupressure, translated as "finger treatment." The acupoints are called *tsubos* and can be stimulated by the fingers, palms of the hands, knees, or feet (*barefoot shiatsu*). During a session with a therapist you will recline while the practitioner stimulates acupoints—however, shiatsu can also be self-applied.

Shiatsu is sometimes accompanied by stretching and specific movements (as in *zen shiatsu* and *acu-yoga*), massage (*Tui Na*), and *amma,* which focuses on points in the head and neck area to relieve tension. *Jin shin jyutsu* and *jin shin do* are other related therapies. Jin shin jyutsu is the skill of awakening the circulation, developed in Japan by Jiro Murai in the early 1900s, and was the basis for jin shin do, which was developed in the United States. Both are pressure-point therapies used to stimulate the flow of ki.

Who Can Be Helped

All types of headache can be treated and prevented with acupressure; of course for serious headaches of organic cause it's strongly urged that you seek professional medical help.

What to Expect

As with acupuncture the approach of the acupressure therapist can vary greatly depending on his or her background and orientation. If you see a doctor trained in traditional Oriental medicine, you may undergo a series of evaluations—tongue and pulse exam, lengthy questionnaire, and so on—to help identify the underlying cause of your headache. Acupressure may be one of several techniques used to treat the disorder.

Whether you see a doctor of Oriental medicine or a practitioner trained only in acupressure (or related) techniques, the therapist will then administer a series of acupressure massages, relying somewhat on trial and error to determine which points evoke the best response. In most cases you will then be taught some techniques to continue on your own.

Treatment Schedule

The treatment schedule depends on the frequency and severity of your headache, as well as the underlying cause. As preventive therapy, acupressure practiced once a day can also help reduce the frequency or lessen the severity of your headaches. In addition acupressure can be used to lessen the symptoms of a headache in progress.

Side Effects

As with acupuncture, slight bruising at the acupressure site may appear.

Warnings

Though simple to practice, acupressure is powerful therapy. Certain points should be avoided if you are pregnant (such as the hand press illustrated on page 178). If you're pregnant, are taking any medications, or have any disease condition, let your therapist know. Don't work on recently healed scars, burns, or fractures.

Finding a Reliable Practitioner

Specialists in traditional Oriental medicine will have a background in acupressure as well—see page 171 for referral sources. See the ''Resources'' section for contacts.

Questions and Answers

• *Does acupressure hurt?* Acupressure should hurt slightly; as described on page 174, it should feel like a twinge—a "good" hurt. But if you feel severe pain at a certain point, use less pressure. If the point is very tender to any touch, try some more deep, rhythmic breathing for relaxation and try again. When pressing one point, some people feel pain at another part of their bodies. Apply pressure to points near to the "referred pain," as they are strong indicators of problems in these areas. To expand your repertoire of acupoints, see the "Resources" section for self-help books on acupressure.

• *How do I know I've got the right acupressure point?* It might take some feeling around to find the point described in the instructions. You'll know if you feel some sensation of pain, or twinging, at the point.

• *My skin is irritated when I do acupressure. Is this normal?* You should not feel any skin stretching or irritation. Remember to direct fingers at a ninety-degree angle (straight up) from your skin surface to get the most out of your treatment. Also keep your fingernails clipped short and remove any jewelry from your hands and wrists.

• *How long do I apply pressure?* Typically one to three minutes.

• *How often should I give myself acupressure treatments?* It's up to you, but for preventive treatment you can apply acupressure every day, or just when you feel a headache coming on. It's a good idea to develop an acupressure regimen that includes general body relaxation—especially for people with tension-type headaches or other tension-related headaches such as eyestrain.

• *What happens if I apply pressure in the wrong place?* As with acupuncture, there is little risk unless you are pregnant or have other health problems. For example you must avoid the hand point recommended on page 178. In most cases the worst that can happen is that you do not experience the benefits. But you should check with a qualified therapist for specific guidelines before doing self-acupressure if you are pregnant or have any underlying health condition.

• *I have some other health problems; is it safe for me to do self-*

acupressure?   If you have any health condition, including pregnancy, or are taking medications for any illness, seek the advice of a professional in acupressure or a doctor of traditional Oriental medicine who can guide you in safe self-acupressure techniques.

• *Is acupressure covered by health insurance?*   The likelihood of coverage is greater if you are under the care of a licensed specialist or have been referred to one by a medical doctor. Check with your insurance company to make sure.

• *Can children receive acupressure?*   Yes, but for infants and very young children it's best to receive guidance from a skilled practitioner.

Ayurvedic Medicine

In Ayurvedic medicine the mapping system for the flow of *prana* (the life force, the Indian equivalent of qi) is related to that of traditional Oriental medicine. The 107 Ayurvedic acupoints, called *marmas,* were recorded in the ancient Indian text *Sushruta Samhita,* which originated before the tenth century B.C.

In the Ayurvedic system injury to the marmas can bring severe illness or death, while therapeutic massage can rejuvenate and heal. For example acupressure applied to the forty-second marma, *simanta,* which is located on the top of the skull, can help control blood circulation in the head. However, if this area is injured, it can cause premature death. The therapeutic means for regulating the marmas are varied, ranging from massage and acupressure to yoga and aromatherapy.

Qigong

Qigong (pronounced "chee-kung") is also referred to as *chi gung, chi kung,* and qi gong. It unites two concepts: *qi,* the life force, and *gong,* the skill of working with qi, and it is a powerful tool for self-healing. The ancient Chinese martial arts *kung fu* and *tai chi* evolved out of qigong.

As with acupuncture and acupressure, the practices of qigong focus on renewing, unblocking, and regulating the flow of qi through the channels of the body. Qigong is a relatively simple practice that uses movement and/or meditation techniques that can be learned by anyone. In addition there are doctors trained in Chinese medicine who practice a form of qigong that involves transmitting qi to ailing subjects.

History

Qigong is thought to predate and lay the groundwork for traditional Oriental medicine. References to qigong predate the *Nei Jing,* the ancient sourcebook of traditional Chinese medicine. Early forms of qigong were practiced and refined by physicians and monks in ancient China. An estimated 100 million people practice qigong throughout the world today. Among them are qigong masters who are reputed to heal masses of people and perform miracle cures. Many hospitals in China routinely include a staff of qigong physicians (different from qigong masters, who are very few in number), who are trained in traditional Chinese medicine with a specialty in qigong. Research from institutes and universities in China has shown qigong potentially effective in treating many diseases. In the United States and Europe enthusiasm for this ancient method of self-healing is growing rapidly.

How It Helps Relieve Headache

There are two categories of qigong: internal and external. Internal qigong can be practiced by anyone for self-regeneration or therapy. External qigong, known as *waiqi,* is the form used by healers to transmit qi to another person. Within the category of internal qigong there are meditational forms, known as *nei dan,* and movement forms, known as *wei dan.* Both share a spiritual component, and a focus on breathing. Today, according to Sheila McNamara and Dr. Song Xuan Ke, authors of *Traditional Chinese Medicine* (HarperCollins Publishers, Inc., 1995), millions of Chinese people "start their day with a form of exercise which does not aim to burn off energy, but rather to accrue, store and reinforce it."

Within the two categories there are hundreds of forms of qigong, and more are evolving even today. Some are widely available for study, while others are reserved for those with special knowledge and skill. Indeed, according to Roger Jahnke, in Santa Barbara, California, and author of many books about qigong, adaptability to personal limits or inclinations is one of qigong's unique characteristics. Catching the *spirit* of qigong is more important and beneficial than precisely mirroring an instructor's movements. He recounts this story to illustrate the point:

> At a conference I recently attended, a woman from the audience told me that she had been taught qigong by a friend who had attended one of my workshops, and had benefited tremendously. Curious, I asked her to show me what she had learned. To my surprise, her movements were very new to me—even though my lessons were the original source of her qigong practice.

Jahnke does not discount the benefits of this pupil's qigong practice just because her movements didn't match his lesson. Quite the contrary, the woman's positive experience serves as vivid testimony to the value of qigong as a self-care practice. Although there are many formalized ways of practicing qigong, at its core it can be a practice without prescribed movements. By following fundamental guidelines, qigong can be practiced virtually anywhere, by anyone, from the most flexible and healthy to the bedridden. In Jahnke's words, "There are no barriers to qigong." It is the responsibility of the practitioner to be "filled with care," as Jahnke puts it; that is, to remain inwardly sensitive to the powers of qigong—and adapt the practice to match one's limitations.

Qigong's effectiveness is rooted in the accumulation and circulation of qi—through either meditation or physical activity—to achieve connectedness with the fundamental healing forces of nature and the universe. Qigong practices can remove qi blockages along meridians in the same way as acupuncture or acupressure. It is said by some that when levels of proficiency are attained, the effects of qigong can be more powerful than those achieved by acupuncture.

Who Can Be Helped

Qigong experts universally agree that the daily practice of qigong can help relieve virtually any physical illness, including all forms of headache. General internal qigong practice is considered a mind-body tonic that can only benefit the body by restoring levels of qi. But as with any condition, it is easier to prevent headache than it is to deal with a migraine in progress. Ongoing qigong practice is a preventive measure. Therapeutic qigong, under the care of a qualified qigong therapist, can have specific health effects.

What to Expect

There are hundreds of forms of qigong, and many ways to practice it. Certain forms can be administered by a qigong therapist, who will almost certainly teach you a series of movements or meditations to perform on your own; self-practice through videos and group or private classes are also available.

A qigong therapist can instruct you on ways to activate qi along certain meridians that have been diagnosed as being obstructed. A qigong doctor may pass his or her hands across your body, often not touching it at all, to transmit qi to certain areas for therapeutic effect.

You might feel sensations of heat, lightness, tingling, or weight— which are generally good signs that qi is being activated in your body.

Qigong Fundamentals

As mentioned, there are many forms of qigong, and they can evolve almost spontaneously. Dr. Jahnke outlines three fundamental features for any qigong practice: regulating the breath, regulating the mind, and regulating the body—referred to as the "three regulations" in China.

Regulating the breath simply means focusing on the breath to make it full and natural, To regulate the mind means to bring the mind to a state of calm and near-stillness, as devoid of thought and worry as possible. Focusing on the breath or the sensation of qi is one way to regulate the mind. To regulate the body means to assume the correct position. There are at least three ways to regulate the body: by assuming a specific supine, sitting, or standing posture; by following a prescribed set of qigong movements or by practicing *spontaneous qigong.*

Spontaneous qigong is a method of movement that aims, in Roger Jahnke's words, "to find a personal and unique combina-

tion of the three regulations that maximize the circulation of qi.''
It is an intuitive movement guided by one's personal connection
with qi. This could mean anything from long periods of stillness
punctuated by micromovements to maintain comfort, to contin-
ual, gentle or radical movement. Basically if the movement connects you with a sense of qi, do it.

An awareness of qi is fundamental to qigong—which is not as
mysterious as it sounds. A typical qigong session will begin with
relaxing the body—regulating the breath and the mind. Either
standing, sitting, or lying down, imagine your body connecting
deeply to the earth, absorbing the earth's qi. Then connect with
the universal energy. With this image firmly rooted in your mind,
you have already begun to access qi.

Your awareness will take the form of a sensation of tingling,
warmth, or circulation. You may feel deeply relaxed and begin to
sway, as if experiencing an invisible breeze. Your qigong practice
could be as simple as taking deliberate steps as you walk—ever
mindful with each step down of the connection to the earth's qi.
Or your practice may be a complicated sequence of precise movements. In either case, a profound sense of qi is the objective. Qi
awareness is subtle and may take months of vigilant practice.

Getting in Touch with Qi

Try this spontaneous qigong exercise: Stand with your feet
shoulder-width apart, with feet pointed inward at a forty-five-
degree angle (pidgeon-toed). Relax your whole body. If you feel
strain at the small of your back, squat slightly until the pressure is
relieved—or sit in an armless chair. Relax your whole body. Focus on your breath. Wriggle your fingers. Then move your body
rhythmically, or in a shaking pattern. Slowly exaggerate the
movements that you started, but keep them slow. Add head and
neck movements to your body's movements. Continue moving,
conscious of your breath. Follow the natural pattern of your
movements wherever they want to go, exaggerating them or slowing them down, shifting your weight, as you see fit.

Practice Schedule

Again your personal practice depends on the type of qigong you choose to practice. However, the effects of self-practiced qigong are very powerful according to proponents. Daily practice for twenty to thirty minutes, with periodic advice from a knowledgeable instructor, can result in very rapid improvement. It is said that daily practice is a way of maintaining health and generating a stronger defense against disease, and even healing difficult disease states.

Effectiveness

There are few controlled studies of the efficacy of qigong in migraine and headache. However, one of the reasons it works probably has to do with the fact that it reduces stress. A recent report revealed that qigong produces the relaxation response—reduced heart rate, blood pressure, and muscle tension.[5]

Side Effects and Warnings

Practiced with mindfulness of one's own limitations, there should be no side effects to qigong practice. And if guided by an experienced qigong practitioner, even people with severe disabilities can safely practice some form of qigong. Indeed qigong can be practiced while lying entirely still by people in hospital beds and adapted for people in wheelchairs. However, some of the qigong movements may create a sense of heat, dizziness, or even fainting. Since qigong movements are readily adaptable to anyone's physical or emotional limitations, any discomfort should be a signal to slow down your practice or change the movements until the sensation passes, advises Roger Jahnke.

Finding a Reliable Teacher or Therapist

As with many complementary healing methods, the recommendations of friends and acquaintances are your best resource. There are many organizations that can refer you to qigong practitioners or teachers in your area. A good start is the International Qi Gong Directory. A list of organizations can be found in the "Resources" section.

Questions and Answers

• *Does qigong hurt?* If performed with care, there should be no ill effects or discomfort from practicing qigong. But, as just mentioned, people with emotional problems or physical disabilities would benefit greatly from the guidance of an experienced qigong instructor.

• *I am not very flexible. Can I practice qigong?* There are many ways to practice qigong. It is as flexible as the practitioner. If the "set" you were taught is causing pain, do not continue. For example people with arthritis of the knees may not be able to practice qigong forms that include a lot of bending. Speak with your qigong instructor about ways to adapt your practice to your needs—or if you are familiar with qigong movements, adapt it yourself. You can do this without sacrificing any benefits.

• *I practice regularly, but I don't feel anything. Am I doing something wrong?* If you are under the care of a therapist or instructor, ask his or her advice. If you have taken a class, review the practices. Make sure you are focusing on the movement or meditation techniques and in time, experts say, you should begin to feel positive effects.

• *Is it normal to feel a little light-headed after my qigong practice?* This is not abnormal. You may also feel warmth, tingling, or other sensations—including the sense of energy traveling across your channels, or meridians. If the feeling becomes uncomfortable, adjust your practice by slowing down, or changing your movements, or simply stopping and regulating your breathing.

• *How long should I practice qigong each day?* For best effects practice the entire set you were taught for thirty minutes a day. But even a few minutes or seconds of qigong will yield some benefit. Qigong can be practiced at any time that you feel you can focus. Even regulating your breathing—while you work, play, or rest—can be a form of qigong. Or sitting in a quiet place with your feet connected to the earth. Or walking slowly, and being mindful of your connection with the ground are also forms of qigong.

• *How often should I practice qigong?* Follow the recommendations of your instructor or use your intuition. For general health daily practice is recommended. But again qigong can be practiced for just a few minutes at any time during the day when you have time to regulate your breath, your mind, and your body.

• *If I'm not sure of the movements and do something wrong, can I hurt myself?*   Generally qigong movements are slow and gentle, and there is no harm in doing them differently from the way you were taught. Some experts might disagree, but instructors believe that if you are sensing the circulation of qi and are not experiencing negative effects, you might just have invented a form of qigong that is right for you.

• *I have some other health problems—is it safe for me to do qigong?*   If you have any health condition, including pregnancy, or are taking medications for any illness, it's a good idea to seek the advice of a person with expertise in qigong or traditional Chinese medicine. Generally, gentle qigong practice may benefit all conditions.

• *Is qigong covered by health insurance?*   The very few policies that cover alternative health practices may cover qigong, particularly if it is recommended by an M.D., osteopathic physician, or physical therapist. Check with your insurer.

• *Can children and the elderly do qigong?*   Yes, anyone who can learn the simple meditations and movements can practice qigong. Children respond very well to the playfulness and spontaneity of certain forms of qigong, such as spontaneous wiggling or forms that use movements that imitate those of animals. The benefits for older people can be especially good, says Roger Jahnke, as long as the practice is adapted to their particular limitations.

Yoga and Breathing

The word *yoga* has its roots in the Sanskrit word *yuj,* which means "to yoke, unite, join, or integrate."

In its traditional Hindu context, yoga is more than a physical discipline: it is a system of philosophy and a way of life. It is a means of disciplining the body, mind, and emotions to unify with the spirit, which is part of all living things. From this philosophical foundation one can see how deeply yoga acknowledges the unity of mind and body.

Yehudi Menuhin confirms this connection in his introduction to B.K.S. Iyengar's classic text on yoga, *Light on Yoga,* ''The practice of yoga over the past fifteen years has convinced me that most of our fundamental attitudes to life have their physical counterparts in the body.''

Traditionally, there are eight stages of yoga, which address physical, ethical, and spiritual aspects of life. But most Westerners are familiar with only three: the postures, or *asanas* (AH-sa-nas); breathing exercises, or *pranayama* (prah-nah-YAH-mah); and meditation. (We'll discuss meditation in Chapter 8.) A wide range of therapeutic benefits of yoga have been proven through clinical study. And its effectiveness as both a general stress-reducing method and a way of reducing headache has also been shown. An estimated five million people in the United States do some form of yoga.

History

The first book to systematize the practice was the *Yoga Sutras* (aphorisms) by Patanjali, which dates to about 200 B.C. There are many yoga asanas, which are coordinated with breathing, and many individual pranayama techniques.

Over the past century investigators in India and the West have conducted numerous research studies to show the therapeutic benefits of both yoga postures and yoga breathing, which are synchronized during yoga sessions. Today yoga is part of many health programs to treat chronic diseases, notably Dean Ornish's method for treating coronary artery disease.

Yoga classes have been avidly embraced by Westerners as a way of calming the mind and toning the body. While many people practice yoga with spiritual intent, others are drawn to its physical and therapeutic benefits. It is common to find classes adapted for all ranges of flexibility, endurance, and overall health. One can find yoga-aerobics, step-yoga, and yoga workouts. There are yoga classes for people with back problems and people with HIV. Physical therapists often base exercises on yoga poses, says Nancy Ford-Kohne, co-founder and director of Yoga and Health Studies Center in Alexandria, Virginia, and American editor of *Yoga for Common Ailments* (Simon & Schuster).

Some yoga traditionalists disparage the popularization of yoga and its adulterations. Others welcome it as a way of reaching more people with specific medical problems.

Asanas

Asana means ''ease'' in Sanskrit. Not because the poses are so easy to achieve but because they help achieve a state of ease—a balance—mentally, physically, and spiritually.

The asanas are very specific postures that involve stretching and holding different parts of the body. Yoga asanas were designed to exercise every muscle, nerve, and gland in the body. Except for props, used on occasion to aid in the postures, the asanas are ingeniously formulated so that the body works with itself to produce therapeutic benefits. These stretches can be very gentle, or quite rigorous, depending on the type of class you take.

Pranayama

Pranayama means ''control of the breath.'' The word comes from *prana,* which means both ''breath'' and ''life force'' in Sanskrit, and *yama,* which means ''control.'' Prana flows throughout the body in a system of *nadi,* or channels. As with qi in traditional Oriental medicine, free circulation of prana is a prerequisite of health. Prana can become blocked due to improper diet, disease, or constitutional imbalances. The objective of pranayama exercises is to encourage the free flow of prana and eliminate blockages.

Yoga teaches that the breath reflects and influences the state of the mind. By focusing on breath, one focuses the mind; by making the breath steady and clear, the same effects are achieved in the mind.

How Yoga Helps Relieve Headache

According to Nancy Ford-Kohne, yoga offers many benefits to people with headache. ''From a physical view, the best thing yoga can do for people with tension-type headache is to increase blood flow and to release tension in the neck and upper body,'' she says. The asanas can also help drain the lymphatic system and remove toxins. Certain poses, such as the twists and the cobra, can help the adrenal glands and kidneys. In addition studies have shown yoga to help balance neural problems, regulate serotonin, and release endorphins—all of which have been shown to help relieve headache. The emphasis on breathing helps oxygenate the blood.

With regular practice of asanas, structural balance, flexibility, and posture can improve dramatically.

In addition yoga practice induces a general sense of relaxation, which may also ward off headaches.

Finally, if practiced with mindful intent, yoga engages the mind and the body; it is a truly holistic practice. One can learn, through awareness of the discomfort of the asanas, how to better manage pain. One also learns, through the experience of trying to master the asanas, how to work with one's limitations and have compassion for the body. Through pranayama and asana practice, one begins to grasp and harness the power of the mind to deal calmly with stressful situations. Says Iyengar in *Light on Yoga,* ''A lamp does not flicker in a place where no winds blow; so it is with a yogi [one who practices yoga], who controls his mind, intellect and self, being absorbed in the spirit within him.''

Who Can Be Helped

People with tension-type and migraine headache can benefit from yoga.

What to Expect

Wear loose clothing or footless leotards and bring a towel or yoga mat. Some classes begin with meditation or chanting; most start with at least a few moments of relaxation, either lying down or sitting in a comfortable position.

Most classes begin with breathing, or focusing awareness on the breath. Pranayama may range from taking complete, full breaths deep into the belly to specific pranayama. Gentle stretching exercises often precede the formal asanas, or postures, to help loosen muscles and joints.

In the asana portion of the class the instructor will guide the group step-by-step into the stance. In some classes the instructor will ask that you breathe through your nose while doing the asanas. The poses are performed with slow, steady motion and then held for several seconds, or minutes, giving attention to full, quiet breath and the sensations that arise.

The form of each asana is very specific and should be practiced correctly to get the full health benefits—and avoid injury. The instructor is there to help. Achieving good form takes time, patience, and practice, so you should not feel bad about not doing it right. It can take many years to do asanas. During the learning process many asanas can be adapted to your level of flexibility. For example some of the balancing poses are difficult for beginners. In most classes the instructor will encourage you to stand against the wall to help you gain a sense of balance. No matter what your ability, the main point is to do the best you can, and to practice the asana with concentration and awareness. Any level you reach will yield some benefit.

Though the word *asana* is Sanskrit for "ease," some of the asanas will be challenging. You will be encouraged to explore your limits. At the same time it's important to honor your "edge." If you cannot touch your hands to your feet, for example, it is better to go only a little beyond your limit and back away to a stage of comfort than to make heroic gestures and risk injury. If a certain pose seems impossible, advises Nancy Ford-Kohne, skip it until you feel comfortable trying it again. Having compassion for your body is a basic tenet of yogic practice. Over time, and with patience, you will find yourself getting closer and closer to the desired goal.

It may be tempting to compare your progress to that of others in the class. But yoga is a not a competitive sport. A main point is to release judgment and, as much as possible, all other mind "chatter." A big part of yoga practice is training the mind to focus, a practice that helps cultivate concentration and mind-body (and spirit) unity.

After completing several asanas, many classes move to pranayama and then to a period of relaxation, usually lying down flat on the back while focusing on the breath or on the contact of your body with the ground.

Classes often end with a short period of meditation and/or chanting of the sound *om.*

While some of the asanas will challenge you physically and mentally, the practice of yoga can bring great rewards. Most people leave classes feeling lighter and more relaxed. It is a practice with some immediate benefits and many subtle, positive qualities that accumulate over time and with practice.

Yoga Approaches to Headache Relief

Coping with Stress

(suggested by Nancy Ford-Kohne)

1. Sit with your spine as straight as possible. (If you need to sit in a chair, make sure your feet are flat on the floor with knees directly over the center of your feet. Use a book or cushion under your feet if they do not rest comfortably on the floor.) Place hands on the tops of your legs.
2. Close your eyes gently and let them rest behind closed lids.
3. Think about your ribs, at the front, back, and sides of your body. Your lungs are behind those ribs.
4. Feel your lungs filling up, your ribs expanding out and up. Feel your lungs emptying, your ribs coming back down and in. Don't push the breath.
5. The first few times do this for two to three minutes, then do it for up to five to ten minutes. At first set aside a time at least once a day to do this. When you learn how good it makes you feel, you'll want to do it at other times as well.

Asana to Help Prevent Tension Headache: Child Pose (Balasana)

This posture gently stretches the muscles of the lower back and helps relieve shoulder tension. It should be avoided by people with migraine or sinus headache. Feel free to use pillows under the head to minimize strain.

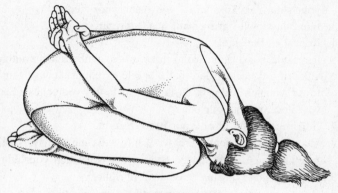

Child pose (balasana)

1. Kneel with your feet behind you and sit on your heels, the top of your feet flat on the ground. Keep your spine straight, but not too rigid.
2. Bend forward slowly. Rest your forehead on the ground, or on pillows (or folded towels) if you cannot reach the ground. Turn your face to one side. Let your arms fall to your side in a relaxed position.
3. Breathe regularly for one to two minutes.
4. Slowly and gently return to sitting.

Asana to Help Prevent Tension: Neck Roll

This exercise is a common warm-up for doing asanas but can also help relieve tension and improve flexibility of the neck muscles.

CAUTION: Avoid neck rolls if you have whiplash, disk disease, or any problem in the bones of the cervical (neck) spine.

1. Sitting in a comfortable position, relax your shoulders, arms, and hands. Remember to breathe regularly and deeply.
2. Take in a deep breath. While exhaling slowly, gently tilt your head to the left, as though you wanted to touch your ear to your shoulder. Stop when you reach your "edge."
3. Inhaling slowly, bring your head upright.
4. Repeat to the right.
5. Repeat left and right two to three times, gently and smoothly.
6. Take in a deep, gentle breath. While exhaling slowly, gently lower your chin down, as though to touch your chest. Stop when you reach your edge.
7. Inhaling slowly, bring your head upright.
8. Take in a deep, gentle breath. While exhaling slowly, gently reach your chin to the sky. Stop when you reach your edge.
9. Inhaling slowly, bring your head upright.
10. Breathing gently and rhythmically, *very slowly* and gently move your head to the left, to the back, to the right and to the front—ever mindful of your limits. Continue rotating two to three times.
11. Repeat step 10 in the opposite direction.

Treatment Schedule

The best way to get health benefits from yoga is by regular practice. Some people take classes once or twice a week for a while and then continue on their own. Instructors of traditional yoga recommend practicing either first thing in the morning or before retiring. Class length varies from twenty minutes to one and a half hours.

Effectiveness

As mentioned, yoga asanas and pranayama have been studied widely and have proved to have wide-ranging health benefits. More than 1,500 studies have shown the effectiveness of yoga and meditation in relieving pain and reducing stress, among other health benefits.[6]

In one study yoga proved to be a successful adjunct to treatment for people with migraine. A survey by the Yoga Biomedical Trust showed that 80 percent of 464 individuals with migraine benefited from yoga therapy.[7]

Side Effects

Yoga asanas, when practiced correctly, should not cause side effects. If you are not used to physical activity and you overdo it, you may experience tender joints or muscles for a few days afterward.

Warnings

If you are over thirty-five, or have high blood pressure or a history of heart disease in your family, you should have a physical exam before starting yoga. Then let your yoga instructor know about any health conditions. Avoid forward-bending asanas if you are in the middle of a headache attack, though these are good to help *prevent* headaches. Also certain asanas should be avoided during pregnancy and menstruation.

Finding a Reliable Yoga Instructor or Therapist

While you can learn yoga asanas and pranayama through books, audiotapes, or videotapes (there are many available), it's wise for beginners to start off with a qualified yoga instructor.

Recommendations from friends, physicians, or physical therapists are the best way to start. A qualified yoga instructor may or may not be certified—it is not a requirement in any state. And certification is not as important as having an instructor who understands your special needs. You can find help in both regards by contacting the International Association of Yoga Therapists. While they do not refer to yoga instructors, the IAYT can provide a list of schools that offer yoga-teacher certification, which can in turn refer you to a certified instructor in your area.

When you speak or write to the school, ask for an instructor who can help with headaches. See addresses in the "Resources" section.

Questions and Answers

• *Does yoga hurt?*   If you do not go beyond your limits, and practice the asanas with awareness, you should not feel pain. While holding some asanas for minutes or seconds, you may experience strong sensations: Your body may urge you to move out of the posture, your mind may fill you with negative thoughts about your abilities. Yoga instructors will ask that you acknowledge these feelings, then move on to focus on the breath and posture. If the sensations are very loud and demanding, honor your body's limitations and back off to a level of comfort or stop entirely.

• *Some of the postures I've seen look like contortions. Will I have to do them?*   The asanas are designed to activate all of the body systems, from the muscles to the internal organs and blood system. To achieve this, some of the asanas may seem awkward-looking. Most beginning yoga classes start with fundamental postures, which help build strength, flexibility, and balance. Over time, instructors will add more challenging asanas. You may be very surprised at how naturally you assume some of the odder-looking postures.

• *Can I do yoga if I am pregnant?*   There is some debate over this. You should definitely seek medical advice before starting any exercise regimen if you are pregnant. Some sources recommend avoiding yoga during the first three months of pregnancy; others recommend practicing only during the first three months. However, yoga can be adapted to the needs of pregnant women, and there are yoga classes specifically for women who are pregnant. If you are in the least concerned, avoid yoga during pregnancy, or limit your practice to gentle, stretching postures.

• *Can older people do yoga?*   Yes, yoga asanas are an excellent way to build strength and flexibility. Be sure to let your instructor know of any physical problems, such as arthritis or osteoporosis. If available, take a gentle yoga class, or one that is designed for older people.

• *Is yoga covered by health insurance?* If recommended by a doctor or physical therapist, it might be covered. Check with your insurance carrier.

PRESSURE-POINT THERAPIES

Trigger-Point Therapy (Myotherapy)

Trigger-point therapy, also known as Myotherapy, is a method of relaxing muscle spasm, improving circulation, and relieving pain. It is based on the concept that there are *trigger points* in muscles that are extremely tender to the touch.

Trigger points are damaged, spasm-prone areas of muscles caused by accidents, disease, postural habits, and other factors. They can lie dormant for many years until physical or emotional stress causes them to flare up and cause pain.

Today there are two techniques used to *defuse,* or neutralize, the trigger point. *Trigger-point injection therapy* (injection of anesthetics into the trigger point) was developed by Janet Travell, M.D., in the 1940s. Some physicians use electrical stimulation on trigger points, which is related to TENS (see page 255). *Myotherapy* (application of pressure by hand to the trigger point) was developed by Bonnie Prudden in the mid 1970s, who discovered that applying strong manual pressure to trigger points worked just as well as injections in relieving pain. Since Myotherapy does not use drugs and is noninvasive, we'll focus on it in this section.

Although these therapies are widely practiced with significant effect in relieving all sorts of pain, including headache, the medical community is still in the dark about why it works.

Others postulate that Myotherapy is a way of teaching the brain to break old patterns of muscle spasm, that it helps reeducate damaged muscles. Any stress to the body will initiate communication with the brain via nerve pathways. With Myotherapy, pressure to trigger points in the muscle initiates a new mode of communication with the brain.

With trigger-point pressure hundreds of thousands of signals are sent from the muscle to the spinal cord and then to the brain. These messages allow the brain to release the spasm and open the door for corrective movement. In essence Myotherapy prepares the muscle for freer movement, which breaks the habitual cycle of spasm. Once freed from the spasm, Bonnie Prudden's Myotherapy method follows up with corrective exercises designed to retrain the muscle into a new, spasm-free pattern of movement.

History

In the 1930s a German physician named Hans Lange discovered that tender areas in muscles are 50 percent harder than surrounding areas. In the 1940s the American physician Janet Travell, M.D., developed trigger-point injection therapy; she found that injecting Lange's "tender points" with an anesthetic helped relieve muscle spasm. In many cases trigger-point injections are followed by muscle-stretching exercises.

In 1976 an exercise specialist named Bonnie Prudden was working with an internist named Desmond Tivy, helping to identify trigger points in patients before injection. By chance she discovered that applying pressure to the trigger points relieved pain. Out of this discovery she developed an integrated system of trigger-point treatments and exercise known as Myotherapy. Today Myotherapy by a Bonnie Prudden therapist is available only through referral from an M.D., osteopathic physician, naturopathic physician, dentist, or other medical professional. Laypeople can learn her method through books available from Bonnie Prudden Pain Erasure.

How It Helps Relieve Headache

Myotherapists believe that trigger points are the cause of most non-organic headaches. With vascular headaches such as migraine and cluster, the pain is purportedly linked with the pressure that spasmodic muscles exert on blood vessels and nerves in and around the head and upper neck. Tension-type headaches are caused by direct muscle spasm in the area of pain. Sinus headaches are caused by blocked sinuses related to muscle spasms around the nose and cheekbones. In addition, headaches can result from trigger points in distant areas, called *matrix trigger points,* which cause referred pain to the head area.

Head muscles, according to Myotherapists, are especially vulnerable to the assaults that create trigger points and muscle spasm. Think of how many times you fell on your head as a child, or chewed gum, or experienced stress that made you clench muscles in the neck and jaw areas. All of these situations according to therapists can set the stage for muscle spasm and trigger points.

By finding, then defusing, trigger points in the head and neck area, Bonnie Prudden Myotherapists, and physicians who use trigger-point injections, help relax muscles, improve circulation, and relieve associated pain.

Who Can Be Helped

Myotherapy and trigger-point injection therapy are used to treat migraine, tension-type, TMJ, and sinus headaches.

What to Expect

There are typically four parts to the first Myotherapy session. First, a history is taken to help determine when and where trigger points were "laid down" in the patient's muscles. You may be asked questions such as how you were delivered as a baby (forceps births may insult head muscles), whether you have ever suffered any accidents or injuries, the type of dental work you have received (e.g., bridges, braces, etc.), and whether or not you have any diseases such as arthritis or lupus.

Second, you will be asked to wear loose clothing and lie down on a comfortable table. Then you will be given a painless test to determine the strength and flexibility of key posture muscles.

Third, the Myotherapist will locate the trigger points believed to be directly responsible for your pain. This step entails drawing a map of the afflicted area and marking off points that are especially sensitive to pressure. Since trigger points often congregate, the Myotherapist will move inch-wise around that area in search for more.

Fourth, the Myotherapist will erase the trigger point. This typically involves applying about fifteen to twenty pounds of manual pressure to the trigger point for seven seconds, then releasing slowly. The pressure will be lower if working on the face and greater if working on the gluteals of the buttocks. Depending on the area being worked on, the Myotherapist will use hands, knuckles, or even elbows to apply pressure.

Finally, the Myotherapist will gently stretch the affected muscles. You will leave with exercises tailored to your specific problem to help keep the muscles free of spasm and pain.

Later sessions focus on continuing to erase your trigger points. Corrective exercises will be reevaluated and you will learn how to apply Myotherapy yourself to prevent pain from recurring.

Office Stress–Release Exercises

According to Myotherapists, the neck, shoulders, arms, upper and lower back, and legs are at risk for spasm-causing tension while sitting at a desk. The following exercises are recommended to be performed regularly—after each phone call, each client, or each trip to another part of the office—to ward off stressful tension.

SHRUG SERIES
Do three sets of each, every hour.

1. Round the shoulders forward.
2. Press the shoulders down.
3. In a neutral position, look left and look right.

1. Press shoulders back.
2. Pull shoulders up.
3. In a neutral position, look up and look down.

LOWER-BACK STRETCH

1. Before you leave your chair, lean forward and let your upper body hang downward in short, gentle bounces.
2. If you are well stretched, open your knees for a better stretch.

© Copyright 1993, Bonnie Prudden, Inc.

Treatment Schedule

To relieve pain, most people need fewer than ten sessions; the average number of sessions is five. Bonnie Prudden Pain Erasure also offers educational aids so that you can learn the technique yourself.

Effectiveness

Based on unpublished experiences, Bonnie Prudden Myotherapists report significant improvement among 90 to 95 percent of headache and TMJ sufferers with Myotherapy and subsequent corrective exercise. Like many complementary therapies, few clinical studies have been performed. However, Ann Naylor, a Bonnie Prudden Myotherapist in San Francisco, has recently concluded a study of 125 people, 72 percent of whom suffered from headache. Overall, 57 percent of patients had 85 percent improvement or better with Myotherapy.

Side Effects

Other than rare cases of minor muscle bruising, Myotherapy is free of side effects.

Warnings

Underlying disease conditions might contraindicate Myotherapy. Since you must receive written clearance for Myotherapy from a doctor (M.D., D.O., chiropractor, dentist, or naturopathic physician), your doctor will know whether you are a candidate. But if you decide to go the self-help route and learn Myotherapy from one of Bonnie Prudden's books, be sure to first seek the advice of your doctor.

Finding a Reliable Myotherapist

Certified Myotherapists must train for 1,300 hours, and undergo 45 hours of continuing education every two years by the Bonnie Prudden School for Physical Fitness and Myotherapy. The school also lists doctors and dentists who know about or use Myotherapy. Ask your doctor, or contact Bonnie Prudden Pain Erasure for a referral and for self-help books and videotapes (see ''Resources'').

Questions and Answers

• *What are the benefits of Myotherapy over trigger-point injection therapy?*   Both achieve a similar effect on the muscle; however, Myotherapy does not involve injections or the use of drugs. It is a hands-on, noninvasive method. In addition Myotherapy can be learned (and self-taught) through Prudden's educational materials.

• *Why are the follow-up exercises important?*   In the words of Ann Naylor, a certified Myotherapist in San Francisco, ''Myotherapy prepares the muscles for movement by releasing the spasm, the exercises help imbed the new pattern of movement in the brain.'' The exercises help retrain the muscles to prevent spasms from recurring.

• *How come I might have a spasm recurrence?*   If you reinjure the muscle, you might reactivate the spasm. The sooner you defuse the trigger point, say Myotherapists, the less treatment it will take to break the pain-spasm cycle. For this reason Myotherapists teach their clients how to recognize and defuse trigger points themselves.

• *Can children receive Myotherapy?*   Yes, but the pressure used to defuse trigger points will be lighter. When children get Myotherapy, parents are taught how to recognize and neutralize trigger points.

• *Is Myotherapy covered by medical insurance?*   When it is recommended by a physician, physical therapist, dentist, osteopathic physician, or chiropractor, Myotherapy is often covered by health insurance. But you should check with your carrier.

Reflexology

Reflexology is a type of pressure-massage therapy that operates by the belief that there are reflex areas in the feet and hands that correspond with other systems of the body. Applying pressure to these points, reflexologists maintain, can release tension, improve circulation, and bring the body into a state of balance.

History

Reflexology's roots can be traced to ancient China, with probable connection to the meridian therapies of acupuncture and acupressure. Historical evidence of reflexology has been found in ancient cultures of Japan, Egypt, as well as some Native American and African groups. Its emergence in modern Western culture took shape as a mapping system of pressure points on the hands and feet that correspond to different points of the body and was developed by Eunice Ingham. Her nephew, Dwight Byers, founded the International Institute of Reflexology, which trains reflexologists and publishes books.

How It Helps Relieve Headache

Reflexology operates by the concept that every part of the body is linked to a reference point, or *reflex point* on the foot, ear, and hand. The foot is the favored therapeutic focus because of its extreme sensitivity. Each foot houses thousands of nerve endings, which, according to reflexology theory, are connected via the nervous system to organs, bones, muscles, and glands throughout the body.

The reflex points corresponding to headaches and sinus problems are found at the tips and sides of the four small toes on both feet. But since headache may originate from neck, face, or shoulder tension—or stress in general—other reflex points may need to be pressed to achieve headache relief.

Reflexologists believe that applying pressure to reflex points helps stimulate the nerve pathways to corresponding body systems, which in turn helps improve circulation. According to reflexologists, ongoing massage with the right degree of pressure—it should "hurt good"—

will also release endorphins, the body's own feel-good messengers, from the bloodstream.

Who Can Be Helped

Theoretically reflexology can benefit people with all sorts of headaches. However, reflexologists do not claim to cure illness—or to diagnose it. The most that a reputable reflexologist will promise is to heighten your sense of relaxation and help improve circulation.

What to Expect

The reflexologist will begin by asking you the purpose for your session. Conventionally he will warm his hands and apply a pleasant-scented cream to your feet, starting off with light massage of the feet. You may feel a tingling sensation as tensions are released. Then, taking your foot in one hand, the therapist will start working on specific areas with the other. Inching his thumb or fingers across your toes (a natural starting point for people with headaches), he will apply pressure that may feel painful.

While the reflexologist might be able to target problem areas by feeling or looking at your feet, your feedback is very critical. It is important that you let him know of any pain, sensitivity, tenderness, or discomfort. These sensations sound the alarm that the therapist has landed on an area that may need work—the area on the foot that should be massaged in order to restore health to the corresponding organ, bone, muscle, or tissue. Other indicators of blockages in the neural pathways (and possible problems in the corresponding body system) are calcium crystal deposits, which feel like grains of sand or salt under the skin. These deposits are massaged until they dissolve or separate.

Pointers for Self-Applied Reflexology

Here are some pointers on do-it-yourself reflexology:

1. Sit in a relaxing place and in a comfortable position on the floor or a bed.

2. With shoes and socks removed, apply a greaseless moisturizer to your feet.
3. Apply some powder and massage until your feet are no longer slippery.
4. Now hold your foot with one hand.
5. With your other hand, starting at the edge of your heel, press your thumb into the bottom of your foot near your heel. Apply pressure at a forty-five-degree angle.
6. Inch your thumb up your foot from the heel to the toe, like an inchworm, a little at a time. This is called thumbwalking.
7. To work the top of your foot, use your fingers in the same way. This is called fingerwalking.
8. Repeat twice.
9. Return to any tender areas and rework them by applying pressure.
10. Repeat on your other foot.

Specific Reflex Points for Headache

The whole-foot reflexology massage serves as a kind of reconnaissance tour for tender reflex points—these are your best guides. Here are some of the more common reflex points for headache:

- For tension-type and sinus headache: the four small toes, *top and bottom of toes*
- For migraine: the webbing between the big toe and the next toe, *top of foot*
- For eyestrain: at the base of your four small toes, in the crevice where the toes meet the ball of the foot, *bottom of foot*
- For neck muscles: the base of your big toe and the toe itself, *bottom of toe*

Treatment Schedule

Your treatment schedule with a reflexologist depends on the nature of your problem. For prevention and relaxation, reflexologists recommend weekly sessions. A more economical way to get preventive help is to heal yourself. Learn reflexology from one of the many books available (see "Resources"); reflexology seminars are often taught at health fairs and YMCAs. Write to the International Institute of Reflexology for a schedule (see page 382).

Effectiveness

Since the mechanism of reflexology is not completely understood, it has not been studied. However, massage therapists, reflexologists, and clients have reported cases of headache relief. Since reflexology is generally considered very safe, there is no harm in trying it for yourself.

Side Effects and Warnings

Reflexology is quite safe—and serves as a good proxy for massage when that method is contraindicated. Be sure to apply pressure only to the point of tenderness, not pain, to avoid damaging your foot.

Finding a Reliable Reflexologist

You should seek a reflexologist who is certified by a reputable organization, such as the International Institute of Reflexology (IIR), which requires two hundred hours of training and one year's practical experience. The IIR can refer you to a certified reflexologist and provide you with a schedule of seminars geared to laypeople for self-application of reflexology. Another organization, the Foot Reflexology Awareness Association, is a source for information and educational aids.

Many licensed massage therapists also practice reflexology and may not require as much training in order to bring effective skills to the practice. See the "Resources" section for information.

Questions and Answers

• *What are the benefits of reflexology over massage?*   Reflexology and massage are two completely different disciplines, but they can complement each other.

Reflexology is sometimes recommended by massage therapists for clients who, for health reasons, cannot receive massage (see "Warnings,'' page 157). It's also a good option for people who feel uncomfortable about taking their clothes off.

In general, both massage and reflexology are methods that provide relaxation and improved circulation. However, whereas the focus of work for the massage therapist is the musculature, reflexologists claim that they can address problems of specific body systems (organs, etc.) through reflex points in the feet, hands, or ears. In short, massage therapists work directly on the area of concern, while reflexologists work indirectly.

• *I'm very ticklish—will I be able to stand reflexology?* The feet are very sensitive because they are so richly endowed with nerve endings. You may feel ticklish at first, but a skilled reflexologist will apply firm, gliding pressure that will feel relaxing, not tickling.

• *Can I receive reflexology if I am pregnant?* Yes. However, avoid points that stimulate the uterus and pelvic area.

• *Is reflexology covered by health insurance?* It is not usually covered, but it's worth checking with your insurance carrier.

BODYWORK THERAPIES

The world of bodywork therapies is vast, and growing all the time. The term embraces a large category of treatments, most devised in the twentieth century, which can be broadly defined as treatments that involve a therapist who works with one's body. They can be divided into several smaller categories, as defined by the Office of Alternative Medicine of the National Institutes of Health. For example, many of the modalities discussed in the following pages can be considered postural-reeducation therapies. This technical-sounding term describes a group of methods that share a basic goal: to help the body relieve chronic tension and achieve freer movement through the teaching of exercises that bring greater awareness of inhibiting postures and movement habits.

The following bodywork therapies share the belief that structural misalignment is a common cause of muscle tension and of many resulting illnesses, such as headache. The body is engineered by nature to move freely against the constant opposing force of gravity. The skull, which weighs twelve to fifteen pounds, rests on the vertebrae, each of which weighs only a few ounces. The spine's curves, and the muscles and connective tissues in the body, work together to keep the body in balance. But balance is easily thrown off by a number of factors, including improper posture, physical trauma (such as breaking a leg), and chronic emotional tension. When this happens, the body compensates for the misalignment by employing muscles that do not need to be used. When this compensating misuse is chronic, the muscles, bones, and the connective tissues that surround them can become distorted, resulting in chronic tension and pain.

These therapies also all agree that emotional tension can produce physical tension and misalignment. Like his mentor Sigmund Freud, the psychiatrist Wilhelm Reich believed that people express and hold their emotions physically. Unlike Freud, who did not believe that the therapist should ever touch the patient, Reich felt that physical therapy was an important route to emotional well-being. His therapy combined psychoanalysis with physical manipulations to release the individual from his or her "armor block"—the physical expression of psychological tension. While not all of the structural-reeducation methods overtly delve into emotional issues, proponents do believe that the body's contortions may reflect the holding of emotional tensions.

Similarly they all hold that conscious awareness of habitual postural patterns plays a key role in relieving them. All of the approaches discussed in this section can be considered experiential; rather than the instructor demonstrating or simply telling you how to achieve ease of movement, you are encouraged to discover it for yourself. Conscious awareness of these patterns enhances your ability to change them.

As we have already discovered, headache is often the result of muscle tension. For example tightening of the upper-body muscles may be linked with migraine or tension-type headache. In migraine, tension of the occipital muscles (near the nape of the neck) contributes to blood-vessel spasm, resulting in auras, which in some people precede head pain. In chronic tension-type headache, tense muscles cause nerve irritation; the muscles become deprived of blood and oxygen, triggering the production of nerve-sensitizing hormones, such as prostaglandin, that contribute to pain. Therefore headache relief may be a secondary benefit of overall ease of movement.

Treatment of specific illness is not the primary goal of these methods; in fact most proponents would strongly assert that their method is not a therapy but an educational process. They make no specific therapeutic claims. For this reason there are rarely any formal clinical studies confirming the effectiveness of these methods in relieving headache. At the same time many of the experts we spoke with have observed relief of all types of chronic headache as a result of the body's general release of tension.

Many of the innovators of these methods were influenced by one another, although with each the result is unique. F. M. Alexander was one of the first to develop a formal method for realigning the body through gentle manipulations. His work was deeply rooted in the idea that the body's innate intelligence can be a powerful tool in changing long-held patterns—if informed of structural problems and new options for overcoming them. Alexander's work provided a springboard for Moshe Feldenkrais. Ida Rolf, the originator of Structural Integration (Rolfing), studied the Alexander Technique and communicated with Feldenkrais. Judith Aston and Joseph Heller were at one time avid followers of Ida Rolf, and have adapted Rolfing techniques as part of their methods. Milton Trager independently came upon many of the concepts that shaped the methods of Alexander and Feldenkrais.

This is not to say that these individuals were one another's sole influences. Ida Rolf, for example, was greatly influenced by yoga and osteopathy (which changed her life). In addition, each can be considered more than innovators of techniques. They were philosophers of human movement, exploring how the conscious mind and physical body are intimately linked.

These similarities notwithstanding, each of the methods is distinctly different in many ways. In the pages that follow we'll give you a taste for how they work, their philosophy of healthy movement, and in certain cases exercises that might help reduce stress to relieve headache.

Alexander Technique

The Alexander Technique is not a therapy; it is an educational process. The method is taught to pupils by instructors who are trained in anatomy and physiology as well as in specific ways to help pupils unlearn tension-producing ways of moving.

History

F. M. Alexander, a Shakespearean actor born in the mid 1800s, tended to lose his voice during performances. When conventional medicine failed to help him, he took on the task of curing himself. By watching himself recite in the mirror, Alexander came to a revelation: In preparing to recite he would unconsciously pull his head back, causing his throat to tighten and creating the need to gasp for air. Somewhere in his past he had come to believe that it was somehow *necessary* to tense his neck muscles in order to perform. In actuality, he realized, the tension was not only unnecessary, it was unnatural and therefore inhibiting to optimal ease of movement—and performance. It was also a very inefficient use of his muscles.

By adjusting the position of his head, Alexander found dramatic improvement in his ability to speak, and noticed his entire body opening up. Heightened awareness of these unconscious, habitual patterns is one philosophical goal of the Alexander Technique.

Another goal is to regain the natural balance that allows freedom of movement, the freedom we all innately experienced before these tension-causing habits took hold.

Over the next several years Alexander explored how these concepts might apply to the rest of the body. He focused his attention on the way the head, neck, and back were anatomically connected and how movements in these areas affected the rest of the body. With his brother, Alexander went on to develop specific lessons that aim to help students uncover habitual tension in all parts of their bodies and rediscover a more efficient, freer way of moving.

The Technique was embraced by many famous people of Alexander's time, including George Bernard Shaw and Aldous Huxley. Today its popularity continues to grow in the United States and Europe.

How It Helps Relieve Headache

Though proponents of the Alexander Technique do not proclaim therapeutic benefits, practitioners report success in relieving a variety of disorders, including headache, as a secondary benefit of the practice. Anecdotal reports of success in headache (it hasn't been formally studied) could be explained by the tension-relieving effects that Alexander-taught practices have on muscles in the neck, shoulder, and occipital area near the base of the skull.

Alexander instructors put much emphasis on regaining a natural balance of the skull on the vertebrae. Here's why. The skull, which weighs twelve to fifteen pounds, is anatomically designed to rest on the first vertebra of the spine, called the atlas. The occipital joint serves as a cushion between the skull and the atlas. The curves of the spine are designed to help keep the body upright and the head balanced comfortably at the top. From this it's obvious that the human structure is an example of exquisite engineering. But considering that the vertebrae weigh only a few ounces each, it's also apparent that this balancing act might be hard to maintain. In many people—due to physical trauma, chronic emotional responses to situations, or bad postural habits—the skull is thrown off balance, causing the muscles in the head, neck, shoulders, and sometimes the entire body to compensate with undue tension. The head, instead of lifting upward in a natural state of balance, gives in to gravity and must be supported by other muscles.

Alexander teachers call this response *compression,* and it results in extra muscle work, which interferes with blood flow, nerve transmission, and muscle tone. The Alexander Technique helps pupils become aware of stimuli that cause downward compression and how to restore one's natural balance periodically during the day.

The Alexander Technique does more than simply relax muscles; that can be achieved with drugs, but it will be only a stopgap measure unless the underlying structural problems are resolved. The goal of the Alexander method is to get to the root of muscle tension—but not by layering new movements over old habits. Instead Alexander believed that this can be achieved by "inhibiting" and "directing." The Alexander lessons teach pupils to become aware of their own individual tension-causing habits, then to "inhibit" that habitual action. The act of inhibiting, or not doing, opens up an opportunity for the body to choose a more efficient, easeful way of accomplishing the same action—which Alexander believed the body will move toward naturally. Gentle manipulations by the Alexander instructor help increase the pupil's awareness of patterns of tension, and help correct them by guiding the pupil toward experiencing movement in a more easeful way.

At the same time Alexander instructors stress that the real work is the responsibility of the pupil. Teaching people how to be responsible for themselves is the instructor's role. In essence Alexander work is a team approach to help individuals learn how to be responsible for their overall health.

Who Can Be Helped

All muscle-tension-related headaches may benefit from Alexander instruction. However, as Alexander trainers clearly state, the method is not intended as a therapy; it is a learning process that may help people with structure- and tension-related disorders. And because these unnecessary tensions put pressure on organs, joints, and the body's vasculature, a host of related problems may be relieved once you remove the tension.

What to Expect

The Alexander Technique is taught in a series of lessons. The subject of the first lesson is the head, neck, and spine—and its relationship to other parts of the body. The rest of the structural anatomy is addressed in subsequent lessons.

Lying down or sitting fully clothed on a massage table, you will be asked by the Alexander teacher to become aware of the table supporting your body. With gentle, guiding movements, he or she will call your attention to different parts of your body, such as the back of your neck. All along, your instructor will explain the structural relationships of the bones, muscles, and tendons.

You will be asked to consciously *inhibit* the tendency to help the instructor cradle your neck, or lift your arm. If this sounds like you're not doing *anything,* think again—indeed "thinking again" is part of the point. You may be surprised at how difficult it is to follow such simple-sounding instruction. To *not do,* to let gravity and the natural balance of your body do the work instead, is a primary Alexander lesson.

Through the guided experience of inhibiting, you will learn where you tend to hold tension. Through the guided direction of letting go, you will experience a new and more relaxed way of accomplishing the same movement, whether it be sitting up or walking across a room. Soon the simple act of lying on your back or standing up becomes a new experience. You will feel your body lengthening and opening; after working on your left arm, for example, you may notice that it has suddenly grown longer. An Alexander instructor can also help you with specific tasks that you regularly perform, such as sitting at a computer or lifting your baby.

At first these "new" movements might feel strange; even though you're actually using your muscles and bones more efficiently, the mere fact that it's a departure from your normal way of moving may make the movement feel unnatural. Breaking bad habits doesn't come easily. However, the Alexander practice is just that: practice. The real work comes when you leave your session; it's then incumbent on you to practice your newfound patterns of moving by being aware of how you move.

Lesson Schedule

Most instructors recommend at least weekly sessions, lasting about forty-five minutes each, until completion of the twenty- to thirty-session course—but the number of lessons varies from person to person. After learning the basics (the instruction doubles as a course in structural anatomy), people may return for refresher sessions, or miniseries, if they feel old tension-causing habits creeping back.

Side Effects and Warnings

The Alexander Technique is a very gentle method of releasing tension; there should be no side effects. If you have an underlying illness or acute pain, seek the advice of a health professional.

Finding a Reliable Alexander Technique Instructor

There are several hundred Alexander Technique teachers in the United States. The North American Society of Teachers of the Alexander Technique (NSTAT) provides certification, which requires sixteen hundred hours of training, most of which is hands-on work. NSTAT can refer you to a trained Alexander instructor. See the "Resources" section.

Questions and Answers

• *Does the Alexander Technique hurt?*   No. Since the focus of the Technique is release of tension, you should feel less pain, not more. The guided movements during sessions are very gentle, never abrupt. You may feel some *emotional* discomfort in practicing new, tension-free movements, or inhibiting your normal habits of movement, but they will not be physically painful.

• *Why does it take so many lessons to learn the Alexander Technique?*   An Alexander Technique instructor might explain it this way: We have spent a lifetime "learning" how to move with tension, which ultimately might have contributed to our headache. A lifetime habit is not easy to erase. It takes time and practice to learn the structure of your body, awareness of your unique patterns of holding tension in different situations, and to allow your body to return to a new "habit" of easeful balance. The more committed you are to the Technique and to applying it to your everyday life, the fewer lessons you will probably need.

• *How long does it take to perfect the Alexander Technique?*   Even F. M. Alexander, the originator of the Technique, never perfected it. As long as we are alive, we will be confronted with new tension-causing situations and, according to people who practice the Alexander Technique, the option for releasing that tension. The Technique is a practice in every sense of the word; practice in awareness of our emotional and physical responses to situations and practice in inhibiting our habitual responses to them.

Feldenkrais Method

Seemingly similar in many ways to the Alexander Technique, the Feldenkrais Method also asserts that recognizing habitual patterns of movement and thinking is the first step toward changing them. But the techniques differ in their approach and in the resulting sensations. Whereas the Alexander Technique focuses on helping students to experience an opening of the body, even this open-ended directive is absent from Feldenkrais teaching.

Where the Alexander Technique puts forth a standard for easeful movement, the Feldenkrais Method puts forth options for *learning;* the method centers on learning how to learn. The resulting sense of movement, according to Feldenkrais, is one that feels right for the individual. The movement may *feel* like an opening or lengthening, but more important to Feldenkrais is that one uses the information in a way that makes a difference in one's life.

History

A Russian-born Israeli physicist, Moshe Feldenkrais originally launched his exploration of movement as he attempted to heal his own knee injuries, and face the behaviors and thinking that produced the injuries.

As a trained scientist, he was thorough in his research, and finally arrived at a model that was inspired greatly by the works of F. M. Alexander (see page 212) and G. I. Gurdjieff, martial arts, hypnosis, and yoga. Alexander's concepts about awareness and inhibition of habitual movements were folded into Feldenkrais's theories.

In simple terms one of Feldenkrais's goals was to learn how to become more aware of habits so that he might use them as he wished, rather than being controlled by them. He maintained that when presented with a choice, the individual will naturally select the motion that is least stressful and most efficient.

Today the Feldenkrais Method is widely practiced in the United States, Canada, New Zealand, Australia, and Europe and is recommended by physicians and physical therapists.

How It Helps Relieve Headache

As with the Alexander Technique, the Feldenkrais Method makes no claims of cure; it's an educational system, communicated through instruction given by teachers to students. It aims to enhance the way individuals experience themselves in the world. As a by-product of an increased awareness, students should discover more harmonious ways of moving, learning to function with more freedom and less pain.

Feldenkrais believed that human beings are born with the possibility of learning all of the countless combinations of movement that make up the human repertoire. But over time we become habitual with our choices; for example we tighten our shoulders while sitting at the computer. The habitual pattern is engaged without thinking and can result in tension that remains constant even during sleep.

When the strain that caused tension is no longer present, people act as though it still is. What ends up happening is that we become accumulations of our adaptations.

For many people that tension results in headache. According to Feldenkrais, human beings are good at adapting but they often do not have the awareness needed to let go of the adaptation after it's no longer useful.

When movement becomes dysfunctional (painful), people naturally seek out ways to minimize it. They can thus readily learn new ways of moving, not by verbal instruction but by experience. And that begins with becoming aware of poor "self-use," as Feldenkrais would say. Headache, or any other kind of pain, is not something that happens to you; it is something integrated with the self, and something an individual can affect. Recognizing habitual patterns of movement and thinking that contribute to headache is the first step toward changing them.

Moshe Feldenkrais maintained that the Feldenkrais Method helps make the impossible possible—and the possible easy. And it makes the easy simple and elegant to do, as well as aesthetically pleasing.

Who Can Be Helped

People with a wide variety of muscle-tension-related headaches may be helped by the Feldenkrais Method.

The benefits of Feldenkrais Method, like many postural-reeducation methods, come as a result of increased awareness and functioning of the entire body. Feldenkrais described this effect as "generalization." When one starts exploring new options for moving, the action takes place on many levels. Feldenkrais therefore does not treat headaches, but helps people realize their desired goals.

What to Expect

There are two ways of learning the Feldenkrais Method: *Awareness Through Movement* (ATM) or *Functional Integration.*

At the core of the practice is Awareness Through Movement, a group approach consisting of hundreds of movement lessons that address the relationship between the mind-body and the environment. The movements can be minutely small, or they can be large gestures that winnow down to small movements, or quick movements becoming increasingly slower, or slow movements becoming quicker. One aim of ATM is to enhance one's awareness of the effects of the movement, and the brain's response to the movement. Does it feel comfortable? Is it unnatural? Why? Does it present a new option for a habitual, dysfunctional movement? Many of the exercises intentionally evoke responses that are not habitual but that may therefore feel uncomfortable; they aim to wake the brain up to new possibilities for the movement it directs.

Functional Integration is the private-lesson form of the Feldenkrais Method. You will lie on a low, padded table while the instructor guides you through different movements. "It's a nonverbal communication between two nervous systems," says Allison Rapp, a Feldenkrais instructor in Alexandria, Virginia. "Together we establish a communication that helps the student enlarge areas of ability until the entire self becomes encorporated in a more harmonious way." Because private lessons are more customized, there is more opportunity to work on problem areas.

Lesson Schedule

The ATM lessons last between forty-five minutes and an hour. They are taught in weekly classes and extended weekend workshops. Functional Integration lessons are also about forty-five minutes long, but the goal is to complete a lesson rather than fill an amount of time. The number of classes is flexible. Feldenkrais recommended that you use your age as a basic guide; if you're thirty years old, take thirty lessons. Add more if you have a specific physical challenge you want to overcome, such as chronic pain.

Side Effects and Warnings

While you should alert your instructor of any illness or limitations, there are no side effects as we generally think of them; the movements are very simple and shouldn't cause injury. The student is always in control of his movements and is encouraged to stop whenever he needs to rest.

Finding a Reliable Feldenkrais Practitioner

Practitioners are certified by the Feldenkrais Guild, a membership organization that establishes standards of practice, sets policy for and certifies training programs, and distributes information to the public. To become certified as a practitioner, one must have successfully completed eight hundred hours of training over thirty-eight months. To maintain their certification status, one must attend twenty hours of advanced training per year. There about 750 certified Feldenkrais practitioners throughout the United States and Canada. To locate one in your area, see the "Resources" section.

Questions and Answers

• *Does the Feldenkrais Method hurt?*   It should never cause pain. The exercises are not designed to strain or even tone muscles; generally they are very gentle and easy to do. However, each individual has different limitations. Be sure to let your instructor know of any physical problems.

• *How do I know if I'm doing it right?*   There is no right or wrong way to do the lesson. Each individual learns how to establish his or her own standards. A person with multiple sclerosis, for example, has physical abilities that are different from those of a person who does not have MS. The only real requirement for participation is the desire to become more in touch with yourself, your abilities, your habits, and the ways in which you stop yourself from living as you wish.

- *Can children learn the Feldenkrais Method?* Many practitioners work with children. Debby Ashton and Stephen Rosenholz have developed programs for children; some of these are available in the form of books, videotapes, and audiotapes, while others are aimed at classroom use.

Rolfing

Rolfing, also known as Structural Integration, is one of several modern bodywork methods that were developed based on the concept that structure determines function—and many painful conditions are the result of the body's structural imbalance. When the imbalance becomes chronic, the connective tissues (fascia) become rigid, which thus inhibits movement and potentially causes muscle tension, which in turn causes an imbalance in the functioning of the rest of the body. (It might be helpful to review Chapter 2, page 47, about the role of connective tissue in the body.)

History

Like many other bodywork innovators of the nineteenth and twentieth centuries, Ida Rolf's own injury initiated her journey into self-healing methods. After an injury, an osteopathic physician adjusted her spine, resulting in an immediate return of normal breathing and reduction of fever. The success of this treatment convinced her of an osteopathic tenet: Body structure determines body function.

Over the next several decades Rolf went on to develop her own methods for establishing proper alignment and health. In 1972 she established the Rolf Institute, and established standards for Rolfing.

Ida Rolf's method was influenced by physical therapy, osteopathic medicine, yoga, and contemporary bodywork originators such as Moshe Feldenkrais. But unlike Feldenkrais, who developed a method of gradual progression toward alignment, Rolf felt that there needed to be a more direct action to achieve major changes.

Rolf believed that the body has an intrinsic order that organizes the body parts to function optimally. When factors disorganize the body, such as tightening or shortening of the fascia, the body does not function in its natural, orderly way.

She also believed that deep manipulation of the fascia—the connective tissue that envelops bones, muscles, and other body tissues—was necessary in order to restore its original flexibility and order. Once the fascia are stretched, the body becomes free to align itself. Rolfers describe this process as one that "organizes" and balances the whole person. The purpose of Rolfing is to "soften the old inhibited order and introduce the client to another order which benefits posture and movement."

How It Helps Relieve Headache

Any local injury or focal point for stress will not only affect the fascia in that area but will have a rippling effect over the entire body. Following this reasoning, chronic tension in the lower back, for example, can result in tightness of the fascia in the upper neck and head; it may cause headache if the rigidity is great enough to cause muscle contraction, vasospasm, and nerve irritation.

What to Expect

As writer Ann Lewis aptly put it in her article on bodywork for *Outside* magazine (March 1994), "Where massage therapists rub, Rolfers sculpt." You will lie down semiclothed on a table and, using fingers and palms, the Rolfer will focus over the course of ten sessions, on the areas that need to be opened and lengthened. The first session will often begin with a deep-tissue massage of the rib cage, which, in addition to addressing the structural problems in that area, will help enhance your breathing. This will serve to help you work through any discomfort in later sessions. Over time the practitioner will systematically move over the body, section by section, until the fascia covering the entire body have been stretched and mobilized.

Rolfing is famous for being a painful process, both physically and emotionally. The physical pain varies, depending on the individual's threshold and the area being massaged. Rosemary Feitis, D.O., an osteopathic physician in New York City who practices Structural Integration, and editor of the book *Ida Rolf Talks About Rolfing and Physical Reality,* describes the pain in two ways: "The pain emerges because the tissue is changing," she explains. "For most people, it's like the Jane Fonda 'burn'—it's a pain that hurts 'good.' Another dimension of the pain is emotional, which is nonetheless very real." Indeed the deep-tissue work of Rolfing taps into the Reichian concept of body armoring: the emotional memories that become lodged in the body.

Others assert that the pain of Rolfing serves a therapeutic purpose. In his book *Planet Medicine* (North Atlantic Books, 1995), Richard Grossinger says, "As in Zen, the pain serves as a reference point for remembering, a way to learn how to inhabit new postures."

Its utility as a mnemonic device notwithstanding, pain is *not* a requisite for successful Rolfing according to Rolfers. Some clients may not experience pain and still be successfully Rolfed. They also mention that the pain is not long-lasting, but rather immediately gives way to a pleasurable sensation of free movement.

Over the ten sessions your Rolfer will photograph you, in order to document your progress.

Rolfing Movement Integration

Based on the concepts developed by Rolf, Rolfing Movement focuses on learning to move harmoniously with gravity, enhancing the opportunity to move without tension or armoring.

In a series of sessions you and your teacher will explore your movement patterns, paying particular attention to habitual movements such as walking and sitting; or occupation- and recreation-related movements, such as desk work, housework, and sports activities. As with Structural Integration, each section of the body is reviewed for holding patterns. Gentle movement exercises are developed to ease pain and stress.

Movement Integration can be practiced alone, or along with Structural Integration. A series of eight sessions is usually recommended, though the number is flexible.

Who Can Be Helped

People with muscle-related tension, especially those with noted structural misalignments, may find that Rolfing helps reduce headaches.

Treatment Schedule

Rolfing is a system that works with the entire body. There are ten standard sessions, each dedicated to a specific area of the body. These sessions can occur at your own pace: once a week, once a month, or whatever; they last an hour each.

Effectiveness

Like the Alexander Technique and Feldenkrais Method, Rolfing does not claim clinical benefits; it is an educational process designed to help its clients gain a better understanding of postures that inhibit their movement and to provide ways of experiencing more freedom. However, some studies have shown Rolfing to be effective in a number of areas, including improvement of muscle tone, psychological function, and stress symptoms. One study confirms the effectiveness of Rolfing in reducing anxiety.[8] Specific studies of people with headache have not been conducted, but anecdotal reports have shown that Rolfing can benefit people with headaches.

Side Effects and Warnings

Rolfing can be uncomfortable. As mentioned on page 223, some people experience no pain, while others find the pain almost intolerable. The first session, which focuses on the chest area and breathing, is designed to help clients work through such pain. Rolfing instructors generally encourage clients to bear the pain as much as possible, but will definitely respond to your wishes to ease up or move to another area. They will also help you find ways of dealing with the pain as it comes up.

Finding a Reliable Rolfer

The Rolf Institute provides a degree training program that requires twenty-eight weeks of class work. There are also three other schools based on Rolf's work. Licensing requirements vary from state to state. (See the "Resources" section.)

Questions and Answers

• *Why does Rolfing hurt?*   The technique used to stretch the fascia is akin to ironing out a wrinkled piece of stiff fabric. Once restored to its original, unwrinkled condition, the fabric becomes more flexible and better fits the wearer. The tissue changes that occur during manipulation of the fascia—the deep connective tissue that envelops muscles, bones, and other internal tissues—are often experienced as pain. The pain varies from individual to individual, and some people never experience it.

• *Should I tell the Rolfer that I'm in pain?*   Definitely. Acknowledging and expressing feelings are integral to the treatment, and essential to helping the Rolfer find a way to minimize discomfort.

• *What will the Rolfer do if I feel the pain is too great?*   Generally Rolfers will try to help you work through the pain, either by focusing your breathing or encouraging you to express it. If the pain is too great, certainly the Rolfer will respect your wishes to stop working on a specific area.

• *Is Rolfing covered by medical insurance?*   If it is performed or recommended by a physician (M.D. or D.O.), Rolfing may be covered; ask your insurance carrier.

Aston-Patterning

Aston-Patterning is a bodywork technique based on the premise that each individual's body is unique and asymmetrical; release of one's patterns of tension and stress—the "holding patterns," to use a term popular among bodywork practitioners—entails working *with* the individual's unique structure in order to achieve balance and freedom of movement rather than trying to change that structure to meet an ideal standard.

History

Judith Aston's interest in movement began in childhood, continued through college, and became translated into a career afterward, when she taught dance to athletes. After suffering two severe automobile accidents, Ms. Aston sought care from Ida Rolf (see page 221), where she found significant relief. She trained with Rolf, and developed movement exercises to accompany the massage of connective tissues that characterize Rolfing. Joseph Heller, also a protégé of Ida Rolf, assimilated some of Ms. Aston's movements into his technique (see page 230).

Over time Ms. Aston's views diverged from those of Rolf. She came to believe that there was no ideal standard for body structure, that bodies are asymmetrical and should not be manipulated to become symmetrical. Instead Aston asserts that easeful movement emerges not by making the body more symmetrical but by respecting an individual's asymmetry and, within that context, allowing it to move as it needs to. In addition she felt that Rolfing was unduly painful. Like Ida Rolf, Ms. Aston believes that distortions of the fascia result from emotional and physical tension, and that release of these tensions can be accomplished by making the fascia more pliable. However, unlike Rolf, Ms. Aston feels that this can be accomplished without pain.

In 1977 Judith Aston formed her own organization. Aston-Patterning, as her technique is called, integrates several types of bodywork (massage techniques) with Movement Education; it also includes customized fitness programs. Ms. Aston has developed specific methods for addressing the special needs of people of all ages, from infants to people of advancing age. Today aspects of Aston-Patterning have been adopted by many physical therapists, biofeedback therapists, and other health professionals to complement their primary work.

How It Helps Relieve Headache

Aston-Patterning works according to the same principles of stretching the fascia as Rolfing (see page 221).

Who Can Be Helped

In theory, people with all types of nonthreatening headache can benefit from an education in Aston-Patterning. However, clinical studies have not been conducted.

What to Expect

Each session of the basic Aston-Patterning technique entails several steps: In the first session your practitioner will ask you many questions relating to your medical history, with a focus on events or practices that have affected your body. You'll be asked about your job, recreational activities, parts of your body that are in pain, accidents, trauma to the body, and so on. In subsequent sessions you will be asked to report any updates.

To get a sense of how you move while engaging in normal activities, you will be asked to perform simple movements (such as sitting and walking), during which the practitioner will call your attention to your body's patterns. At this time your practitioner will chart the sources or areas of tension in your body for future reference, and as a guide for areas that need work. In some cases the entire session will be videotaped.

The core of the session involves bodywork and movement education. Several concepts guide Aston-Patterning bodywork. First, muscle tissue naturally follows a spiral pattern. Second, the integrity of muscle tissue should always be honored—tissue should never be compressed by force. Instead body tissue should be gently stretched and manipulated following and restoring its natural direction, an approach Aston called matching, or spiraling. In these ways Aston-Patterning practitioners uphold Aston's primary goal of honoring the body's integrity.

There are three bodywork techniques, one or more of which may be employed for you:

• *Massage:* Since Aston believed that the body's tissues follow a pattern of spirals, the double-handed massage traces the direction of the tissue. Massage is generally used as a tension-releasing method, working on large areas of tension, or as a calming technique after deep-tissue bodywork.

• *Myo-kinetics:* A firm, pressing movement with the fingertips is used to work on very small areas of tense muscles; though firmer than the massage technique, it is still gentle. Aston believed in stretching, rather than compressing, the deep tissue. The deep connective tissue of muscles is reached not by penetrating the superficial layers (as is done with Rolfing and Hellerwork) but by gently manipulating the superficial tissue to gain access to the deep connective tissue.

• *Arthro-kinetics:* Addresses joints and soft tissue that has hardened. A specialized technique that requires specific training, not all Aston-Patterning practitioners are trained in arthro-kinetics. Often preceded by myo-kinetics to loosen the surrounding muscles, arthro-kinetics involves mobilizing the joints in spiral patterns.

Aston Movement Education is a part of all Aston-Patterning sessions. Once the muscles and joints are open, movement exercises are performed; these movements are customized to the specific needs of the client based on his or her own movement patterns, "holding patterns," occupation, and so forth. The main lesson in each session is to call one's attention to the shifting of weight during movement and its relationship with gravity.

In addition to movement education, clients receive an education in how to make their environment more compatible with their body, for example evaluating and changing the ergonomics of their workspace.

As with many bodywork and movement techniques, especially those that reach deep tissue, Aston-Patterning may evoke emotions that have become ingrained, and possibly helped shape, muscle tensions and movement patterns. While Aston-Patterning practitioners are sensitive to emotional responses, and expect them, they are not trained to help you cope with them in a psychotherapeutic way.

Treatment Schedule

The initial session lasts two hours, with subsequent sessions going from two and a half to three hours each. Eight to twelve sessions are generally needed before clients learn how apply what they have learned to their life.

Effectiveness

As mentioned, Aston-Patterning is an educational process, not a therapy. However, there have been reports of headache relief from people who practice Aston-Patterning, though these claims have not been substantiated by clinical study.

Side Effects and Warnings

Some people experience soreness after Aston-Patterning sessions, particularly with the arthro-kinetics bodywork. In addition your newly learned ways of moving might at first feel uncomfortable; although they may be more attuned to your individual body structure, their newness may initially produce a sense of awkwardness.

Finding a Reliable Aston-Patterning Practitioner

Certification requirements for Aston-Patterning involve at least eighteen weeks of coursework, including annual continuing-education courses. See "Resources."

Questions and Answers

• *How does Aston-Patterning differ from Rolfing?*   Proponents of both methods believe that the body's deep connective tissue thickens and becomes rigid when chronically stressed (either emotionally or physically) or when subject to physical trauma. They also concur that distortion of the fascia can have negative effects on the body's ability to function in a healthy, integrated way. And they agree that restoring the suppleness and moistness of the fascia helps release pressure on muscles, blood vessels, and other body tissues—and helps restore freedom of movement and health. But this is where the similarities fundamentally end. Whereas Rolfers believe that the goal of treatment is to achieve an ideal standard of symmetry for body structure, Aston-Patterning practitioners assert that the body is naturally asymmetrical and that the integrity of the body's unique structure should be honored. Thus excessive force should not be used to manipulate the fascia; this would violate the structure of the muscles. As a result Aston-Patterning bodywork techniques are not known to cause discomfort.

• *Can children benefit from Aston-Patterning?*   Yes. Judith Aston has developed specific methods for addressing the unique needs of infants and children.

• *Why might I have an emotional response to Aston-Patterning, and how will the practitioner handle it?*   Ida Rolf, Judith Aston, and many other modern bodywork innovators were strongly influenced by the work of the psychiatrist Wilhelm Reich, who asserted that many of the tensions we hold in our bodies have an emotional source. This effect is known as armoring. In essence the body holds memories of emotional stress that in some cases the conscious mind has "forgotten." Rolfers and practitioners of Aston-Patterning believe that this emotional tension is manifested in distortion of the fascia. Manipulation of the fascia dislodges these memories and brings them to consciousness.

If you experience an emotional response to Aston-Patterning bodywork, your practitioner is trained to allow you to experience and listen to it. If the emotional response is very troubling to you, he or she will respect your wishes to stop working on that area. However, practitioners are not trained to help you work through the emotions in any psychotherapeutic way—and may suggest that you seek the help of a trained counselor.

Hellerwork

Hellerwork comprises a series of one-and-a-half-hour sessions of deep-tissue bodywork, movement education, and verbal dialogue that aims to realign the body in order to release chronic tension and stress. Like other bodywork methods, it is not a remedy for a specific illness but a way of helping the body gain overall balance and health.

History
Born in wartime Poland, Joseph Heller (no relation to the novelist) immigrated to the United States in his midteens and ultimately pursued a career as an aerospace engineer. Under the guidance of Ida Rolf, the originator of Structural Integration, also known as Rolfing, Heller became trained in the technique of manipulating the fas-

cia (see page 221). Later he studied with Judith Aston, also a protégée of Rolf, and became trained in Aston-Patterning—a movement discipline that helps individuals to "reclaim" their unique, and often asymmetrical, way of moving with ease (see "Aston-Patterning," page 225, and "Rolfing" page 221).

The synthesis of these two strong influences resulted in Hellerwork in the 1970s.

Who Can Be Helped

Anyone with headaches related to muscular (or connective-tissue) tension may benefit from Hellerwork.

What to Expect

There are three related components of Hellerwork, all of which aim to align the body, release it of rigidity and tension, and increase awareness of the physical and emotional patterns that contribute to the imbalance and, possibly, headache:

• *Deep connective-tissue bodywork:* Virtually identical to Rolfing, this hands-on massage works to release tension in the fascia and stretch it back to its normal position.

• *Movement education:* To prevent the body from returning to a state of misalignment, movement education seeks to enhance your awareness of your body-use patterns and help you explore easier ways of moving. Video feedback is used to show how you move; visualizations are used to help find easier movement patterns.

• *Verbal dialogue:* A focus is placed on helping you become aware of how your emotions and attitudes shape your movement patterns.

To benefit fully from Hellerwork, be prepared to explore the sources of your physical and emotional tension—which can be painful. The bodywork involves massage of deep connective tissue. Some people experience no discomfort, whereas others experience pain in certain areas. However, Hellerwork strongly encourages a dialogue between the practitioner and the client. The practitioner is trained to be sensitive to the client's concerns, and responsive to needs for less pressure.

Practitioners are trained to be encouraging their clients' emotional expressions. The relationship you develop with your practitioner will be close, though the focus is on the client, not the practitioner.

Treatment Schedule

Hellerwork is structured in eleven sections, each of which has a theme, which relates to and links the bodywork, movement education, and verbal dialogue that comprise each section. Two thirds of the hour-and-a-half session is devoted to bodywork (connective-tissue massage).

Section 1: Inspiration
- Bodywork: muscles near the surface of the body
- Movement: breathing
- Verbal dialogue: what inspires you?

Section 2: Standing on your own two feet
- Bodywork: muscles and connective tissue of the legs and feet
- Movement: walking
- Verbal dialogue: security, self-support

Section 3: Reaching out
- Bodywork: arms, hands, and torso
- Movement: breathing, arm relaxation
- Verbal dialogue: giving, receiving, asserting yourself, anger

Section 4: Control and surrender
- Bodywork: inside of legs, pelvic floor
- Movement: relaxing the pelvic "core"
- Verbal dialogue: sensitivity to feedback, creativity, flexibility, trust

Section 5: The guts
- Bodywork: front of the core, deep muscles of the pelvis
- Movement: relaxing pelvis and abdominal area
- Verbal dialogue: relationship with food, intuition, courage, and strength

Section 6: Holding back
- Bodywork: spine and back muscles
- Movement: flexibility in the spine
- Verbal dialogue: self-expression and power

Section 7: Losing your head
- Bodywork: facial muscles, alignment of head, and release of tension in head, face, and neck
- Movement: releasing the head from tension
- Verbal dialogue: balance of reason and feeling

Section 8: The feminine
- Bodywork: lower half of the body
- Movement: walking from the core of your body, the pelvis
- Verbal dialogue: receptivity, attraction, complementing the masculine

Section 9: The masculine
- Bodywork: Upper half of body
- Movement: upper-body movement
- Verbal dialogue: initiation, insight, action

Section 10: Integration
- Bodywork: overall integrity of body through joints
- Movement: moving body as an entire, integrated whole
- Verbal dialogue: being in touch with self, sense of completeness

Section 11: Coming out
- Review of the sessions and how to apply them to daily life
- Feedback to the practitioner

Side Effects and Warnings

There are no known side effects of Hellerwork. However, as mentioned, the bodywork (like Rolfing) and verbal dialogue can uncover painful areas, both physical and emotional. But Hellerwork practitioners quickly point out that the client is in control; if you want the practitioner to stop or slow down, simply say so.

Finding a Reliable Hellerwork Practitioner

Look for someone who is certified in Hellerwork, which entails more than twelve hundred hours of coursework in addition to continuing education. See "Resources" section.

Questions and Answers

• *Does Hellerwork hurt?*   Since it involves deep massage of connective tissues, Hellerwork may be painful. It's important to let your practitioner know if you experience pain. This dialogue is encouraged with Hellerwork. However, the work is not dangerous and, like deep stretching or massage, the pain can be lessened by asking the practitioner to work more slowly on areas of discomfort, or by your breathing deeply into it—or stopping entirely.

• *Why is it important to explore emotions with Hellerwork?*   Like many bodywork innovators who were influenced by the psychiatrist Wilhelm Reich, Joseph Heller believed that emotions help shape the body; the body may hold and express emotional stress as rigidity in the fascia, which can distort muscles and cause physical imbalance. The process of Hellerwork bodywork massage of the fascia may bring out deeply lodged emotions; the themes of the sections explore emotions as well. By uncovering emotions, Hellerwork helps the client to explore those that cause tension and offers ways to help release them. The bodywork, movement education, and verbal dialogue work synergistically toward this end.

• *What if I don't like my practitioner?*   Liking your practitioner is not as important as trusting him or her. You must trust your Hellerwork practitioner enough to freely express emotions and feelings of discomfort. If you don't, you should find another practitioner. Your experience during the first session will inform you whether you want to continue with the full eleven-session course.

Brief Review of Other Bodywork Approaches

Polarity Therapy

Born in Austria, Randolph Stone moved to the United States, where he obtained training as a chiropractor, osteopath, and naturopath. He studied in the Far East and was influenced by Ayurveda. Out of his travels and research, Stone came to believe that life is energy in motion. In the body the energy circulates in five currents, moving down the right side of the body and up the left side. The bodywork that Polarity Therapists perform is designed to free the flow of blocked energy, conceptually in much the same way as traditional Oriental therapies. The mapping system for energy is guided by the five chakras (of Ayurvedic medicine and yoga), each of which holds sway over different energy categories. Instead of applying needles, pressure, or heat, however, the Polarity Therapist tugs and pulls at different points of the body. In this way, by unblocking body energy, Polarity adherents claim to balance the body and relieve pain. Other methods employed to release and balance energy include exercise and diet therapy. See ''Resources'' section.

Trager Psychophysical Integration and Mentastics

Developed by Hawaiian physician Milton Trager, the Trager Psychophysical Integration is a hands-on process whereby a practitioner uses shaking, rocking, and other rhythmic movements to loosen joints and muscles, ease movement, and release chronic tension in clients. The mind, remembering the sensation of this ''softening'' of tensed-up muscles and joints, will return to the state of relaxation when needed. The goal is to interrupt deep-seated emotional and physical patterns. The process includes a meditative state that is designed to enhance the newfound experience of free, pleasurable movement that results from interrupting the habitual patterns. Another aspect of Trager's method is *Mentastics,* a system of physical movements designed to enhance the results of Psychophysical Integration.

There are more than eight hundred Trager practitioners worldwide. See ''Resources'' section.

PhysicalMind Therapy

PhysicalMind Therapy is a method based on Pilates—a mind-body exercise program developed by Joseph Pilates. Pilates is a system of physical exercise that strengthens muscles and realigns the body. Many of the exercises are done flat on the back and usually entail repetitive movements. Some are performed using machinery, others with weights, some without any props at all. The exercises are typically customized to meet individual needs.

Like Rolfing, Hellerwork, and Aston-Patterning, PhysicalMind Therapy aims to alter the body's dysfunctional holding patterns by releasing the fascia. However, unlike these methods, PhysicalMind employs very slow, deliberate, mind-directed movements and breathing in order to accomplish that same goal. The belief is that the mind and the body are vitally related. Even people who have no range of movement can generate healing effects through imagery, according to Michelle Larson, cofounder of the PhysicalMind Institute in Santa Fe, New Mexico. For example one of the exercises for improving alignment entails coordinating breath with the lifting of the vertebrae, one at a time, from spine to skull. Once you reach the skull, imagine a circle floating above your head and trace the circle with your nose. This exercise, says Ms. Larson, serves to realign the vertebrae. "And it can be adapted to the needs of people with limited, or no, range of movement," she says. "For example people with migraine who do not want to move at all can perform the exercise through imagery until they regain enough confidence and ability in their movement to perform it physically." The effectiveness of PhysicalMind Therapy, according to proponents, is rooted in the mind—as a result, mind exercises help imprint new patterns of movement in the nervous system that eventually become translated into actual movement.

There are currently more than seven hundred PhysicalMind Therapists around the world (see the "Resources" section).

JOINT AND BONE MANIPULATION

If the body were a tree, the nervous system would be the root. Without a healthy spine—the nervous system's main artery—you cannot have a healthy body. This is the belief shared by proponents of chiropractic, osteopathic medicine, craniosacral therapy and applied kinesiology. The route to identifying and correcting an unhealthy spine—that is, one plagued by misalignments—differs from one discipline to the other.

Osteopathic Medicine

Osteopathic medicine parallels conventional medicine in many ways. Osteopathic physicians (titled Doctor of Osteopathy, or D.O.) must go through four years of medical training. They can go on to practice a specialty, such as cardiology or obstetrics. They must pass comparable state licensing examinations. Board-certified D.O.'s are found in accredited and licensed hospitals in the United States. Like M.D.'s, D.O.'s can prescribe medicine and perform surgery.

Philosophically, however, most osteopathic physicians take a more holistic approach to medicine, and put more emphasis on prevention and treatment of the underlying cause of disease than on symptom management.

Looking at the roots of the word—*osteopathic* refers to a disease process (*patho*) that derives from the bones (*osteo*)—one can see why D.O.'s focus special attention on the bone and muscle systems of the body, which make up about 60 percent of the body's mass. A routine part of the osteopathic medical examination is an evaluation of the bone and muscle systems. Many D.O.'s practice *manual methods,* also known as *osteopathic medical manipulations* (OMMs) in selected situations. In addition you are more apt to find osteopathic physicians with training in other holistic medical disciplines, such as homeopathy.

History

Andrew Taylor Still, M.D., founded the first medical school for osteopathy in Missouri in 1874. Frustrated with the limitations of the surgical techniques and drugs he was taught to use, and the failure of these methods to save members of his own family, he founded a philosophy of medicine that harkened back to the Hippocratic concept of the body as an integrated unit: Illness in one part of the body will affect other parts as well—and the musculoskeletal system, he felt, was a key to good health. In addition he strongly believed in the body's ability to heal itself, and stressed the importance of preventive health habits.

Today osteopathic medicine represents a synthesis of Dr. Still's experience: full medical-care knowledge and skills (prescription medications and surgery), emphasis on manipulation of the musculoskeletal system, holistic/self-healing modalities, and disease prevention. Americans make 100 million visits to D.O.'s each year. Today, according to the American Osteopathic Association, there are osteopathic physicians in each of the fifty states, numbering approximately thirty thousand.

How It Works

As mentioned, osteopathic physicians receive a classic medical education and are licensed to prescribe medicine and perform surgery in all states. One of the distinctions between D.O.'s and mainstream M.D.'s is the emphasis on structural manipulation—called *osteopathic manual manipulations* (OMMs), or manual therapy. While all osteopathic physicians are trained in manual therapy, not all of them use it. An estimated 60 percent of osteopathic physicians use OMMs for selected situations, and only about 5 percent use it routinely. Approximately five hundred D.O.'s nationwide have received special certification in manual therapy, requiring five hundred hours of extra training.

The OMMs emerge from the principal that the body's structure and its function are interdependent. When the musculoskeletal system undergoes negative change, other body systems will suffer as well. There are several manual methods that osteopathic physicians use:

• *Hands-on contact.*   D.O.'s believe that touch is central to healing; the contact of the physician's hands on the body initiates the treatment process.

• *Soft-tissue technique.*   Rhythmic stroking and pressing of the muscles surrounding the spine are designed to move excess fluid and to relax muscles.

• *Myofascial release.*   This technique aims to treat the myofascial (fibrous) muscle structures—the muscles and the surrounding fascia. There are two types of myofascial release: direct and indirect. With direct myofascial release, the tissues are restricted with constant force until movement returns. With indirect myofascial release the tissues are guided toward free movement on the path of least resistance.

• *Cranial osteopathy.*   This is a specific discipline within osteopathy (see page 240). The belief is that the structure and fluid surrounding the brain can be manipulated to initiate a self-healing effect throughout the body. It involves pressure and massage of the muscles and fascia surrounding the skull.

• *Lymphatic technique.*   There are several ways with which osteopaths help promote circulation of lymphatic fluids. In one the D.O. will apply pressure to the chest wall, forcing the patient to exhale as much air as possible, then rapidly release the pressure.

• *Thrust technique.*   Fast, light thrusts on specific dysfunctional joints are used in this technique in an effort to help the joint "reset" its reflexes.

• *Muscle energy technique.*   The D.O. applies pressure to a muscle in a specific direction while the patient resists.

• *Counterstrain.*   Suppose a patient has a frozen shoulder. With counterstrain the D.O. will slowly guide the shoulder out of the restrained position to the area of greatest comfort.

• *Visceral.*   This is a type of fascial release of viscera—fascia release and craniosacral work—to rest of body.

There are several ways the muscles and bones can affect organic function, according to osteopathic physicians. Since the nervous system helps keep the circulatory system moving, any impairment in the spine (which supports the main line of the nervous system) can influence the ability of blood vessels to do their work. Muscle spasms, for example, will cut off blood circulation to surrounding areas. In one recent study, scanning of muscles using MRI (magnetic resonance imaging) showed that muscles in spasm have reduced blood flow and that manual therapy helped restore it.

Chronic muscle spasm will also cause the nerve muscles to transmit continuous signals to the spine, resulting in an overload of messages in the spinal cord; the cross-circuiting of messages could result in problems in other parts of the body, according to some osteopathic researchers. Manual therapies are designed to restore the soft and hard tissues of the body to normal structure and improve blood flow and the flow of cerebrospinal fluid.

Cranial Osteopathy

Janet Xenos, an osteopathic physician in Santa Ana, California, who teaches cranial osteopathy at the College of Osteopathic Medicine of the Pacific, explains that there are five ways that cranial therapy can help headache: By (1) increasing the mobility of the bones in and near the head and (2) increasing the mobility and motility of the strutwork within the cranium, manual therapy helps to (3) take pressure off the nerves of the skull, (4) improve blood flow, and (5) improve the flow of cerebrospinal fluid inside the head.

Who Can Be Helped

Since osteopathic-medicine training parallels conventional medical education, D.O.'s can address the same scope of problems handled by M.D.'s. Manual methods can be used to treat and help prevent all types of nonthreatening headaches, according to Janet Xenos, D.O. "Even people in the midst of a severe migraine attack can be helped with manual therapy," she says. "The body is an integrated unit, connected by a fabric of fascia throughout. Since the head will probably be extremely sensitive, I would start working on other areas of the body to help relieve related stresses in the connective tissue and, once the pain is reduced, work directly on the head."

What to Expect

If you're used to seeing a conventional M.D., your visit to an osteopathic physician is likely to look and feel familiar. After taking a medical history and ruling out threatening causes of headache, osteopathic physicians who specialize in manual methods and cranial osteopathy will start with manipulations. In the case of headache, twenty minutes of the half-hour manipulation will be devoted to cranial work. However, most specialists in cranial osteopathy will do some work on the rest of the body as well—based on the belief that the organs and bones of the body are unified by a three-dimensional "stocking" of connective tissue. If the connective tissue or muscle becomes rigid in the head area, causing headaches, there is likely to be a reciprocal pull of connective tissue—possibly the underlying cause of the headache—in other parts of the body. D.O.'s who specialize in manual therapy and cranial manipulations will use any number of manual methods that are appropriate for the individual.

What does a cranial manipulation feel like? Patients report that cranial manipulations feel like a gentle pressure, a pushing and pulling, on various regions of the head. Some of the intra-oral methods—working from inside the mouth to manipulate the bones inside the skull—can be somewhat painful.

Treatment Schedule for Manual Method

The treatment schedule will be heavier at the beginning and then taper off. Generally practitioners will start patients with once-weekly treatments for three to five sessions. This may yield significant improvement in about 50 percent of patients. Then the frequency will be reduced to every two weeks, then every three weeks. Patients can then return as needed for preventive "tune-ups," or if they start having more frequent headaches, or if they have an injury.

Effectiveness

Studies on the effects of OMM in general are scarce. And studies on the effectiveness of OMM in the treatment of headache are even less common. Like many other mainstream and holistic medical groups, the American Osteopathic Association is stepping up research efforts in order to continue justifying their procedures to health insurance carriers. In years to come, says the AOA, the medical and lay communities can expect to see more hard data about the efficacy of osteopathic practices.

Variations on Osteopathic Medicine

There are a number of osteopathic subspecialties. As mentioned, about five hundred D.O.'s have received intensive training in manual methods, and use them regularly. An even smaller percentage specialize in *cranial osteopathy,* which focuses on the kind of cranial manipulations just described.

A discipline related to cranial osteopathy was developed by an osteopathic physicians, John Upledger. His approach, trademarked as *craniosacral therapy,* is based on osteopathic manipulations that focus exclusively on the cranium (head) and sacrum (pelvic area).

Craniosacral therapy arises from the concept that the twenty-nine bones of the head can move. This concept defies conventional medical wisdom, which asserts that these bones are immobile. However, a turn-of-the century osteopathic physician, William Sutherland, believed that the fluid that circulates inside the brain—the cerebrospinal fluid—moves rhythmically and causes the skull bones to expand and contract. To prove his theory, he performed an experiment by wrapping the skull tightly with bandages and believed that the flow of cerebrospinal fluid was reduced.

In addition adherents of craniosacral theory maintain that the membrane that envelopes the brain, spinal cord, and spinal nerve routes—the dura mater—is a key link between the sacrum and the head and neck muscles. Headache may result from chronic muscle contraction and joint restrictions in the sacral area. It could be due to tension of the dura inside the head, pulled tight by dysfunction of the sacrum. And it could be caused by compression of the nerves leading into the head (trigeminal nerves) due to compression in the lower back/sacrum.

These concepts are shared by "classic" osteopathic physicians, but the difference is that D.O.'s believe that restrictions in the connective tissue and bones affecting the head are not limited to problems of the sacrum. These reciprocal restrictions could happen anywhere in the body. So while a small percentage of D.O.'s and M.D.'s practice cranial manipulation, they do not limit their treatment to the craniosacral area.

One might say that craniosacral therapy is a very focused subspecialty of osteopathy—except that craniosacral therapists are not required to undergo the same extensive medical training as osteopathic physicians. Certification requirements vary from institution to institution. The Upledger Institute requires about twenty days, or 150 hours, of training, interspersed with hands-on work. The Colorado Cranial Institute follows a training format similar to that of the Upledger Institute. Craniosacral therapy is popular among massage therapists who want to expand their services and expertise, but can be learned by anyone; chiropractors, osteopathic physicians, dentists, and a few medical doctors (M.D.'s) have also received training in craniosacral therapy as an adjunct to their primary approach.

Side Effects and Warnings

Assuming that you have ruled out organic causes (tumors or broken bones), there are no contraindications to osteopathic manipulations or craniosacral therapy.

Finding a Reliable Osteopathic Physician (D.O.)

Your best resource to find a licensed doctor of osteopathy is word of mouth or the American Osteopathic Association, which can refer you to an osteopath in your region.

The fifteen schools of osteopathic medicine in the United States accept only college graduates who have passed the Medical College Examination Tests and, through a personal interview "exhibit a genuine concern for people." The governing organization, the American Osteopathic Association, sets standards for the schools of osteopathic medicine that include four years of medical training, with an emphasis on the muscle and skeletal systems and preventive care. After graduating they must complete a year-long internship; many then select a residency program in a specialty area. They must also complete a certain amount of continuing education each year. Licensing requirements differ from state to state; in some cases the tests for licensing are the same as they are for M.D.'s. See the "Resources" section.

Questions and Answers

• *Do osteopathic manual manipulations hurt?*   No. The manual methods rarely cause pain, though they may be somewhat uncomfortable; for example the intra-oral manipulation used in cranial osteopathy can be painful. You should let the osteopathic physician know if you experience any pain.

• *What other types of treatment will an osteopathic physician give me?*   Osteopathic physicians are licensed to do everything that an M.D. can do, such as prescribe drugs and perform surgery. Like M.D.'s, osteopathic physicians may also specialize in certain areas, such as obstetrics or neurology. Depending on your condition and preferences, other treatments may be given. In addition some D.O.'s complement their practices with holistic modalities, such as homeopathy or herbal therapy. Osteopathic physicians often recommend nutritional therapy and other self-healing methods more often than M.D.'s, and offer more drug-free options.

• *Can children receive OMMs?*   Yes, osteopathic physicians are trained to perform manual methods on children and the elderly.

• *Are osteopathic procedures covered by medical insurance?*   Osteopathic procedures are covered by most insurance plans, but you should certainly check to make sure.

Chiropractic

Chiropractic is an approach to healing based on manipulation of the spine. In keeping with the Greek roots of the term, manipulations are "done by hand." Like many holistic disciplines, chiropractors believe that the body holds the ability to heal itself. The spinal column and the nerves within it are key players in maintaining the balance of health.

History

"Bonesetting" techniques, as rudimentary chiropractic was widely referred to before the 1800s, date back to the ancient Chinese, Greeks, and many Native American cultures. In the Middle Ages it was a skill handed down from generation to generation. Its transformation into a formal discipline can be attributed to the Iowa grocer David Palmer, whose healing abilities were confirmed when he performed a spinal manipulation on a deaf customer and restored his hearing. He came to believe that misalignments (*fixations*) in the vertebrae—the bones of the spine—interfere with the functioning of the nervous system, causing *subluxations.*

Fixations are often marked by lack of mobility or hypermobility (overextended movement) in the vertebrae. A joint fixation can feel painful and tender without necessarily affecting the spinal nerves. But when a fixation causes a defect in a joint and the surrounding bones, muscles, tissues, and nerves, this is called *subluxation.* A pinched nerve can be caused by a misaligned vertebrae owing to subluxation.

By correcting subluxations, Palmer believed, chiropractors could improve the mobility of fixated joints, restore balanced movement, and restore health to the nervous system. Toward that end different types of *manipulations,* or *adjustments,* are employed, which entail applying controlled, quick, forceful pressure to the subluxated areas. Usually the manipulations are made on the spine, but can be applied to any joint in the body.

Early on, chiropractors split off into two groups, known as the "straights" and the "mixers." Straights uphold classical chiropractic theories and focus almost exclusively on manual manipulations. Mixers blend other treatments, such as nutritional counseling, with manual manipulations.

In addition there are now two broader groups of chiropractors. One group asserts that chiropractic can help alleviate any illness in the body; in general they believe in preventive adjustments to keep overall health. Their governing organization is the American Chiropractic Association. The other group, represented by the National Association of Chiropractic Medicine (NACM), maintains that chiropractic is useful mainly for musculoskeletal problems, and focus their skills on treating head, neck, and back pain.

Among these groups there are a total of more than fifty thousand licensed chiropractors in the United States today, and they make up the third largest group of health practitioners after medical doctors and dentists.

How It Works

Chiropractors believe that most forms of tension-type, migraine, and cluster headache ultimately arise from the musculoskeletal system. The blood supply and nerve supply to the head are closely linked to spinal anatomy and function. According to chiropractors, there are three ways that headache can result from fixations of the vertebrae of the cervical spine:

• Pain-sensitive nerve fibers in the joints, which are plentiful, can activate headaches *directly,* due to compression or subluxation, or *indirectly,* by causing spasm of the muscles surrounding the spine. This can happen due to an injury, such as whiplash, or chronic postural problems.

• Neck and head muscles are chronically damaged. In this case the muscles are the main instigator of nerve pain, not the spine. Again, injury or bad posture can cause these problems.

• Misalignment and fixation of the joints can irritate the nerves, which causes a chronic mix-up or overload of pain messages. In this way chronic fixations, chiropractors say, can interfere with the vascular (blood vessel) system and cause headaches.

If the pain seems to come from fixated joints (not organic causes), then the chiropractor will make an *adjustment,* or manipulation. Most often adjustments for headache focus on the neck area of the spine, or the *cervical* spine, but this may vary. (The spine is an integrated unit, and problems in one area can lead to pain in others. In one study migraine pain was attributed to fixations in the lower back.)

As just mentioned, the chiropractor achieves this by applying fast, forceful pressure with her hands to the area of subluxation. In this way, according to chiropractic theory, the joint is freed from its restriction, allowing the nerves and muscles to return to normal functioning.

Who Can Be Helped

Chiropractors from both schools—the "treat every problem" school and the "treat only musculoskeletal problems" school—will assert that many chronic, nonthreatening headaches can be helped by chiropractic manipulations. The *Textbook of Clinical Chiropractic* points to specific treatments for headaches due to migraine, cluster, hypertension, digestive problems, sinuses, TMJ, and whiplash. Eyestrain headaches are often referred to an optometrist or ophthalmologist. There are studies to support its effectiveness in migraine and tension-type headache (see page 248).

What to Expect

The chiropractor will first take a detailed history, asking questions about the nature, severity, and frequency of your pain, as well as general questions about your health, your occupation and level of exercise, and about other methods you've tried for pain relief. Some chiropractors will also ask about your diet.

After a routine physical exam, like the one you're used to from a conventional doctor, the chiropractor will spend some time examining your spine. You'll be asked to bend forward, backward, and from side to side. These movements give the chiropractor an idea of your range of movement and the shape of your spine. Then, with both hands placed on the spine, the chiropractor will feel how you move, a procedure called *motion palpation,* to help locate joints that do not move well enough or that move too far out of the normal range of motion.

The chiropractor will also feel the muscles and tissues surrounding the spine—sometimes with the aid of a metal gauge—to get a sense of muscle tone and health and help determine the type of manipulation that might be right for you.

In many cases chiropractors will want to take an X ray to get a baseline picture of your spine against which to monitor future progress. The initial X ray also helps rule out problems such as tumors or fractures that would require a different type of treatment.

The X rays are usually ready right away, and the chiropractor will review them with you, pointing out the overall shape of your spine, areas of fixation and subluxation, and disk degeneration, as well as goals for treatment. For example, if you have migraines, the chiropractor might find fixations in the cervical, thoracic, or lumbar regions of the spine—basically the upper neck, throat, and mid-to-lower back. Observing these problems, chiropractors would mark the spots on the X ray (and the corresponding points on your back) and explain how the chiropractic adjustments will help resolve them.

Finally, the chiropractor will perform the adjustment(s). You will sit or lie down on a padded table, semiclothed. The chiropractor will first lightly massage the muscles surrounding the spine to help relax you. Then he or she will make the adjustment, which involves applying quick, forceful pressure to the spine. You might hear a cracking noise— which might resonate especially loudly if your neck is being adjusted. This is more alarming than it is painful, something akin to cracking your knuckles. In fact the adjustment is rarely painful. In some cases head pain is immediately alleviated.

In my opinion good chiropractors routinely recommend an exercise regimen to complement the adjustments. Exercise helps improve flexibility and maintain mobility, and builds muscles to support the spine.

In addition many chiropractors emphasize dietary changes and vitamin supplementation. People with headaches may be prescribed an elimination diet to uncover hidden food sensitivities that might be triggering headaches.

Treatment Schedule

The treatment schedule depends on the severity of your headache— and the orientation of your chiropractor. Some may initially recommend a few weeks of intensive adjustments, two to three per week. As needed, weekly sessions might be required to produce the necessary spinal changes. However, some chiropractors will recommend ongoing preventive maintenance. The value of this treatment approach is under debate in the medical community, and even among chiropractors. In studies of people with headache, ongoing preventive treatment was not needed to produce long-term benefits.

Effectiveness

There are several studies showing the effectiveness of chiropractic for migraine and tension-type headache. Relief of migraine with and without aura is reported to range from 72 to 90 percent.[9] In one study eighty-seven individuals reported an average 74 percent improvement in migraine pain, which was maintained for two years after treatment had ended.[10] However, these were all uncontrolled studies, that is, there was no control group for comparison.

Side Effects and Warnings

Chiropractic is generally considered safe, though there is a slight risk (less than 1%) of stroke due to compression of arteries leading to the brain, though evidence gathered by the medical community suggests that this risk is underestimated. The risk is higher when the spine is rotated during adjustments.

With certain chiropractic techniques, such as the Gonstead method, the spine is not rotated before an adjustment, and there have been no reports of stroke among people treated by this method. To be absolutely safe, chiropractic should be avoided in people at risk of stroke, including those with high blood pressure, high cholesterol, ischemic heart disease, the elderly or people taking blood-thinning drugs.

In addition there is also a small risk of ruptured disks and paralysis.

The common use of X rays in chiropractic also presents the risk of cancer. Some chiropractors use X rays more liberally than others, and their value as a way of monitoring progress is under debate.

Chiropractic is not recommended for people with severe osteoporosis, rheumatoid arthritis, fractures, tumors, infection, or malignancies of the spine.

Finding a Reliable Chiropractor

Chiropractic is licensed in all fifty states. The American Chiropractic Association is the governing organization for chiropractors, who view themselves as the equivalents of primary-care physicians—treating a wide range of conditions. Chiropractors who are members of the National Association of Chiropractic Medicine generally focus on musculoskeletal problems. The Orthopractic Society focuses on manipulations to improve joint mobility, and does not adhere to the concept of subluxations. For referrals and more information, contact the organizations listed in the "Resources" section.

Questions and Answers

• *Is chiropractic painful?*   The adjustments should not hurt—however, there are reports in rare cases of chiropractic adjustments producing more pain due to ruptured disks. Make sure that your chiropractor has received adequate training and hands-on experience.

• *What causes the cracking sound of an adjustment?*   The movement of joints can make a cracking noise; this is normal and nothing to worry about.

• *Can chiropractic be done in children?*   Yes—it is generally a safe practice for children and could be of benefit if headaches are related to structural problems. Children generally need fewer adjustments to correct fixations because their vertebrae have not endured as many years of degeneration as adults'.

• *How about older adults?*   Chiropractic can be of benefit to people of advanced age. However, people with osteoporosis (bone thinning), osteoarthritis, and rheumatoid arthritis should not receive chiropractic therapy.

• *Can I get chiropractic adjustments if I'm pregnant?*   Yes, an experienced chiropractor will know how to focus the adjustment to make sure it's safe during pregnancy. However, you should avoid all X rays during this time.

• *Is chiropractic covered by medical insurance?*   This depends on your carrier, but forty-one states now require coverage for chiropractic.

Variations on Chiropractic: Applied Kinesiology and Touch for Health

The word *kinesiology* means the study of body movement. Today it is a method practiced by many chiropractors based on manual muscle testing. Touch for Health is a self-education approach based on kinesiology methods. A hands-on therapy, kinesiology blends concepts from chiropractic, osteopathy, traditional Chinese meridian therapy, and naturopathy. It was developed by chiropractor George Goodheart in the mid 1960s, who found that muscle evaluation enhanced his diagnosis of spinal problems. With further research Goodheart came to believe that muscle tone reflects the health of corresponding organs and body systems.

Kinesiology treatment is geared toward restoring total health—as measured through muscle response—through a triad of balancing approaches: nutrition, structural adjustments, and mental attitude.

The evaluation takes shape as a series of muscle-strength tests that at first may make you feel like the main act of a magic show. You will hold your arm or leg while resisting pressure from the kinesiologist. One moment you succeed with little effort. But after pressing a point on your chest, putting salt on your tongue, inhaling fumes, or simply thinking about an emotionally draining experience, your limb turns to jelly. The reason? According to kinesiologists, muscles that are "switched off" and weak indicate a blockage or imbalance in the corresponding body system—and the need for restoring energy flow. For example, a muscle's response to certain foods or supplements placed in the mouth (or near the mouth) help determine the body's needs for that nutrient. If the body needs that food, its "neurolingual" (brain-to-tongue) reflex will almost instantly reflect it with muscle changes.

Like other holistic disciplines, kinesiology views the body as an integrated whole. What makes kinesiology unique among Western complementary disciplines is its reliance on many body techniques to help the body achieve integrated wholeness, or balance. These include (a) nutritional therapy, as determined by muscle response to contact with certain nutrients; (b) reflex therapies—neurolymphatic massage, neurovascular holding points, meridian tracing, acupressure holding points, and massage. Reflex therapies consist of the following:

- Neurolymphatic massage stimulates reflex points that trigger the flow of lymphatic fluids to different areas of the body.
- Neurovascular holding points, activated by very light touch, help stimulate blood flow and enhance circulation.
- Meridian tracing, based on the traditional Chinese meridians, involves lightly following the meridian line to enhance the flow of energy (qi).
- Massage of muscles helps stretch and strengthen them.

In addition to these primary techniques, kinesiologists may use chiropractic adjustments, acupuncture, acupressure, aromatherapy, homeopathy, and other adjunctive treatments to help relieve head pain.

Kinesiology is mainly available through chiropractors (an estimated 37 percent practice applied kinesiology), though some are M.D.'s, osteopathic physicians, and dentists. For referrals to certified kinesiologists or Touch for Health courses and/or information in your area, see the ''Resources'' section.

Touch for Health Tension Headache Relief Exercise

The following exercise, actually an acupressure technique, accesses the gallbladder meridian (of traditional Oriental acupuncture).

1. Standing erect, drop your hands to the sides of your legs. Press with your middle finger, looking for a sore or tender point in that area. It may take a little searching, but the point will be there.
2. Once you have found a sore or tender point on one or both sides of your thigh, massage these points with your fingertip with firm pressure until the headache goes away.
3. Concentrate on the headache disappearing while you do this. It is okay to rub on one side at a time. It may be sufficient to rub on one side only to get rid of the headache.
4. Sometimes the headache will disappear in just a few seconds. Other times you may have to rub one or both points for a minute or so.

Copyright © 1994 Touch for Health Association. Elizabeth and Hap Barhydt. All rights reserved. 6955 Fernhill Drive, Suite 5A, Malibu, CA 90265

OTHER PHYSICAL APPROACHES

Exercise

The health virtues of regular exercise have been extolled for thousands of years. It keeps your weight down, improves circulation, strengthens cardiac muscles, and tempers the ravages of gravity and age on muscle tone.

But researchers have recently been finding that the effects of aerobic exercise on stress are not what they once thought. Back in the 1980s scientists believed that aerobic exercise was an unmitigated boon. By increasing heart rate, aerobic exercise stimulates the body to release endorphins, the body's own mood-elevators. In addition it helps to oxygenate the body. Finally, by raising body temperature an intense workout was believed to help relax tense muscles. All of these effects can indeed be of benefit to people with chronic headache.

However, new evidence suggests that aerobic exercise is not the only route to the tension-relieving benefits of exercise. An analysis of more than one hundred studies by Steven Petruzzello from the University of Illinois showed that relaxation is equally effective in reducing anxiety.[11]

The message here is not to stop exercising. All of the physical health benefits of aerobic exercise remain valid. But the mind- and body-relaxing benefits of exercise—which are among the primary goals in helping prevent headache—can be accomplished with any type of regular exercise that you enjoy. Even dance, which combines physical activity with rhythmic movement to enhance the relaxation effect, can be of benefit in relieving stress. Walking and swimming are also excellent exercises for people with chronic headache.

According to Herbert Benson, cardiologist and director of the Mind/Body Institute at New England Deaconess Hospital, combining exercise with a simple mantra—a word or phrase that helps focus your mind away from worrisome thoughts—can bring the stress-releasing benefits of meditation to your routine. (For more on meditation, see Chapter 8.)

Exercise is generally a preventive tool; you should avoid exercise during a headache attack although I have had some patients who stopped a headache early in its course by exercising. Also be sure to stop exercising if a headache comes on in the middle of your routine.

As with any physical method, be sure to consult your physician before embarking on an exercise program.

Dance/Movement Therapy

Dance is an expression of body and mind. For people with headaches its physical benefits include relief of body tension and body armoring. Mentally dance can help reduce stress.

It is the belief of some dance therapists that dance method can promote the inner healing process by improving mood states and awakening stored feelings. By stimulating the circulatory, respiratory, skeletal, and neuromuscular systems of the body, dance therapy has been clinically shown to decrease anxiety, reduce body tension, and reduce chronic pain.

The American Dance Therapy Association sets standards for professional practice. It also serves as a referral resource for certified dance therapists (who carry the initials D.T.R. after their names), who have completed a master's degree and 700 hours of supervised clinical internship. The title of Academy of Dance Therapists Registered (A.D.T.R.) means that the therapist has completed 3,640 hours of supervised clinical work.

Hydrotherapy

Hydrotherapy is the use of water, of varying temperatures and pressures, to alleviate pain and relieve tension. Whirlpools, directed water pressure, hot and cold compresses, and saunas are all examples of hydrotherapy.

With tension-type headache it has been shown that application of heat to the neck and head area for ten to twenty minutes can relieve headache by opening blood vessels and relaxing muscles.

With migraine, which is initiated by dilation of blood vessels, *alternating cold with hot compresses* has been effective with some people at the onset of a migraine attack. *Regular use of hot compresses* can help prevent tension headaches by relaxing muscles.

As a preventive measure warm baths, whirlpools, and saunas may help provide overall relaxation and release tension. *Note:* Avoid very high temperatures if you have high blood pressure, are pregnant, or have circulatory problems. If you have any health problems, consult your doctor before starting hydrotherapy.

To locate sources for hydrotherapy, ask your doctor or physical therapist for a recommendation. Or contact a naturopathic physician who practices hydrotherapy (see "Resources").

Head Band Therapy

A recent small study of people in the middle of a migraine attack showed that using an elastic band to put pressure on the head, particularly the temple area, helped 87 percent of the study group relieve pain by more than 80 percent.[12] The band they used was made of elastic, secured with Velcro, with rubber disks inserted underneath to apply direct pressure to the area that hurt the most.

Transcutaneous Electrical Stimulation

It has been shown in some studies that electrical stimulation of nerves can help people with headache. This concept is based on a theory of pain developed by Ronald Melzack and Patrick Wall, M.D., in the 1960s. They maintained that there is a group of cells that regulates pain signals; some transmit pain, some close the gateway to pain. This theory is known as the gate-control theory. Based on this concept, proponents believe that stimulating the cells that inhibit pain will get them to travel to the brain and close the gate before the pain-transmitting cells get there. The most common method for achieving this goal is by *transcutaneous electrical nerve stimulation* (*TENS*). For headache, there are special low-level electrical devices known as transcranial electrostimulation devices.

With TENS, two electrodes are placed on the head wherever it hurts. The wires from the electrodes are attached to an electricity-generating device, which can be regulated. The device sends measured pulses of electricity through the wires to the electrodes, which are then transmitted through the skin to the cells.

There are more than one hundred FDA-approved TENS devices

available. Some are small and portable so that they can hook onto a
belt.

Studies have shown possible effectiveness of TENS and transcranial
electrostimulation in reducing headache. You do not need a doctor's
authority to purchase TENS devices, but it is a good idea to get a
physician's guidance.

Posture

The way we hold our bodies can have a dramatic effect on our
health—so say most bodywork therapists and many headache experts.
As discussed in this and other chapters, chronic patterns of bad posture
put undue tension on the muscles and connective tissue around the head
and neck, reduce blood circulation, deprive the blood of oxygen, and
compress nerves—which can lead to headache. Good posture is often a
matter of eliminating bad habits. What follow are some tips for improving your posture (you might also want to investigate some of the structural-reeducation methods described earlier to carry your postural
awareness to a deeper level).

Standing

Standing with your back against a wall and your heels about three
inches from the base, distribute your weight evenly on both feet. Your
ears, shoulders, and hips should be aligned in a straight line. The curves
of your back and neck should be slight and balanced.

To test your posture, put one hand behind your neck, palm inward.
Now put one hand behind the small of your back, palm toward the wall.
Your hands should fit easily, without much extra room.

From the front, check to see whether your hips line up; one should
not be higher or lower than the other. Kneecaps should face straight
ahead. Your ankles should be straight.

Here are some general tips that can help improve standing posture:

- When standing for long periods of time, shift your weight every so
  often from one foot to the other.
- Strengthen your abdominals three or four times a day with this

isometric exercise: Flatten your stomach muscles and hold for a few seconds, then relax.
- Imagine that your head is suspended by a thread, floating effortlessly on the top of your spine. Relax your back and stomach muscles.

Sitting

To test your sitting posture, sit down in a straightback chair. Shoulders should be at the same height. The head should rest directly over the shoulders, without straining either forward or backward. They should be slightly elevated from your hips. The neck should be relaxed, shoulders kept down. The back should be upright or slightly angled from the hips, keeping a slight natural curve of the lower back. Knees should be slightly lower than hips. Feet should be planted firmly on the floor or on a footrest.

Try to pay attention to the following:

- If your feet don't reach the floor, use a footrest or phone book so that they rest on a firm surface.
- Change positions often.
- Stretch every half hour or so.
- Roll your neck very gently every so often.

Working at a Computer

When working at a computer, follow the above recommendations for sitting. In addition make sure of the following:

- Elbows: relaxed and at right angles to the arms
- Wrists: relaxed and in a neutral, floating position—without flexing up or down
- The computer screen: at eye level or slightly lower
- Fingers: gently curved
- Keyboard: should be flat and level with, or just below, the elbow. Keys should be reached by moving the entire arm, from the shoulder down, rather than twisting the wrists or straining the fingers. Take frequent breaks.

Sleeping

Make sure you have a firm mattress. Avoid sleeping on your stomach. If you sleep on your side, support your neck with a pillow so that the head and middle of your chest are aligned in a straight line.

Walking

Avoid carrying packages, briefcases, or purses on one side all the time, and avoid high heels and platform shoes for long walks. This can put strain on your muscles. Wear a backpack, distribute the weight to both hands, or alternate hands.

Lifting

Lift heavy loads by using your legs to lift you up, keeping your back straight. Never bend your back or shoulders.

Driving

Position your seat so that you can reach the steering wheel and foot pads easily. Support your lower back with a rolled towel or pillow. Adjust the seat so that your knees are just a little higher than your hips. For long trips stop every few hours and walk around.

Isometric Exercise

To help keep your neck muscles strong and prevent spasm, do this isometric exercise, illustrated on page 259, several times a day:

1. Sit in a neutral, balanced position (see page 257). Throughout these exercises breathe slowly and deeply.
2. With palm on your forehead, begin to press against your head. Gradually press harder, but resist with your neck muscles so that your head remains in the same place.
3. Hold for five seconds, then relax.
4. Repeat five times.
5. Follow steps 2 through 4, pressing on each side of the head. Repeat five times on each side.
6. Follow steps 2 through 4, pressing from the back of the head.

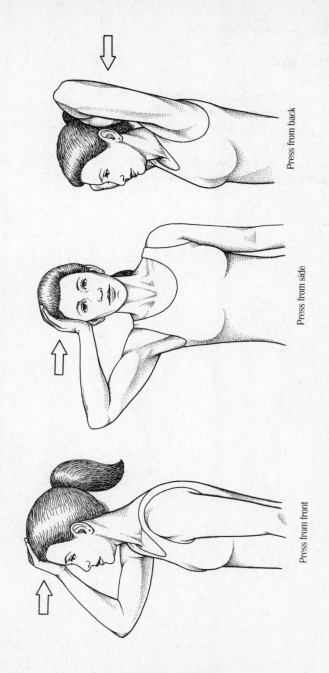

Press from back

Press from side

Press from front

For TMJ

- When not chewing, teeth should never touch.
- Monitor your jaw for signs of clenching.
- Place your tongue lightly on the top of your mouth behind your front, upper teeth.
- Avoid habits that put tension on jaw muscles, such as biting cheeks or lips, pushing tongue against teeth, clenching jaws.

CHAPTER 8

Mind-Body Therapies

A new world is only a new mind.
—WILLIAM CARLOS WILLIAMS

━━━━━━

"Where does the mind end and the body begin? Where does the body end and the mind begin?"

Not too long ago the answers to these questions, posed by B.K.S. Iyengar in *Light on Yoga,* would have been clear to most Western physicians. The body and mind were thought of as distinct entities: Disease was caused by physical stimuli and improved by physical interventions—period. The concept that the mind can influence the health of the body, though not new to some systems of medicine, was certainly not entertained by most serious medical researchers. Today there is mounting evidence from renowned research institutions that supports the mind-body connection—and the use of techniques using the mind to influence the health of the body.

That the body reflects what the mind perceives is a physiological fact widely accepted by modern medicine. If the brain is the seat of the mind, it is also home base for almost all physical responses and expressions. Twenty-four hours a day the brain and the body interact through a vast network of lightning-quick biochemical and neural (nerve) messengers. Modern science can acknowledge that this interaction happens on an unconscious level—but it has a harder time accepting that willful, conscious thought can create specific changes in the body.

The advent of psychiatry and behavioral sciences in the twentieth century has done much to bring the mind-body connection into the clinical spotlight. Through studies we have learned that the way patients *perceive* their conditions can influence their "quality of life," regardless of the severity of the disease. An optimistic and relaxed outlook, it is widely believed (and has been proved), helps improve quality of life, and may also make pain more bearable.

Why do patients who feel better emotionally also fare better physically? In search of answers medical research has used sophisticated tools to look closely at the brain and how the nervous system interacts with the rest of the body. As we've begun to penetrate the mysteries of the brain, we have started to see that its influence extends beyond the skull. A relatively new medical science, *psychoneuroimmunology,* has done much to advance our understanding of the mind-body link.

Psychoneuroimmunology, also known as PNI, is the study of the interactions between the mind (*psycho*), the nervous and endocrine system (*neuro*), and the immune system (*immuno*). PNI got its start with the work of psychologist Robert Adler, who found in the 1970s that the immune system could be conditioned to react to brain-generated stimuli. Since then a number of other studies in PNI and other medical disciplines show that the immune system harbors nerve tissues that are connected to the brain, that chronic stress may impair the immune system, and that psychological and social attitudes shape not only the way one perceives illness but can physically redirect the course of it.

Another important, and related, area of mind-body research focuses on the physical effects of relaxation (see Chapter 2). In the late 1960s Herbert Benson, M.D., and coworkers monitored the physiological functions of people in a state of meditation. They found that meditation induced a variety of measurable physical effects: Breathing and brain wave patterns slowed down. In future work Dr. Benson and colleagues found that meditation and other mind-body activities induced a condition that he called *the relaxation response,* which is the inverse of the fight-or-flight response described decades earlier (see table, page 263).

A variety of methods have been used to induce this response by Dr. Benson, who founded the Mind/Body Medical Institute at Harvard Medical School, including progressive muscle relaxation, hypnosis, prayer, yoga, and meditation.

The Effects of Stress and Relaxation on Different Body Functions

Body System	Fight-or-Flight Response	Relaxation Response
Heart rate and blood pressure	Increased	Decreased
Blood flow	Directed toward muscles, lung, and heart	Directed toward internal organs
Breathing rate	Increased to supply heart, muscles, and lungs	Decreased due to reduced oxygen demand
Digestive enzymes	Reduced	Increased
Blood sugar levels	Increased	Unchanged

Finally, the field of energy-based medicine, or biofield therapeutics, which has its origins in age-old concepts that all living things are imbued with a vital life force, has been making quiet strides along the formal alternative road to health. Examples of these methods include Therapeutic Touch, prayer, and Reiki—although some forms of external qigong (see Chapter 7) are also considered biofield healing methods.

What all mind-body techniques have in common, and what makes them so extraordinary in the context of modern medicine, is the use of the mind to *willfully* direct healthful effects in the body.

Mind-body approaches are generally safe and free of side effects. But those interested in these techniques should pursue them with one caveat: Make sure to first rule out other serious causes for your headache.

RELAXATION METHODS

Can something as basic as relaxation really be effective? The answer is in clinical proof. Relaxation is thought to be the primary power behind the effectiveness of mind-body techniques for preventing headache.

- In one recent study tension-headache sufferers had up to 98.2 percent *fewer* headaches with the use of relaxation—and they remained virtually headache-free for one year.[1]
- At the State University of New York at Albany, progressive relaxation helped 96 percent of headache sufferers reduce the number, duration, and severity of headache after ten therapy sessions.[2]
- In a review of several studies relaxation combined with cognitive therapy or biofeedback was shown effective in up to 75 percent of headache sufferers.[3]
- Relaxation helped people with TMJ disorder reduce pain by 56 percent.

Many studies have also confirmed the value of mind-body methods in children with headaches. In one, progressive relaxation and/or autogenic relaxation helped reduce headaches in children over long periods of time.[4]

One of the most appealing qualities of these methods is that you can practice them on your own—though at first you might benefit from qualified instruction.

Progressive Relaxation Exercise

We know that muscle and vascular tension trigger headaches. Progressive relaxation, developed by Edmund Jacobsen in the 1920s, is a simple way to relax the muscles. You need no training or special skills—just the ability to tense and relax muscles. Tensing and relaxing your muscles one by one teaches the mind and body how to recognize when stress creates muscle tension, and a method for releasing it.

Here is how progressive relaxation works:

1. Get comfortable. Wear loose clothing, remove your shoes. Make sure you are neither too warm nor too cold. Find a quiet room where you won't be distracted for fifteen minutes.
2. Sit in a comfortable chair, or lie down on the ground on your back, using an exercise mat or soft carpet.
3. Take a few deep, easy breaths.
4. Tense all of the muscles in your body, from head to toe. Hold the tension for several seconds. Let your mind feel the sensation of this tension.
5. Holding on to the tension, inhale deeply and hold your breath for several seconds. Let your mind and body register the sensation of this tension.
6. Exhale slowly as you let the tension go. Let your mind and body register the sensation of this relaxation.

Now, work on individual muscle groups. As you tense the following muscles, try to keep the rest of your muscles as relaxed as possible. Repeat each of the following exercises three times:

1. Tighten your fists. Feel the tension radiating up your arms. Inhale deeply and hold the tension for several seconds. Exhale and let your hands relax.
2. Press your arms down against the ground or chair. Inhale and hold the tension for several seconds, concentrating on the sensation. Exhale and let your arms relax.
3. Shrug your shoulders up to your ears. Experience the tension in your neck and shoulders. Inhale and hold. Exhale and let your shoulders drop.
4. Frown and raise your eyebrows. Study the tightness in your face. Inhale and hold the tension. Exhale and release.
5. Press your eyelids closed as tightly as possible. Inhale and hold. Exhale and open your eyes gently.

6. Open your mouth as wide as possible. Inhale and hold. Exhale and release your jaw.
7. Clench your jaw, biting down with your teeth. Feel the tension spread across your skull. Inhale and hold. Exhale and release.
8. Inhale deeply into your belly, letting your chest expand. Hold the chest tension. Exhale and let your breath return to normal.
9. Tighten your abdominal muscles. Hold, then relax.
10. Arch your back, chest up and hips down. Inhale and hold. Exhale and release your back gently.
11. Tighten your hips and buttocks. Inhale and hold. Exhale and relax.
12. Tense your left leg, from thigh to heel. Inhale and hold. Exhale and relax.
13. Tense your right leg, from thigh to heel. Inhale and hold. Exhale and relax.
14. Curl your toes under. Inhale and hold. Exhale and relax.
15. Remaining still, scan your body. Experience the relaxation over your entire body. If you need to, return to areas of tension and repeat the exercise for that muscle group. Breathe naturally and deeply for several moments, experiencing the relaxed state. Gently and slowly stand up.

Hypnotherapy

Hypnotherapy has come a long way since the days of Svengali. More than opening act entertainment, hypnosis has earned solid scientific status as a medical treatment approved by the American Medical Association (AMA).

Coming from the Greek word, hypnos, which means "sleep," hypnosis is a state of focused concentration that makes the participant highly receptive to suggestion. In its therapeutic application, hypnotic suggestion allows the participant to get in touch with thoughts and actions of the mind that are difficult to access consciously.

The World Health Organization reports that 90 percent of the general population can be hypnotized, about a third of whom are highly responsive to hypnotic suggestion. Hypnosis can be self-applied, or induced by a hypnotherapist.[5]

History

Hypnosis has been around since ancient times. There is evidence that hypnotic trances were part of early Greek religious rituals. Hypnosis was introduced to modern medicine in the late 1700s by Franz Anton Mesmer, a German physician.

As a therapeutic practice, hypnotherapy fell in and out of favor until the early 1900s, when Sigmund Freud used it in conjunction with psychoanalysis. In 1958 the American Medical Association approved hypnosis as a therapeutic modality. Today the American Society of Clinical Hypnosis is the governing body for more than four thousand physicians, dentists, and psychologists who use hypnotherapy as a healing technique—but its use also extends to other physicians.

How It Works

Hypnotherapists assert that hypnotic states can occur at any time: People fall in and out of hypnosis while watching TV, reading, or other focused activities. During states of controlled hypnosis, research has shown physical changes similar to those observed during states of deep relaxation: decrease in nervous-system activity, decrease in oxygen consumption, lowering of blood pressure and heart rate, and changes in brain wave activity.[6]

Once one enters the deep state of concentration found in hypnosis, the mind becomes more receptive to suggestions. The suggestions often involve imagery that call upon any of the five senses—sight, sound, taste, smell, or touch (see page 270). The imagery used is tailored to the individual to help control the mechanisms of pain. For example, for a person with tension-type headache who loves music, hypnotic suggestion may involve associating neck muscle relaxation and pain relief with a certain piece of music. Biofeedback techniques (page 280) have been used successfully in conjunction with hypnosis to reinforce the feeling of relaxation.

Who Can Be Helped

People with chronic pain of many types can benefit from hypnotherapy, if only by its ability to induce relaxation, release tension, and improve tolerance of pain. It has proven particularly useful in children with headaches.

What to Expect

You can either learn self-hypnosis or go to a hypnotherapist. If you decide to learn it yourself, you could benefit greatly from instruction from a reliable hypnotherapist.

The hypnotherapist will often begin by helping you understand what hypnotherapy is about and what feelings you can expect during hypnotic trance. He or she will also ask about your specific problem and the patterns of your head pain. You may undergo some tests to determine how easily you can be hypnotized.

Then the hypnotherapist will guide you through relaxation, images, and suggestions. The images, as discussed, are tailored to your personality and problems. Alternatively the hypnotherapist may teach you how to do this yourself. Some hypnotherapists will make audiotapes for you to use at home.

Treatment Schedule

Success with hypnotherapy does not happen overnight. Persistence and a desire to make changes are critical. Children seem to have more success with hypnosis. Karen Olness, M.D., in *Mind/Body Medicine* (Consumer Reports Books), asserts that this may be due to children's greater facility with imagination and that, during play, they are more apt to move in and out of different states of awareness. As a result children often learn pain-control strategies in just a few sessions, where it may take the average adult two months of daily practice to learn pain control.

Effectiveness

Hypnotherapy has proved effective in reducing the frequency and severity of tension-type and migraine headache in people of all ages. It has proved particularly helpful for children.

In twelve controlled studies of children and teenagers with migraine, hypnosis proved superior to a variety of methods, including drug therapy, in controlling headache. Some of the studies included biofeedback. Adults with migraine have also benefited from hypnotherapy.[7]

Side Effects and Warnings

Hypnosis is generally safe, but it is powerful. Instruction should be received by or learned only from a qualified professional (see below).

Finding a Reliable Hypnotherapist

Because hypnotherapy is a potent tool, you should seek out a therapist who is not only adequately trained and certified but who has an understanding of how to tailor the technique to your specific problem. For referrals to a reliable hypnotherapist in your area, contact the organizations listed in "Resources."

Questions and Answers

• *Will I lose control during hypnosis?* This is a myth about hypnotherapy. It is true that you may be open to suggestions to do things that you might normally not do—but this is partly why hypnotherapy works. By inducing you to suspend conscious critical judgments, hypnotherapy opens access to your inner mind. Rather than lose control, you gain relaxation.

However, hypnosis is not a passive state. You must *want* to achieve the suggested goal—and *want* to be hypnotized to begin with. Nor will you be walled off from outside influences; if a threatening situation arises, you will react the same way you would while in a nonhypnotic state.

• *I'm pretty stubborn. Can I be hypnotized?* You may be stubborn about some things, but if you *want* hypnosis to work for you and believe that you have a good imagination, your general stubborn qualities will not get in the way. However, the World Health Organization estimates that about 10 percent of the population is hypnosis immune. This may be due to fear of and strong resistance to losing control, or to difficulty "going with" your imagination and following imagery.

- *Can I be made to do things I wouldn't normally do?*   Yes—and that's the point of hypnosis—but you can't be forced to do things you don't *want* to do. By entering a very relaxed, highly attentive state, you can access parts of your brain that normally cannot be reached while operating on a conscious level. If you work with a professional, qualified hypnotherapist, this power will be directed toward improving your health.

- *Is hypnosis covered by medical insurance?*   Hypnosis is recognized by the American Medical Association, but it may not be fully covered by all insurance companies—even if administered by an M.D. Check with your carrier.

Imagery and Visualization

Imagery is the use of the mind to call upon specific images to help change attitudes, behavior, or physical health. Used as a vehicle for focused concentration, imagery can affect physiological functions that are not normally altered consciously.

If you read about hypnotherapy (page 266), you will see similarities. The difference is that hypnosis is a state of mind, whereas imagery is an activity. Indeed imagery is often used to help bring people into a hypnotic state and, while in that state, to effect a physical change. They are complementary and may be used either together or individually along with biofeedback. They are also used in meditation.

Visualization is a form of imagery. Whereas imagery can make use of the full range of senses, visualization employs the visual sense.

A common imagery exercise involves imagining in exquisite detail the characteristics of a lemon—its scent, color, texture. Normally it's difficult to induce salivation by conscious will. But by vividly imagining the sensations associated with a lemon, most participants start to salivate.

Imagery has two therapeutic uses—*active* and *receptive*. Active guided imagery is used to directly relieve symptoms. For example, in the case of tension headache you might imagine your neck muscles, then imagine them melting like honey, which relieves pressure on your blood vessels, which in turn allows the nerve endings to relax and the pain to disappear.

Receptive guided imagery is more like association: When thinking about your headache, what images come to mind? Does it feel like a vise around your head? What does a vise mean to you? This level of inquiry into your personal associations can be revealing about your emotional feelings about headache. As we know, emotional stress is often a trigger for chronic headaches. Receptive imagery can help individuals understand the link between stress and headache—and find ways to interrupt it.

History

Imagery has been a traditional part of the healing arts of many cultures throughout the world. It has been used in a formal, therapeutic way since the early 1970s. Today guided imagery is widely used in pain clinics and wellness programs.

How It Works

Researchers are not exactly sure how imagery works to help relieve pain. They believe that sensory information is housed in the part of the brain called the *cerebral cortex.* Martin Rossman, M.D., co-director of the Academy for Guided Imagery, reports that through the use of a diagnostic imaging method called *positron emission tomography* (*PET*), scientists can see that imagining a thing, place, or situation elicits the same changes in the cerebral cortex as experiencing it. And any physiological changes associated with that image may also occur. The more vividly you imagine a situation—through visual images, odors, physical sensations, sounds—the stronger the physical response.[8]

This is a very powerful idea. What it means is that *imagining* a relaxing situation—a languorous day at the beach for example—may bring on the same *physical* reactions as actually being there.

Guided imagery helps people with headache in two ways:

- *Relaxation.* The first step in imagery exercises is learning to relax. The healthful effects of relaxation have been well described, including reduced muscle tension, improved blood flow, lower blood pressure, and reduced need for oxygen. Relaxation alone may be a helpful way of preventing stress-induced headaches.

• *Direct physiological effects.* Guided imagery can also be used to reverse physical effects. If you have a headache that feels like a rock pounding the inside of your skull, for example, you might imagine that the boulder is turning into a sponge—or that the boulder is disintegrating.

Guided Imagery Exercise for Relaxation

Though it is best to use images that are personally meaningful to you, there are some images that evoke relaxation almost universally, such as the following:

With your eyes closed, imagine that you are lying down on a beach on a sunny afternoon. Feel the sun radiating over your skin. It is warm and comforting but not too hot. You can hear the waves lapping gently and rhythmically against the shore. You are alone, but completely safe. You can hear people in the near distance enjoying the beach. Move your feet through the sand. Feel the warm grains of sand massaging them. Smell the fresh sea air. The temperature is perfect and your mind is as free of worry as the clear blue sky.

Who Can Be Helped

As a general relaxation technique, guided imagery can help people with all types of headache.

What to Expect

The guided-imagery session typically begins with relaxation exercises to help focus the mind. Hypnosis may be used to induce this state. Then you will concentrate on a specific image that has been individually designed to help you relieve or prevent headache.

Treatment Schedule

The sessions last between twenty minutes and an hour. As with hypnosis, guided imagery can be self-taught.

Practice makes perfect. The more often you practice, the more "real" your imagery will become and the more effective it will be in relieving your pain—and the more accessible it will be when you are in pain.

Effectiveness

There have been few controlled clinical trials with guided imagery—in part because imagery is so individualized. However, anecdotal reports have shown imagery to be effective in reducing pain due to headaches.

Side Effects and Warnings

Guided imagery is very safe, and there are no specific contraindications. However, you should rule out any potentially life-threatening situations in order to receive necessary treatment before relying on imagery.

Finding a Reliable Imagery Therapist

It is recommended that you learn imagery from a reliable professional. Seek out a mental health professional or holistic medical practitioner with experience in guided imagery. Or contact one of the organizations listed in "Resources," which can refer you to health professionals with certification or training in guided imagery.

Questions and Answers

• *Can imagery be used by children with headaches?*   Children are especially receptive to imagery—and it is particularly effective when used in conjunction with hypnosis (see "Hypnotherapy," page 266, or "Biofeedback," page 280).

• *I don't think I have a very good imagination. Will imagery work for me?*   You may be surprised by the power of your imagination, even if you think you don't have a good one. Staunch realists may need more practice in developing ease with imagery.

Also consider that imagery should be relaxing, not work. If it requires too much effort and you get anxious trying to induce images, imagery may not be right for you.

• *Is guided imagery covered by medical insurance?* Like many alternative treatments, guided imagery may be covered if recommended or performed by a health care professional.

Meditation

A look at the linguistic origins of the word *meditation* reveals its close link to healing. In Latin both *medicine* and *meditation* share the same root, which means "to cure" and "to measure." *Measure,* in this context, refers to the platonic concept of measure—that is, according to Jon Kabat-Zinn, founder and director of the Stress Reduction Clinic at the University of Massachusetts Medical Center, its inherent quality of wholeness. Bringing the body and mind to its "right inward measure" means achieving a state of health, balance, and wholeness that is in keeping with one's essential being (*Healing and the Mind,* edited by Bill Moyers, Doubleday).

By stilling the mind of its myriad earthly concerns, meditation offers access to the unconscious mind—to some it is a vehicle for spiritual unity. Sogyal Rinpoche, in *The Tibetan Book of Living and Dying,* defines meditation as "bringing the mind home." But in recent years studies have revealed significant health benefits of meditation, and nonreligious techniques have been developed to exploit them.

In the late 1960s Herbert Benson conducted successful studies with people using meditation to lower high blood pressure. Since that time a large body of research has accumulated supporting the value of meditation in helping to treat a number of health problems, ranging from anxiety and chronic pain to high cholesterol and substance abuse.

Some researchers assert that meditation's effects are less complicated. By helping to tame the mind, they maintain, meditation helps us cope with the stressors we face every day; it gives us control over the way we react to events that used to control us. And by lessening our reactivity to stress, we reduce the physical effects—such as headache.

History

Meditation is as old as religion. Indeed meditation is part of almost every spiritual discipline.

In the 1960s researchers became intrigued by reports from India of meditators who could control functions of the autonomic nervous system such as blood pressure, which normally cannot be consciously altered. This led to research, which has been considerable, into the health effects of meditation.

In some practices people meditate on a specific phrase or on the breath, the aim of which is to clear the mind of distracting thoughts and to achieve mental stillness and clarity. Some techniques are very complex and disciplined, while others rely on very simple mental or breathing exercises.

Today meditation is used by many health clinics, notably the Mind/Body Medical Institute at Harvard Medical School and Dean Ornish's Stress Reduction Clinic at the University of Massachusetts Medical Center. It is advocated by many well-known physicians, including Deepak Chopra and Bernie Siegal. It is now on the curriculum of hundreds of colleges and universities. An estimated six thousand physicians practice Transcendental Meditation, a relatively new and popular form of meditation.

How It Works

As mentioned, it appears that meditation induces the "relaxation response"—decreased heart rate, lower blood pressure, and reduced levels of the stress hormone cortisol, among other positive effects. With regular practice meditation can produce generalized benefits—that is, benefits that extend beyond the time of meditation into one's daily life.

Meditation offers a tool for dodging the effects of stressful events. Instead of reacting to the stress, people who meditate often find they can handle it more easily by returning to the still, calm place in the mind created by regular meditation. In this way meditation can help interrupt the stress-headache cycle.

Recent studies suggest that by reducing stress, meditation helps balance serotonin metabolism and "retune" an overstimulated nervous system.

Who Can Be Helped

Though meditation should not replace care from a professional (especially if the cause of headache has not been investigated), it can help people with all types of headache to control their pain.

What to Expect

There are many forms of meditation. It can be practiced while sitting (Transcendental Meditation), standing or lying down (qigong), or moving (Buddhist mindfulness meditation). It can involve focusing the mind on the breath (yoga), a word (any word will do), or a phrase (a prayer). It can be spiritually oriented or nonsecular. In terms of health benefits the type of meditation you choose to practice is less important than the amount of time you devote to it.

In general the practice of meditation begins with sitting or standing in a comfortable position in a place with as few distractions as possible. Plan to meditate for fifteen to twenty minutes. Some meditation instructors recommend closing your eyes, others advise keeping the eyes open; it's up to you.

Then you will either silently (or out loud) repeat a single word or phrase. Or simply focus on the breath. Or imagine a specific peaceful image. During this time many distracting thoughts and images will cross your mind's eye. Do not actively try to block them out. Imagine that these thoughts are floating on a river passing before you—here one second, gone the next. Simply continue to return to your point of focus.

Simple Meditation Exercise

This simple meditation exercise can be practiced by anyone:

1. Find a comfortable position—lying down or sitting either on the floor or in a straight-backed chair. If sitting, keep your

back straight without being rigid and let your hands rest in your lap. If your feet don't reach the floor, place a stool or books beneath them so that they rest on a firm surface.

2. Scan your body for tension from head to toe and relax your muscles. Unknit your eyebrows and unclench your jaw. Release your shoulders, arms, and belly. Let your spine lengthen, without becoming rigid, and your chin pull gently inward. Let your pelvis sink into the chair or ground.

3. Be aware of the sensation of your body touching the earth (or firm surface).

4. Close your eyes if you feel it's more comfortable.

5. Focus your mind on your breath as you inhale naturally. Breathe through your nose if you can. Feel the breath fill your chest and then your belly. Keep focused on the breath as you exhale, feeling it leave your belly and your chest. Alternately you can focus on the sensation of breath entering and leaving your nostrils.

6. Keep your eyes directed toward the end of your nose.

7. Keep your mind focused on your breath.

8. When thoughts cross your mind, gently note them, let them pass, and return to your breathing. Each time this happens, simply return to the breath.

9. Continue for fifteen minutes. It's okay to check the clock every so often.

10. Sit quietly for a few minutes.

You can use the breath as a focus, or select a word. Any simple, positive word or name will suffice.

Practice Schedule

Daily meditation is generally recommended to achieve the best results in health improvement. Try to practice once or twice a day, fifteen or twenty minutes at a time. But it is better to sacrifice time for consistency; if you only have five minutes, do it. Just as long as you do it every day.

Effectiveness

Meditation has been proven effective in many people with chronic pain, including headache. One study showed that 72 percent of meditators with chronic pain experienced a 33 percent reduction in pain after eight weeks of meditation, and 61 percent of meditators had a 50 percent reduction.[9]

Side Effects and Warnings

Though meditation is generally safe, there have been rare reports of negative psychological feelings after extended meditation retreats, and in schizophrenics reports of acute psychosis.

Finding a Reliable Meditation Instructor

Anyone can learn to meditate, and many people without certification or training teach it. Many continuing-education services, YMCAs, religious organizations, and universities offer courses in meditation. Check your community bulletin board. See the "Resources" section under "Meditation and Prayer" or "Yoga."

Questions and Answers

• *I am not very spiritual or religious; is meditation for me?*   While meditation is a spiritual practice for many people, you do not need to be spiritually oriented to benefit from its health benefits. You might want to seek out instruction from alternative health clinics or educational programs, such as those offered by the YMCA.

• *Will I become less rational if I meditate?*   Meditation is not known to erode the rational capabilities of the mind; rather its relaxing effects may help sharpen mental acuity.

• *I don't have time to meditate twice a day for fifteen minutes. What should I do?*   A shorter period of meditation every day is better than missing days. Consistency is the key to the health benefits.

• *Is meditation instruction covered by health insurance?*   It depends on your source of instruction. The likelihood of reimbursement is greater if meditation is part of a health program, for example at a stress-reduction or pain clinic, or if recommended by your health professional. Check with your insurance carrier.

Autogenic Training—Another Route to Relaxation

Autogenic training, developed by German physician Johannes H. Schultz, means "coming from" (*genic*) the self (*auto*). It is a simple exercise that combines verbal, visual, and sensory imagery to bring forth feelings of relaxation to different parts of the body.

Autogenic training exercises can be used to divert your attention away from your pain—for example focusing on your hands or legs while you have a headache—or as a regular practice to achieve general relaxation.

To begin, sit or lie down in a comfortable place. Close your eyes and direct your mind to your breathing. Use imagery that helps your breathing become more regulated. Many people use the image of waves rolling gently against a shore. As you imagine this, silently give your breath verbal messages, such as "My breath is free and relaxed." Repeat this message as you imagine your breath flowing like rolling waves through your body.

Use this same technique to relax the rest of your body, using whatever imagery you feel will bring you to a state of relaxation. Many people envision heat or heaviness ("My arms are heavy and warm, like melting honey"), while others might feel more relaxed with coolness and lightness ("My head is cool and light as a balloon").

You may want to spend more time on areas of tension, such as your neck and face muscles ("My neck muscles are opening and softening"). End the session with more breathing, and with suggestions of calmness ("I am peaceful and calm").

BIOFEEDBACK

It was once thought that involuntary body responses (in medical parlance, *autonomic* responses)—such as heart rate, blood flow, temperature, and brain wave activity—could not be consciously controlled. We now know that people can learn how to willfully control them. Biofeedback vividly reflects this mind-body effect.

Biofeedback is a term used to describe methods that measure specific autonomic responses and feed them back to the participant. When you use a thermometer to take your temperature, you're using a basic form of biofeedback. Typically the biofeedback instrument, when attached to the skin surface, amplifies and converts a physical response such as muscle tension into accessible information such as a flash of light or a line on a computer screen, thus making conscious the normally subliminal physical response. The participant can then use this information to regulate his or her own responses.

The most common types of biofeedback measures include

- *Electromyograph (EMG)*—electrical activity of muscles
- *Thermal (blood flow)*—blood flow and temperature
- *Electrocardiogram (EKG)*—heart rate
- *Electrodermal*—skin parameters, such as perspiration

The goal of biofeedback is to learn how to consciously regulate your own mental and physical processes for better health. Biofeedback has been used with great success in adults and children in relieving stress-related headache. Today many health professionals who treat headache commonly use biofeedback.

History

Biofeedback dates back to the 1930s, when O. Hobart Mowrer used a liquid-sensitive alarm system to help children with bedwetting problems. But it gained national notoriety in the 1960s when EEG feedback was employed to monitor how yogis regulated autonomic functions during meditation. While still considered an alternative therapy, biofeedback is widely used in a number of applications, including pain control, by physicians, behavioral psychologists, and pain experts.

How It Works

For people with headache, two types of biofeedback are mainly used.

- The *EMG* feedback can be used to regulate muscle tension, which is a known contributor to migraine, TMJ, and tension-type headache.
- *Thermal* biofeedback, used for people with vascular headaches such as migraine, redirects blood flow away from the head and toward the hands. The fingers are particularly sensitive to stress (blood vessel constriction) and relaxation (vasodilation).

However, researchers are still unsure about the mechanisms of biofeedback. Some believe its effectiveness stems from its ability to reduce stress. But others think that the success of biofeedback goes beyond stress reduction. With biofeedback therapy headache sufferers have been able to work specifically to increase blood flow and relax tense muscles that trigger headaches.

Who Can Be Helped

People with all types of headache may be helped by biofeedback— though it is important to make sure that the headache doesn't pose an immediate health risk before starting biofeedback. Children are particularly receptive to the effects of biofeedback.

What to Expect

A reliable biofeedback therapist will first ask that you get a full medical workup to rule out organic causes of your headache. Therapists may also rule out dietary causes as well.

Some therapists will obtain a "stress profile" through biofeedback techniques, which offers a dynamic view of how the body responds under stressful situations. Using either thermal, skin responses or EMG biofeedback, electrodes from the biofeedback instrument will be placed on your skin—either at your fingertips (for thermal feedback) or on specific muscles (for EMG). The machine will take a few seconds to equal out. Then you will be asked to relax. This helps the therapist understand the relaxation skills you already have. You will then be asked to evoke different emotions—think of something upsetting, something pleasurable and relaxing, something stressful. To gauge your stress level, you may be asked to do mental arithmetic.

During this time you will get "fed back" your physical responses to these emotional challenges—through either visual images or tones (or a combination) that reflect changes in your temperature, skin, or muscle tension. The therapist or practitioner will then teach you relaxation techniques you can use in conjunction with biofeedback. By seeing or hearing how your body causes these responses, you will acquire skills to change the rate of flashes or tones and alter your response.

The biofeedback images or tones can be computer manipulated. There are graphic images, for example, that make biofeedback more engaging and easier for children to use.

After you understand how to use biofeedback, you will often be asked to practice on your own at home and to keep a daily log of your progress. Some practitioners will make a personally tailored audiotape for you and ask that you practice twice a day with it, often in conjunction with relaxation techniques. The more you practice, the more effective biofeedback is. Practice not only helps improve skills, it helps create a *generalized* response, whereby the effects can be applied to different settings and situations.

Biofeedback can also be used as a springboard for examining your emotions and how they contribute to stress. In some practices counseling is an important complement to biofeedback—and family therapy may be particularly useful for children.

While biofeedback can be performed alone, having a therapist involved can be very useful in providing motivation and structure. Knowing that you have to report to someone may help improve your likelihood to practice throughout the week.

Treatment Schedule
The biofeedback sessions with a therapist may continue until you learn how to use biofeedback on your own, or experience relief of your

headache. They last thirty minutes to an hour. In some cases the thera-pist will use one type of biofeedback—usually muscle relaxation—for several weeks and, if there is no response, will try a different kind, such as thermal training.

Children are extremely receptive to biofeedback and can learn within five to six sessions. The patterns are less entrenched in children. They also don't have as many biases against psychological or behav-ioral approaches as adults. Because biofeedback is so successful in children, if they fail to respond quickly, therapists usually move to a different approach entirely, such as family therapy.

With adults the physical patterns are more embedded, and it may take ten or more sessions before they learn to "retrain" their headache patterns.

Effectiveness

Biofeedback has proved very effective for adults and children in managing a variety of types of headache, including TMJ. In general about 50 percent of people with headache will improve by between 50 and 80 percent.[10]

As stated above, children are generally the most receptive to this technique. Reports indicate that biofeedback is successful in treating up to 93 percent of children with chronic headaches. In one recent study all children with tension headache between the ages of twelve and fifteen who went twice a week for twelve sessions had significantly less headache pain, and this continued for at least one year.[11]

A number of studies have shown that biofeedback helps adults man-age their headache pain as well. In one study an eight-week program of biofeedback and autogenic training in people with a variety of headache types produced reductions in headache that lasted for up to one year.[12] Indeed, both migraine and tension headaches have proved responsive to biofeedback, either alone or combined with other relaxation tech-niques.[13]

Side Effects and Warnings

There are no known side effects to biofeedback. However, people with a cardiac pacemaker or heart problems should check with their doctor before embarking on a program.

Finding a Reliable Biofeedback Practitioner

While you can learn biofeedback on your own (see "Resources"), the level of effectiveness may be better with the initial guidance of a trained biofeedback practitioner or therapist. There are about ten thousand biofeedback practitioners in the United States, two thousand of whom have received certification from governing institutions. See the "Resources" section.

Questions and Answers

• *Isn't it dangerous to have electricity flowing into the body?*   Electricity doesn't actually course through your body; it only penetrates the top skin level to pick up surface responses. There have been no reports of adverse effects with biofeedback, although people with pacemakers or serious cardiac problems should get their doctor's okay before starting on a program.

• *Is biofeedback covered by medical insurance?*   Many insurance companies cover expenses for biofeedback, but not all. Check before starting.

PSYCHOTHERAPY

With a chronic illness like headache, distinguishing emotional from physical causes can be like untangling a knot of silk threads. Briefly here are a few of the ways they interact:

• *Stress and anxiety are common headache triggers.*
• *Chronic pain can erode emotional stability.*   Feeling unable to control pain can give rise to many negative feelings—helplessness,

anxiety, vulnerability, and in some cases depression are just a few examples.

- *Negative emotional states can lower the threshold to pain.*   When we feel good emotionally, we can generally tolerate more physical pain. Feeling bad emotionally makes pain feel more intense.
- *Pain may be a symptom of negative emotions.*   Emotions are sometimes translated into physical symptoms. This effect is called *somatization.* Headache, for example, is a common symptom of depression. But this does not mean that the headache is any less real or worthy of attention.

Stress is subjective. What determines whether an event is stressful or not is how we perceive it. It is the goal of many psychotherapeutic methods to increase our awareness of how we react to life events and to find ways of making them work better for us.

The word *psychotherapy* is a Greek word meaning "healing of the soul." In recent years psychotherapy has taken on many forms—but all aim to guide the individual toward better self-understanding, harmony, or physical health through examination of the mind's patterns.

There are many types of psychotherapy. While psychoanalysis, counseling, and family therapy may be useful in relieving headache, *cognitive therapy, behavioral therapy,* and *support groups* have proved particularly helpful for people suffering from chronic pain.

Cognitive Therapy

In essence *cognitive therapy* is a fancy term for giving yourself "a good talking to." Originated by Aaron Beck, a psychotherapist, in the 1960s, cognitive restructuring operates on the idea that cognition—or perception—is a powerful influence on the way we experience events, such as pain. Rather than focus on actions, as behavioral modification does, cognitive restructuring homes in on thoughts and attitudes that *create* behaviors. For example negative attitudes about headache can be self-fulfilling; if you believe that you will be in pain, you are more apt to be. In addition these negative attitudes can contribute to stress and muscle tension.

Cognitive therapy allows us to reevaluate the events in life as opportunities rather than setbacks. In this way cognitive therapy can defuse a stressful event of its power to cause physical or emotional pain. For example, just as we may talk ourselves into pain by having anxiety about it before an important event ("I have to make a big presentation tomorrow. I know I'll get a migraine"), we can reevaluate our feelings and find ways of making it a positive situation ("I have nothing to worry about because I'm well prepared for the presentation, so there's no reason for me to get a migraine tomorrow"). In essence, cognitive restructuring helps you create a more positive internal dialogue.

To achieve this, you may be asked to keep a headache diary, noting when you experienced pain, your thoughts about it, and the actions you took. Looking at this diary will help you find patterns in the way you "talk to yourself" about headaches, or even how stressful events contribute to their onset. Then you and your therapist (though you can do this alone too), will devise constructive ways of breaking those patterns, such as relaxation training to cope with stress, or positive new thoughts to replace negative ones.

Giving yourself a good talking to can be very effective. In one study people who suffered chronic tension headaches who did cognitive therapy found between 43 and 100 percent improvement, compared with no improvement among people who did not.[14] And its success can be enhanced by combining it with behavioral therapy, relaxation techniques, or biofeedback.

Behavioral Modification

The main tenet of behavioral therapy is that all behaviors are learned or conditioned through positive reinforcement—and they can be unlearned and replaced through positive reinforcement.

According to behavioral therapists, habitual, counterproductive ways of coping with chronic pain can become embedded in the brain due to positive reinforcement. Following this reasoning, it's easy to see how some people become dependent on pain-relieving drugs: The pain relief becomes the positive reinforcement for the behavior of taking drugs.

Behavioral therapy aims to break negative patterns by first identifying your "pain behavior"—how you consciously and unconsciously manage pain. Second, behavioral therapy helps you pinpoint ways of breaking those patterns with individually tailored exercises or tasks. Positive reinforcement is given for achieving these tasks and is withheld when they are not performed.

Cognitive therapy and behavior modification have been used hand-in-hand, with much success for people with tension-related or migraine headaches.

Support Groups

The positive power of support groups claimed widespread attention with a study by David Spiegel, a psychiatrist at Stanford University, who found that women with breast cancer attending support groups lived twice as long as those who did not. Though increased longevity is a goal most desire, it is not necessarily a top-of-mind issue for people with chronic benign headache—but the other benefits of social support may be.

Support groups can help people cope with pain in several ways. For example many people feel isolated by their pain. Spending time with people who have similar problems can feel like a safe way of socializing. It's also a good way to pick up tips on coping with pain, to share experiences, and to vent emotions.

The Healthful Effects of Helping

A variation of getting social support is being *supportive*. Compassion and engaging in altruistic efforts has been shown to produce a "helper's high"—a feel-good effect that can translate into relief from a number of chronic conditions. At least that's what was seen in a large study of volunteers for Big Brother/Big Sister of New York. In his study executive director Allan Luks found that volunteers reported fewer symptoms of chronic headache, back pain, and stomachache.

Why does helping help? Some observers suggest that taking part in a cause that is bigger than yourself elicits some of the same physical "relaxation" responses as meditation and yoga. Other early research seems to indicate that social bonding releases endorphins.

Helping can take many forms, but the most effective, healthwise, are efforts that involve regular, personal contact with people who are not family members.

Finding a Reliable Therapist, Counselor, or Support Group

Ask your doctor or health care professional for a referral. Or contact one of the organizations listed in the "Resources" section.

ENERGY/SPIRITUAL METHODS

Energy therapy, or laying on of hands, is as old as healing. Hieroglyphics, ancient Chinese texts, and Hippocratic writings all make reference to the therapeutic power that emits from the healer's hands. Some believe that this power is mediated by a higher force; faith healing is an example. Others explain the human energy field as the mechanism of healing.

While the latter theory suggests a physical effect, the power of these healing methods originates in the mind, in the intent, of the healer. In this way more direct healing methods such as Therapeutic Touch and Reiki intersect with nondirect methods such as prayer—all of which depend on the intended thoughts and energies of an individual.

Prayer

Meaning "to beseech or implore," prayer is central to virtually every spiritual discipline. Its link with healing is almost implicit: In this religious context prayer is often used to connect with a higher power.

But prayer can also be a vehicle for self-generating health. Though religious sources may prescribe specific prayers, it does not seem to matter *how* one prays. It can be a social or an individual effort, spoken out loud or silently, directed to a specific deity or not. Herbert Benson, a founder of the Mind/Body Institute at Harvard University Medical School, found that prayer, like meditation and other mind-focusing techniques, can induce the relaxation response.

However, prayer may also engage another dimension, which is termed ''nonlocal'' by Larry Dossey, M.D., author of *Healing Words: The Power of Prayer and the Practice of Medicine* (HarperSan-Francisco). That is, the intent of prayer is often directed to the healing of another being at a distance.

That prayer can be effective in helping another person has been shown (albeit inconsistently); why it works has not. The concept of a universal energy, or energy fields, that transport the healing intent of one person to the next has been used to explain the power of prayer and other nonlocal or ''at a distance'' healing methods. This ''naturalistic'' explanation is countered by those who endorse a ''supernatural'' medium for healing—that is, the belief in the existence of a supernatural being.

Scientific research into the effects of prayer are few, but growing. A compilation of this research on spiritual healing can be found in a book by David J. Benor, M.D., called *Healing Research* (Helix Verlag GmBH, 1993). In it Dr. Benor documents over 131 controlled trials of people who intentionally tried to exert influence on the physical nature of another being. Some of the studies include effects on life-forms such as bacteria, but there is one study documenting the efficacy of Therapeutic Touch (see below) on tension headache.

Therapeutic Touch

Therapeutic Touch is a modern method of healing based on some of the same energy concepts that guide many ancient systems of medicine.

As with traditional Oriental and Indian approaches, Therapeutic Touch adheres to the belief that there is an invisible energy (qi, prana) within us all that can be accessed and directed to therapeutic benefit. A nonreligious and common expression of this concept is the soothing effects of touch to the ailing infant. Therapeutic Touch is a formal way of harnessing that natural phenomenon.

The term *Therapeutic Touch,* as it exists today, is something of a misnomer. While originally the practitioner made physical contact with the subject, now the hands generally rest several inches away from the ailing person's body.

History

Therapeutic Touch has its roots in the ancient healing method known as *laying on of hands.* It was not until the mid 1970s that Dolores "Dee" Kreiger, Ph.D., R.N., and Dora Kunz, a clairvoyant and healer, formalized this age-old method and called it Therapeutic Touch. Though originally a method linked with religious ritual and beliefs, Therapeutic Touch today is a nonsecular approach, practiced and received by people without religious overtones. Refinements on the technique (described below) and research into its clinical benefits are under way.

Today Therapeutic Touch is widely used by clinicians, nurses, therapists, massage therapists, and psychologists as well as laypeople without any kind of formal medical background. It was one of the first courses in healing to appear on the curriculum of an accredited college or university. Therapeutic Touch has been taught to more than forty-two thousand people, and exists on more than one hundred college and university curricula.

How It Works

That Therapeutic Touch works to relieve muscle tension, reduce swelling, and eliminate headaches has been shown in an uncontrolled study and anecdotal reports; the reasons why it works has not. It is postulated that through the transfer of energy from one person to another, Therapeutic Touch helps restore balance to the immune system, thus laying the foundation for the body to generate its own healing abilities.

Therapeutic Touch does not aim to relieve symptoms but to help the entire person. A true holistic modality, Therapeutic Touch engages the whole individual to help bring about a state of health.

Who Can Be Helped

As a completely safe and noninvasive method there are no limits to the type of headache that can theoretically be helped with Therapeutic Touch. However, it is very important that you seek medical attention to rule out life-threatening causes of headache before turning to Therapeutic Touch.

What to Expect

There are four phases to a Therapeutic Touch session: centering, assessment, balancing, and reassessment.

For your session with a Therapeutic Touch practitioner wear loose, comfortable clothing. You will lie down on a table or a mat on the floor while the practitioner stands or sits near you. In most cases the practitioner will never touch you; for most of the session her hands will be suspended several inches away from your body.

• *Centering.* The practitioner will first sit silently beside you for a few moments. During this time she is directing her energy inward to a state of stillness, awareness of her own and your energy field, receptivity, and empathy.

• *Assessment.* Once centered, the practitioner will suspend her hands three to five inches over a part of your body. During this phase she is trying to pick up sensations that might indicate energy imbalance—roughness in the energy field, changes in temperature, and so on—and signs of balanced energy, which may be experienced as a gentle vibration. At the same time you might feel similar sensations.

• *Balancing.* As with traditional Eastern systems, Therapeutic Touch aims to balance excesses in energy and remove blockages. Toward this end the practitioner, through directed thought and movement of her hands, will "smooth out" roughness, reduce heat with coolness (or vice versa), and so on. During this time you may feel sensations of energy movement, such as a release of tension or changes in temperature, or relaxation, or pain relief.

• *Reassessment.*   At this point the practitioner determines whether the energy has been balanced and whether to move on to another area of the body.

Treatment Schedule

Each Therapeutic Touch session lasts about half an hour. The number of sessions you need depends on many factors. The treatment schedule depends on your results, your connection with the practitioner, and your commitment to the approach.

Effectiveness

The effectiveness of Therapeutic Touch in the prevention or treatment of headache is still anecdotal. However, several studies have shown Therapeutic Touch to effectively reduce stress; in more than one study the results were statistically significant.[15] In another study of people with tension headache, five minutes of Therapeutic Touch significantly reduced headache.[16]

Side Effects

A completely noninvasive method, Therapeutic Touch is free from side effects.

Warnings

There are no warnings associated with treatment with Therapeutic Touch; however, there may be danger in delaying care for a life-threatening condition. Be sure to rule out organic causes of disease before starting any alternative modality.

Finding a Reliable Therapeutic Touch Practitioner

Anyone can learn Therapeutic Touch because, according to proponents, anyone with awareness has the basic "tools" needed for healing.

There are numerous seminars, books, and tapes available. Anyone can practice Therapeutic Touch. If you feel more comfortable with a practitioner associated with a professional organization, contact the Nurse Healers Professional Associates—a good source for information on books, seminars, and referrals to practitioners who have undergone some formal training. Not all members of the organization are nurses. See the "Resources" section.

Questions and Answers

• *How do I know if Therapeutic Touch is working?* The best sign is relief from your headaches. If used as a preventive measure, it may take some time to recognize an improvement in your pattern of headaches.

• *How do I know if the practitioner is qualified?* Since you do not need to be licensed or certified to practice Therapeutic Touch, you have to rely on your instincts and results. Some practitioners have received training; ask about it. By the same token, you could learn Therapeutic Touch, or take some courses with a partner or friend, so that you can practice it on each other.

• *Is Therapeutic Touch covered by health insurance?* Many practitioners of Therapeutic Touch also perform other types of therapy—many are nurses, physical therapists, massage therapists. If the type of treatment your practitioner generally offers is covered by health insurance, and Therapeutic Touch is one of the modalities he or she uses, it may be covered. Check with your practitioner.

Reiki

Reiki is a Tibetan healing art; the word means "universal life energy." While it recognizes the presence of a higher intelligence, Reiki is not a religion. Like Therapeutic Touch, Reiki is used by people of all religious (or nonspiritual) backgrounds and is regarded as an adjunct to other healing practices by a growing number of health care professionals. Yet unlike other methods that draw on universal energy (such as traditional Oriental medicine and Ayurveda), Reiki students are formally initiated into the practice through ceremonies that can have distinct spiritual overtones.

History

Reiki's sources trace back to ancient Tibetan writings. But it was not until the mid 1800s that Mikau Usui, the head of a Christian seminary in Kyoto, Japan, uncovered, in ancient Buddhist texts called *sutras,* a series of healing methods he termed Reiki.

Usui passed his learnings on to a Japanese physician, who in turn treated and initiated Madame Hawayo Takata into Reiki. It was through the work of Madame Takata that Reiki became introduced to the West.

How It Works

The mechanism for Reiki healing is very similar to that of Therapeutic Touch (see page 289). However, the initiation into Reiki practice is often much more elaborate.

The initiation, or *attunement* process, involves a series of steps and rituals designed to open the chakras, or energy centers, of the body in order to receive and fine-tune the universal healing energy.

The initiate in Reiki goes through up to Four Degrees, or steps, of training. In the First Degree, students learn ways of healing themselves and others through physical or near-physical touch. In the Second Degree, attunement is directed toward intensifying the flow of energy and the practitioner's commitment to the concepts of Reiki practice. The Third Degree is available only to students who are seriously committed to Reiki, for they are exposed to a more powerful degree of Reiki energy; in some schools, Third Degree graduates are called Master Therapists. The Fourth Degree is that of Master Teacher, available only to select individuals who want to dedicate their lives to the preservation of Reiki.

Who Can Be Helped

Since Reiki does not purport to treat specific illness but rather the individual, anyone may theoretically benefit from Reiki.

What to Expect

The experience of Reiki may feel very similar to that described for Therapeutic Touch. The therapist rests his or her hands on or above the body to access specific energy centers, or chakras. In Reiki the positioning of the hands is very specifically prescribed and is usually held for five minutes, or until the therapist perceives a change in energy flow. As with Therapeutic Touch, you may experience changes in temperature or sensation.

Treatment Schedule

The sessions last between sixty and ninety minutes and can be continued for as many sessions as you think necessary.

Effectiveness

Though there are many anecdotal reports that Reiki helps relieve pain and headache, it has not been subject to much formal study.

Side Effects and Warnings

There are no known side effects to Reiki. As with all alternative treatments, make sure your doctor rules out any potentially dangerous causes of your headache before pursuing Reiki.

Finding a Reliable Reiki Therapist

There are several organizations that give training for Reiki practitioners (see "Resources").

Questions and Answers

• *Do I need to have strong spiritual beliefs to benefit from Reiki?*   Reiki is a healing process, and while the practitioner may have strongly held spiritual beliefs, it is not necessary that you uphold them in order to benefit. Like Therapeutic Touch, Reiki practitioners believe that the universal healing energy is accessible to everyone, regardless of his or her spiritual belief system or lack thereof.

• *Is Reiki covered by medical insurance?*   Like Therapeutic Touch, it depends on who administers Reiki—it's more likely to be covered if a nurse or physical therapist performs it—and the limitations of your specific insurance plan.

CHAPTER 9

Botanical Remedies

The green gifts of Mother Earth are
individual, singular, unique.
—*SUSUN WEED,* Healing Wise

——————

Of all the healing methods used by humankind, none have been more consistent or universal than plant remedies. In contrast with the pharmaceutical industry, which extracts and synthesizes the purported *active ingredient* of a plant into drugs, herbalists generally believe that the power of herbs extends beyond their extractable essences. In their whole form therapeutic plants often have complementary qualities that may help protect against side effects and, according to some schools of thought, help balance and restore harmony in awareness.

In this chapter we will look at two forms of botanical remedies: herbal therapy and aromatherapy. At the end of each section you will find guidelines for preparing remedies.

Important Cautionary Information

The scientific information presented in this chapter is usually considered preliminary and is not meant as a recommendation to take or use particular substances.

Not all herbs are safe. By law therapeutic claims cannot be made for herbal preparations that have not gone through the review process of the Food and Drug Administration. This means that herbs are not considered medicine and should not be touted as such. You should be wary of any herb resources that make fantastic claims for cures.

In this section we provide information from published sources about the potential benefits of plants. Most reports of their success in helping people with headache are anecdotal or traditional—the herbs have not undergone clinical study. I urge you to exercise caution in taking plant-derived herbs on your own.

HERBAL THERAPY

Though botanists may define herbs as the leafy part of a plant, herbal preparations may use the leaf, flower, berry, stem, bark, or root—in short, any part of the plant. Depending on the herb and its use, plants can be taken in a variety of forms—dried in their whole form, teas, capsules, tinctures, oils, or ointments.

The roots of herbal therapy trace back to the earliest days of humankind. It is the foundation of all medical systems; about 80 percent of the world's population still relies on traditional therapies, and herbal treatments are a mainstay.

Today India leads the world in the use of plant-based medicinals, according to the American Herb Association. In the Ayurvedic medical tradition, herbs are characterized by their taste, or essence, and are used to bring harmony to constitutional imbalances that contribute to illness. Classic Ayurvedic texts describe more than five hundred plants with therapeutic value. Often the plant preparations take the form of herbs in foods or oils applied to the body in massage.

Herbal therapy is also a central healing modality in traditional Chinese medicine. Like dietary prescriptions, Chinese herbal medicines aim to bring balance to blockages in the circulation of qi, the universal life force. A recent compilation of medicinal plants contains 5,767 entries. Traditional Japanese medicine, called *kampo,* combines Chinese herbal traditions with Japanese folk medicine.

These are just a few of the medical systems that rely on herbal therapies. A long tradition of herbal medicine in Native American cultures still thrives among many groups today. Naturopathic medicine, which advocates the healing power of nature to treat the whole individual, makes ample use of herbal medicine.

The modern Western application of herbs has largely taken the form of pharmaceutical preparations. However, a more naturalistic approach to the use of herbs is now experiencing a renaissance. Many organizations have sprung up over recent years to formally study the medicinal qualities of plants. In addition herbal approaches dovetail with the revival of holistic, environmental, and spiritual movements.

History

There is evidence of herbal medicine in the burial site of a Neanderthal man dating back sixty thousand years. Throughout history plants have been extolled not only for their medicinal value but for use as foods and dyes and in religious ceremonies. Written records of herbal therapies can be found in Sumerian texts over seven thousand years old. Ancient Chinese medical texts dating to 2,500 B.C. document more than three hundred herbal remedies. Hippocrates extolled the virtues of plants as a way to preserve the life force. Hundreds of *herbals* (herb books) have been written since the Middle Ages. The tradition of herbal healing continued, virtually uninterrupted, until the seventeenth century, when rationalism began to supplant folkloric medical approaches in favor of chemical medicine.

The pharmaceutical industry, which has disparaged the use of herbal and "unproven" therapies, actually owes a great debt to traditional herbal medicine; an estimated 25 percent of the drugs in use today were either derived directly from or synthesized to imitate natural plants[1]— and 74 percent of these were discovered based on traditional uses. Indeed in their search for more products many pharmaceutical companies are now investing time and money to investigate the chemical properties of plants.

Today, as the limitations of pharmaceuticals become more apparent—side effects and the inability to effectively manage chronic ill-ness—there has been a renewed interest in less invasive and more natural approaches, such as herbal therapy. In Germany, for example, an estimated 40 to 80 percent of physicians regularly prescribe herbal medicines. In France, herbal medicines are reimbursed 40 percent by the national health plan.

How It Works

There are several views on how herbal medicines work. The scientific tradition sees herbal remedies like drugs: They have chemical qualities that exert biological effects on different parts of the body to treat specific disorders. From this perspective herbs fit nicely into the allopathic view of medicine, which advocates treating a disease with an opposing agent (e.g., treat bacterial infection with an antibacterial).

Naturopathic physicians and many herbalists endow herbal remedies with wider-ranging properties. For while the end results of herbal remedies may be measurable on specific body systems, the route toward these effects is not the same as that of allopathic drugs, and this is what makes the difference in their safety and overall health value. Rather than working directly *against* a specific condition, herbal preparations purportedly work *with* the body to stimulate its own healing abilities, say naturalistic herbalists. As expressions of life themselves, plant remedies may be more gentle on the body than drugs—more easily absorbed, metabolized, and excreted. As unpurified compounds that contain a variety of complementary qualities, herbal therapies may be used to treat more than one type of condition at a time. And as indirect methods of achieving a result, they may take longer to take action.

General Guidelines for Taking Herbs

• *Not all herbs are harmless.*   Herbs may be very potent and in some cases very harmful. It's important that you follow directions as closely as possible to get the best effect. Start out by seeking the advice of a qualified professional with a background in herbology.

• *Find good sources for your herbs.*   Some of the herbs come from your kitchen pantry, such as ginger. Other must be ordered or bought from a store. Make sure that your herbs come from reliable sources (we'll list organizations to help you find them in the "Resources" section). Avoid herbal capsules or pills, which often have been stored for long periods. Herbs should optimally be:

Fresh dried and locally grown—helps ensure that they have not been stored for long periods
Organic (free of pesticides)
Bought in small amounts at a time to preserve freshness
Have a pungent aroma and firm texture; avoid herbs that look brown and crumble easily

• *Proper storage preserves potency.* Store herbs in dark-colored, sealed containers away from light and heat.

• *Dosages for children should be reduced.* The doses we recommend in the following pages are for adults. Consult with a reliable herbalist for children's dosages.

• *If you are pregnant, exercise greater care.* Before taking any herb, seek the advice of your doctor or someone who specializes in women's health.

• *Essential oils of herbs are often more potent.* Some herbs, such as pennyroyal, can be very toxic or even lethal when taken internally in the form of essential oils. Consult the "Aromatherapy" section for guidelines on effective herbal preparations for headache.

What follows is a compendium of herbal remedies that may be of help for people with headaches. Wherever possible, we will include studies that confirm their effectiveness, however most of the reports are anecdotal and their use in headache remains unproven by modern medical standards.

Ayurvedic Herbals for Headache

Note: Avoid these if you have very sensitive skin.

- *General headache remedy:* Mix ½ teaspoon ginger powder with water to form a paste; heat and apply to forehead. May cause a slight burning sensation.
- *Sinus headache:* Apply ginger paste to forehead.
- *Headache at the base of the skull:* Mix 1 teaspoon flaxseed with a warm glass of water and drink before bedtime. Also apply ginger paste behind the ears.

Burdock Root (*Articum lappa*)

Burdock root is a popular vegetable and a remedy that is harvested in the spring.

Effectiveness
Burdock root has a wide range of qualities that may be of benefit to the headache sufferer. It is thought to be a potent blood purifier and immune-system booster (useful for people with food allergies). Long-term use of burdock *root* may help stabilize blood sugar in people with hypoglycemia, though short-term use may lower blood sugar. In combination with dandelion, burdock *root* or *leaf* may help headaches around the top of the head and forehead and assuage PMS-related headaches.

Dosage
Infusion of dry burdock *root:* 1–2 cups a day.
Tea of burdock *leaf:* ¼–4 cups day.

Cayenne Pepper (*Capsicum frutescens*)

Capsaicin is the main ingredient in hot peppers.

Effectiveness

Capsaicin has a long history of pain relief. It has been shown to stimulate and block pain fibers by depleting them of substance P, in this way inhibiting platelet aggregation and pain. In a few studies, capsaicin has been shown effective in the treatment of cluster headaches.[2,3]

In one study with intranasal use of a capsaicin ointment, cluster headaches were reduced not only in quantity but also in severity when compared with a placebo.

Dosage

Capsaicin can be made at home by mixing cayenne pepper with water to form an ointment and applied inside the nostrils, or a commercial ointment containing 0.025 or 0.075 percent capsaicin can be bought over the counter.

Side Effects and Warnings

Capsaicin may cause burning or irritation of the skin and the sensitive mucous membranes of the nose. Also avoid excessive and prolonged use, which may cause intestinal, liver, or kidney problems.

Chamomile (*Anthemis nobilis*)

English chamomile, also known as Roman chamomile, is the type of chamomile used for headache disorders—not to be confused with German chamomile. The *flowers* of this pretty and pleasant-scented herb have traditionally been used therapeutically. The *essential oil* of chamomile can be used as well (see ''Aromatherapy,'' page 312).

Effectiveness

Chamomile tea is a known sedative, offering bodywide relaxing effects. It has also been shown to have antihistamine effects, so it may be of help in allergies. In addition chamomile has relaxing effects on the smooth muscles of the intestine. It has traditionally been useful in relieving nausea associated with migraine.

Dosage

Chamomile *tea:* ½ ounce flowers steeped in 2 cups water for up to 20 minutes.

Chamomile *oil:* See "Aromatherapy," page 312.

Side Effects and Warnings

There are no known side effects or warnings associated with chamomile tea in moderation (no more than two cups a day); however, people with hayfever or allergies to plants may have an allergic reaction.

Dandelion (*Taraxacum officinale*)

This scourge of suburban lawn-tenders is one of the most vital of herbs; virtually every part of the dandelion may have healthful benefits. The zesty leaves make a good salad and are filled with minerals and vitamins that are good for the headache sufferer, including *magnesium* and *B vitamins.*

Effectiveness

Dandelion is a mild laxative and digestive, thus offering help for people with constipation-related headaches. In combination with burdock root, long-term use of dandelion can help relieve headaches and PMS-related disorders.

Dosage

Dandelion leaf infusion: ½ to 2 cups a day.

Feverfew (*Tinacetum parthenium*)

The benefits of feverfew as a headache remedy date to the early seventeenth century. A close cousin of Roman chamomile, it is referred to in Europe as *grande camomile* and *matricaria parthenium.*

Effectiveness

Feverfew has gained much attention for the studies that show it as a well-tolerated way of preventing and treating migraine headache—though there are suggestions that it may be of help for people with cluster and menstrual-related headaches as well.

Its purported effectiveness is attributed to a group of compounds called *sequiterpene lactones,* which inhibit platelet clumping, serotonin, and prostaglandins (which cause inflammation), and improve blood vessel tone. It has been studied in the laboratory, both in animals and in humans.

The first known report of its use, from *Prevention* magazine, was of a sixty-eight-year-old woman who had suffered migraines for fifty-two years. After chewing three feverfew leaves every day for ten months, her migraines disappeared.

There have been several studies of feverfew in people with migraine. In one, a survey of 270 migraine sufferers who chewed feverfew leaves, 70 percent found relief in the number and severity of their attacks.[4]

In another, a well-controlled clinical study, fifty-nine people with migraine took either dried feverfew leaves in capsules or a placebo. The results were reported in the medical journal *The Lancet.*[5] After four months they switched regimens. Feverfew reduced the number of migraine attacks by 32 percent, and the severity of attacks by 26 percent in people who had migraine with aura. Among those who suffered migraine without aura, the number of attacks was reduced by 23 percent and the severity by 13 percent. The main side effect was mouth ulceration, but there were more reports of this effect among people taking the placebo.

Dosage

Based on the above studies, some researchers recommend taking 125 mg of a dried feverfew-leaf preparation that contains at least 0.2 percent parthenolide. But there is some debate over this. In investigating feverfew, the head of the Natural Products Bureau of Drug Research in Canada found that dried feverfew leaves lose up to 20 percent of their potency if left at room temperature for a year, and 50 percent after two years. However, there have been reports that the flowerheads contain up to four times as much parthenolide as the leaves.

Since the effectiveness of feverfew flowers has not been studied, and they may contain pollens that cause allergies, it's recommended that people use the leaves. Chewing two fresh or freeze-dried leaves will give you about 170 mg of feverfew; alternately you can take 125 mg of prepared, dried feverfew that contains at least 0.2 percent parthenolide. Make sure that the preparation or the fresh leaf is *authenticated* feverfew, that is, *Tinacetum parthenium*.

Side Effects and Warnings

Though relatively safe, feverfew may cause mouth sores or stomach upset, which caused 7 to 8 percent of people in studies to stop taking it. The mouth sores are *not* caused by contact direct with fresh or dried leaf—they've been seen in people taking encapsulated forms as well. Some researchers do not recommend feverfew for pregnant or lactating mothers, or for children under two. Consult your physician, herbalist, or naturopathic physician if you want to take feverfew for more than four months in a row.

Ginger (*Zingiber officinale*)

Ginger has been used medicinally in China for thousands of years and is a common ingredient in many foods in China, Japan, and India for its taste and digestion-enhancing qualities. It is also an Ayurvedic medicinal for treating pain and related conditions.

Effectiveness

Ginger has anti-inflammatory qualities; it not only reduces inflammation of blood vessels, and the pain-sensitizing chemical prostaglandin, but helps reduce platelet clumping. It may also help improve circulation.

There is anecdotal and folkloric information about the effectiveness of ginger in relieving headache. In one recent report a forty-two-year-old woman with migraine took ginger at the beginning of an aura and found relief within thirty minutes. The dose she took was 500 to 600 mg powdered ginger in water. She then started adding fresh ginger to her meals and found marked reductions in her pattern of migraine.

Dosage

As a *tea:* 1 ounce fresh grated gingerroot (rhizome) to 2 cups water.

As a *paste:* Use fresh ginger cut up finely or powdered ginger with water to form a paste. Apply directly to the head.

Side Effects and Warnings

Ginger should be avoided by pregnant women.

Gingko (*Gingko biloba*)

Gingko is mentioned in the traditional Chinese herb texts and has been extracted into drugs in Germany and France.

Effectiveness

In a recent report in the *Lancet* gingko was shown to help increase blood flow to the brain and to inhibit platelet clumping. In Germany it is licensed for use for headaches and memory disorders.

Dosage

Taken as an extract, it has been shown by most studies to be safe at 120 to 160 mg a day, in three divided doses. It can take up to six weeks before people start experiencing relief.

Goldenseal (*Hydrastis canadensis*)

Goldenseal has been traditionally used by many Native Americans for skin diseases. Recently it has been found to lower blood pressure. It is also of value in relieving headaches related to sinusitis.

Effectiveness

Goldenseal contains chemical compounds known as alkaloids that have an astringent effect, drying out mucous membranes and reducing inflammation.

Dosage

It's best to drink goldenseal as an infusion, of ¼ part goldenseal root with 1 part each echinacea, eyebright, and peppermint. Drink no more than 1 cup for no longer than 1 week.

Side Effects and Warnings

Goldenseal stimulates the uterus and must be avoided by pregnant women. Due to its blood-pressure-lowering effects, it should also be avoided if you have low blood pressure.

Guarana (*Paullinia cupana*)

The seeds from guarana are powdered and used to make a beverage that is popular in Brazil for relieving chronic headaches and migraines.

Effectiveness

Guarana has been shown in studies to inhibit platelet clumping. Its traditional use for headache is probably attributed to the high caffeine content. As we know, caffeine can be a double-edged sword for the headache sufferer; it can relieve headache in moderate doses—it's part of several headache drugs—or trigger them when used daily for some sensitive individuals.

Dosage

Guarana *tea:* 1 teaspoon guarana seeds to 1 cup water.

Side Effects and Warnings

Guarana is high in caffeine and should not be taken by individuals who are sensitive to caffeine. Nor should it be given to young children or taken by pregnant or lactating mothers. It should not be taken for prolonged periods, since daily caffeine consumption can trigger head-aches.

Nettle (*Urtica dioica*)

Stinging nettle has traditionally been used for everything from asthma to hair care. Its value as a general tonic for women is widely known today, though its benefits extend to men as well.

Effectiveness
Nettle has been shown to reduce inflammation. As an infusion nettle leaves and stalks are thought to normalize adrenal function. Over time and at low doses it may also help relieve allergies, chronic headaches, and nerve inflammation. Its nutritive effects on the endocrine and hormonal systems may help relieve headaches associated with menstruation.

Dosage
One to 2 cups of infusion daily.

Side Effects and Warnings
None.

Valerian (*Valeriana officinalis*)

The root of valerian has been used traditionally for a variety of medicinal reasons, including the treatment of epilepsy, fevers, and to provide general relaxation.

Effectiveness
Valerian is a gentle, non-narcotic, natural tranquilizer when taken in moderate doses (see page 310), having relaxing effects on the central nervous system. These antianxiety effects may make it useful in preventing tension-related headaches and migraines.

Dosage

Valerian *root tea:* 1 teaspoon valerian root in 1 cup water once a day, when feeling nervous or anxious.

Side Effects and Warnings

Do not take more than the recommended dose, and do not take for prolonged periods, as valerian may actually *cause* its opposite effect—headaches and muscle spasm—at high doses. If you experience strange sensations, discontinue.

White Willow Bark (*Salix alba*)

The Pomo, Natchez, Alabama, Creek, and Penobscot Indians knew of willow bark's pain-relieving qualities long before it became that medicine-chest standby, aspirin.

Effectiveness

Willow bark contains salicin, an aspirinlike compound that inhibits prostaglandin (the pain-sensitizing chemical in the body) and works on the immune system to reduce fever. However, because it does not act in the stomach, willow bark does not cause the stomach upset common with its synthesized counterpart. In fact it is known to be good for heartburn and stomach disorders.

Dosage

Willow bark *tea:* 1 cup per day.

Side Effects and Warnings

At recommended doses, willow bark is quite safe.

Other Herbs That May Be of Help in Headache

• *Garlic* and *onion* help improve circulation and reduce platelet aggregation and may be helpful for migraine (taken raw or in enteric-coated capsules to reduce odor), but they should be avoided in people taking anticoagulants (blood-thinning medications).

• *Rescue Remedy* is a widely available Bach Flower Remedy that contains the flowers star-of-Bethlehem, rock rose, impatiens, cherry plum, and clematis. It is available in concentrated form, which is then added, drop by drop, to water or used externally in compresses or creams. For a headache in progress, add 4 drops to 1 cup water and sip slowly until finished. After that take a sip every fifteen, thirty, or sixty minutes. For prevention try 4 drops in water four times a day.

How to Prepare Herbs

We have referred to several methods of preparing herbs. What follows are directions for preparing herbal medicines.

Tea

Pour hot water over herbs. For best results let the water cool for a minute before pouring into the cup. Let sit for five to twenty minutes, depending on the strength you want.

Infusion

More potent than tea, since an infusion must steep for a while in a closed container and is often stored between doses. Use a close-fitting pot or a canning jar.

• *Leaves:* 1 ounce dried leaves to 1 quart boiling water. Infuse at least four hours at room temperature.

• *Bark and roots:* 1 ounce dried root or dried bark (cut up in 6-inch pieces) with 2 cups water. Infuse at room temperature for up to eight hours.

• *Flowers:* 1 ounce dried flowers and 1 quart water. Infuse for up to two hours at room temperature.

• *Combination infusions:* Brew each component separately and then combine, unless the combination is all leaves or all roots.

To Dry Your Own Herbs

One way to ensure the quality of herbs is to grow and dry them yourself. To retain their medicinal value, harvest flowering herbs when they are in bud, before they have opened. If cutting leaves, do so early in the day on a dry day—they should not be wet or damp. Be careful not to crush or bruise the plant. Gently shake off any insects. Discard any discolored weeds.

Hang herbs in small bunches or in a paper bag in a dark, open room. Allow the seeds to dry on the plant for three to seven days; it should still smell and look like the fresh plant. The leaves will be brittle, but not crumbly, to the touch. Flowers should rustle slightly.

Harvest roots in the fall, at the end of the growing season. To prepare roots, wipe off dirt but do not wash. Either string up or dry flat, turning often. Roots may take longer to dry than herbs, about five to seven days. They should be dry enough to snap in half or chip.

Finding a Reliable Herbalist

There is no standard licensing for herbalists. The following organizations may refer you to others that offer instruction in herbal therapy or to professionally trained individuals in alternative disciplines—traditional Oriental medicine, Ayurveda, naturopathy—who may have background in herbal therapy. We refer you to the ''Resources'' section for educational books and tapes on herbal therapies.

AROMATHERAPY

The name of this close cousin of herbal medicine implies that it works by virtue of its scent, but aromatherapy's medicinal effects can be attributed to other properties as well.

Defined as the art and science of using essential plant oils in medical treatments, the effects of aromatherapy derive from the potency and small size of the molecules, which make them readily absorbed through the skin and bronchial passages into the bloodstream to produce body-wide effects. Some of the effects may occur via stimulation of the olfactory (smell sense) nerve. This nerve, though not large, is widely connected to the rest of the brain.

Aromatherapy belies its name in that its essential oils are not just inhaled but can be used in massage, in aromatic baths, as hot or cold compresses, or as simple skin applications. In keeping with its name, however, aromatherapy does employ volatile oils that are indeed often inhaled.

The seriousness of aromatherapy as a clinical approach has been somewhat undermined in the United States. *Aromatherapy* has become a marketing catchword, giving a ''new age'' cachet to cosmetic and personal-care products. And since the Food and Drug Administration does not acknowledge these forms of herbs as having therapeutic qualities, manufacturers are not allowed to make medicinal claims. However, this is changing. The FDA has recently given clearance for me to proceed with a controlled trial of an aromatherapy preparation for migraine. This remedy was developed by Edward Butler, who, after many years of experimentation, discovered that a seven-herb extract stopped debilitating headaches.

In Europe, particularly France and England, aromatherapy is a respected clinical approach to the treatment of a number of disorders, including chronic headache.

Getting to the Essence of Aromatherapy

The most potent forms of aromatherapy come from plants that have been steam distilled to their essential oils. It can take hundreds of pounds of fresh plant material to make just a few ounces of essential oil.

In their distilled form essential oils are too potent for use directly on the skin and could cause sensitivity reactions. For this reason aromatherapy essences must be diluted in a carrying medium before use. Most trained aromatherapists recommend oils that have no competing aromas, enhance the essence's characteristics, and are smooth (not thick) to the touch. Good oils for diluting plant essences are sweet almond or peach kernel oil. We will provide instructions under each entry.

Selecting and Storing Aromatherapy Preparations

- Select only essences that are labeled "pure, distilled."
- Select only essences packaged in dark brown glass bottles.
- Essences may be stored in a dark glass container, in a shelf out of sunlight and in a cool area (and out of reach of children). One-third ounce will last for up to three years.
- Except for massage oils, do not buy essences that are prediluted in oil, as the oil may go rancid if stored for long periods.

Cautions About Aromatherapy

- Never take internally.
- Never give to children, except when distributed through an air diffuser.
- Store out of reach of children.

The Ways of Aromatherapy

Aromatherapy can take several forms:

- Cold or warm compresses
- Diffused into the room through a vaporizer
- Applied directly to the skin and massaged
- Inhaled through a clean cloth
- Added to a bath

History

Aromatherapy can be traced to ancient times. Most likely, as with the effects of herbs, early humans discovered by trial and error that certain plants provided different therapeutic benefits. Religious offerings and ceremonies were (and some still are) accompanied by burning strongly scented plants. Over three thousand years ago Egyptian mummies were found embalmed with aromatics. The process of distilling plants to their essential oils—the basis for modern aromatherapy—is attributed to physician Avicenna. Today France and England and, in following with Ayurvedic tradition, India, employ essential plant extracts with great seriousness for a wide variety of disorders.

Aromatherapy Profiles

Here are the profiles of some aromatherapy essences useful for people with headache. We will provide some specific recommendations for their use in the section below.

Caution: Never take essential oils internally.

Lavender (*Lavendula officinalis*)

Lavender has been popular medicinally and cosmetically since ancient times. Abundant in Mediterranean countries, lavender leaves are especially potent when picked after dry, hot summers. Lavenders grown in high altitudes contain higher amounts of the aromatic chemicals.

The aromatic oils of lavender flowers are well known for their ability to relieve muscle spasm and have been used successfully when applied on the skin or inhaled. Due to its calming effects, lavender is a mainstay for people with headache. It can be helpful for people with tension-type headache, at the very beginnings of a migraine (if scents are tolerated), and for cluster headaches. See recipes on page 317.

Chamomile (*Roman or English*) (*Anthemis nobilis*)

English chamomile, also known as Roman chamomile, is the type of chamomile used for headache disorders—not to be confused with German chamomile. The flowers of this pretty and pleasant-scented herb have traditionally been used therapeutically.

Like lavender, chamomile is known for its gentle sedative effects, offering bodywide relaxation. In addition chamomile has relaxing effects on the smooth muscles of the intestine. It has been traditionally used in relieving nausea associated with migraine and in relieving the stress associated with PMS.

Rosemary (*Rosemarinus officinalis*)

Rosemary has been known to ward off evil spirits, to improve memory, and even to prevent the plague. Its therapeutic uses are traditionally related to its antibacterial effects, but in recent years other qualities have been discovered.

Rosemary has been shown to improve circulation and strengthen blood vessels. Its tested ability to improve digestion has made it useful in treating hangover headaches.

Peppermint (*Mentha piperita*)

Peppermint has been traditionally used as a digestive aid and to relieve stomach cramps; its effectiveness has been proven in research studies. The mentholating effects of this potent aromatic have made it useful as a massage oil or cream to increase blood flow to specific areas of the skin. A combination of peppermint and eucalyptus was shown in a placebo-compared study to relax temporal muscles (implicated in tension-type and TMJ-related headache), elevate mood, and reduce head pain by 40 percent. Alone, peppermint oil, when applied to the forehead, was shown to be effective for relief of tension-type headaches in a double-blind study by well-respected German researchers.[6] This study compared peppermint to 1,000 mg of acetaminophen and found them to be equally effective.

Caution: Avoid prolonged inhalation of peppermint, and never expose babies or infants to peppermint.

Geranium (*Pelargonium graveolens*)

Known traditionally for its relaxing effects, geranium has been shown to be useful in balancing hormones and may be helpful for PMS-related headaches.

Rose (*Rosa damascena, R. centifolia,* and *R. gallica*)

These most common varieties of rose for aromatherapy oil are mild laxatives, but they are often recommended for tension-related problems in women, such as PMS headaches.

Eucalyptus (*Eucalyptus globulus*)

Though traditionally used for treating breathing-related illness, eucalyptus has been shown to have pain-relieving effects when used along with peppermint. It is sometimes recommended by aromatherapists for sinus headaches. But it has also been shown, along with peppermint, to relieve tension-type and migraine headache.

Tiger Balm

This ancient Chinese herbal ointment is composed of camphor, menthol, and clove oil, among other ingredients. In a recent study in an Australian medical journal, Tiger Balm applied in small amounts to the temples within minutes provided strong and effective relief for 75 percent of twenty-two people with tension-type headache. The pain-relieving effects lasted for more than three hours. Note: Avoid contact with eyes and wash hands thoroughly after application.

Aromatherapy Recipes

Here are some aromatherapy recipes for specific types of headaches:

Tension-Type Headache

- *Plant essences:* Lavender or Roman chamomile; you can use one or the other depending on personal preference.
- *Inhalant:* Sprinkle tissue with one drop lavender and inhale deeply.
- *Massage:* Dilute one drop lavender or chamomile with 1 teaspoon almond oil and massage over forehead, neck, and shoulder area.
- *Warm bath:* Dilute five to six drops lavender or chamomile in a warm bath; if you have sensitive skin, first dilute in a carrier oil (1 teaspoon almond oil for every drop of oil).

Migraine

- *Plant essence:* Lavender.
- *Massage:* Dilute 1 drop lavender in 1 teaspoon almond oil. Massage neck and shoulder area.

(Note: Treat at the very beginning of a migraine, as odors may provoke nausea or increase severity.)

PMS-Related Headache

- *Plant essences:* Rose and geranium.
- *Massage:* One week before menstruation get a whole-body massage with geranium or rose oil.
- *Bath:* Take a bath with 5 to 6 drops of rose or geranium oil in the bathwater.

Cluster Headache

- *Plant essences:* Lavender and chamomile.
- *Massage:* One drop of both lavender and chamomile diluted in 1 teaspoon carrier oil; massage the temples and lower neck.

Sinus Headache

- *Plant essence:* Eucalyptus.
- *Inhale:* Add 1 to 2 drops eucalyptus oil to a pot of hot water and inhale deeply.

Finding a Reliable Aromatherapist

As with herbalists, aromatherapists are currently unlicensed in the United States—anyone can claim expertise in aromatherapy. The best thing you can do is to become somewhat familiar with the principles of aromatherapy yourself, then interview "therapists."

CHAPTER 10

Homeopathy

Like—but oh how different!
—*William Wordsworth*, "Yes, It was the Mountain Echo"

BACKGROUND

The origins of homeopathy can be traced to the eighteenth-century German physician Samuel Hahnemann, who became intrigued by the effectiveness of chinchona bark in curing malaria—and noticed a confounding effect: Taking chinchona created many of the same symptoms of malaria. From this experience Hahnemann developed his theory of *like cures like,* known as the *Law of Similars,* which asserts that the ability of a substance to cure a disease emerges from its power to cause symptoms in a healthy person that are similar to those of the disease itself.

Hahnemann's tireless investigations with different substances resulted in a long list of medicines and case studies, which are compiled in a series of reference books called the *materia medica*—in this case, the homeopath's guidebook to remedies and the psychological/physical symptoms that they produce. The symptoms are cross-referenced under *repertories,* which list all of the medications known to cause those symptoms.

Since its invention, homeopathy has become a popular method for treating illness. About two and a half million Americans have received care from homeopathic doctors, and an estimated 3,000 physicians and other health care practitioners administer homeopathy.[1] Homeopathy is more widely practiced in Europe, Latin America, and Asia. In France 32 percent of family physicians use homeopathy[2]; in India there are more than 100,000 homeopathic physicians.[3]

HOMEOPATHIC PRINCIPLES

Like Cures Like

According to homeopathic theory, the symptoms of a disease are an outward expression of the body's natural self-healing mechanism; they are signs that the body is responding to the stress of the disease. Using drugs to suppress the symptoms (as is done in conventional Western medicine) only masks the real problem and suppresses the body's own healing powers. In contrast, using agents with effects that are similar (*homios*) to the suffering or symptoms of disease (*pathos*), homeopathic remedies act as catalysts for the body's natural abilities, or *vital force*. The principle that like cures like, labeled the *Law of Similars,* is a distinguishing tenet of homeopathic philosophy.

No Part of the Body Is Separate from the Rest

That the mind and body are closely intertwined is another fundamental homeopathic belief. Remedies are matched not only to the individual's physical symptoms but to his or her personality or state of mind as well. An illness in one part of the body (or suffering in the mind) does not exist alone; it will almost always create a problem in other parts of the body.

If symptoms are the body's way of sounding the alarm for disease, as homeopaths assert, then *all* symptoms must be addressed. In the homeopathic interview a person will be encouraged to reveal in exquisite detail all major and minor symptoms. From this elaborate questioning, or *profiling*, emerges a blueprint for the remedy that is right for that person.

Layers of Symptoms: Hering's Laws of Cure

In many cases the major symptoms may mask deeper, older symptoms and problems, according to homeopaths. The initial remedy may help relieve one set of symptoms, only to uncover another layer.

However, homeopaths also believe that while a person may express a number of symptoms, they all stem from a single constitutional susceptibility that is unique to that individual.

The pattern of symptom progression after taking a prescribed remedy was described by German homeopath Constantine Hering and is called Hering's Laws of Cure. They are as follows:

1. Healing begins at the deepest levels (mind and organs) and progresses to the external parts (skin). With the correct similum, one often feels better mentally before feeling better physically.
2. Remedies peel away at layers of symptoms. For example, a person's headache may disappear, making way for other symptoms to emerge.
3. Healing progresses from the upper part of the body to the lower. A headache may wane, only for problems in the gastrointestinal tract to come forth.
4. Symptoms get worse before they get better. If symptoms reflect the body's fight against disease, then the proof of a good similum would be, at first, a better fight with stronger symptoms. When other signs show progress—such as generally improved mental condition, relief of other recent symptoms, or healing higher in the body—the temporary worsening of symptoms is considered a good sign.

Potentized Doses: Dilute and Dilute Again

One of the most controversial aspects of homeopathy is its use of remedies that are substances diluted to the point where no actual material substance exists anymore—in homeopathic parlance, they are *potentized.* Deriving from natural sources—plant, mineral, or animal—homeopathic remedies are potentized by diluting them between 3 to 100,000 times and shaking them after each dilution. The medicine is first diluted in 99 parts water or alcohol. One part of that dilution is then diluted again in 99 parts water or alcohol. The process is repeated until the remedy reaches the desired potency. Originally Hahnemann devised this method in an effort to quell the toxic effects of potent substances. But a certain logic emerged from this process. Since homeopathic remedies aim to jump-start the body's own healing powers, Hahnemann believed that only small doses were needed.

In addition Hahnemann advocated highly diluted doses for only short periods of time. Indeed homeopathic remedies are generally not administered for long periods of time; if the body's natural powers do not take over soon, the similum was wrong.

Chronic Conditions Need More Care

Given the highly individualized nature of homeopathic remedies, the success of the treatment rests heavily on the artful skill of a knowledgeable and perceptive homeopath. This is particularly the need among people with chronic problems, such as chronic headache. Such conditions suggest a constitutional vulnerability or susceptibility that, after years of embedding itself, can create a complex web of symptoms.

HOW IT WORKS

There is much dispute over the general effectiveness of homeopathic remedies.

With no measurable evidence that the remedies are anything more than water or alcohol, homeopathy rankles many of today's physicians, who view its remedies as nothing more than placebos.

However, while medical science cannot explain why it works, there is mounting evidence that homeopathy does indeed work. For example a review of homeopathic studies in the *British Medical Journal,* a highly regarded medical journal by conventional Western standards, showed that fifteen out of twenty-two well-designed studies of homeopathic remedies had positive results.[4] These findings were strong enough for the authors to call for more rigorous clinical research into homeopathy.

Two studies have shown the efficacy of homeopathy in the treatment of chronic headache—one of which was double-blind, which means that neither the homeopath nor the patients knew whether migraine sufferers were taking a remedy or a placebo. After four months 93 percent of the migraine sufferers who took the homeopathic remedy reported "sufficient" to "very good improvement." This compared very favorably with the 30 percent of people taking placebo. (The 30 percent placebo effect is very common in drug trials as well.[5])

COMMON REMEDIES FOR HEADACHE

It goes against all the tenets of homeopathy to recommend one or another remedy for general use. Homeopathic treatments are highly individualized. However, for the prevention and treatment of tension-type and migraine headache, several remedies are widely used. Here are some that are recommended by homeopathic practitioners such as Dana Ullman, director of the Homeopathic Educational Services, who has just authored *The Consumer's Guide to Homeopathic Medicines.* The recommended dose for all remedies is 6, 12, or 30 potency. Take every hour during severe pain and discontinue as soon as you feel some relief.

Aconite

Indicated for:

• Early stages of migraine

Characteristics of headache:

• Sudden onset
• Triggered by cold or sudden tension

Individual's characteristics while ill:

• Restless or even panicky
• Stomach pain

Belladonna

Indicated for:

• Tension-type headaches
• Right-sided migraines

Characteristics of headache:

• Appears and leaves very suddenly
• Throbbing or pulsating
• Focused in the forehead
• Confusion
• Visual disturbances and hallucinations
• Tension-type headaches come on very quickly

Individual's characteristics while ill:

• Sensitive to touch, light, sound, or motion (though pressure may provide some relief)

- Prefers sitting still
- Throbbing

Bryonia

Indicated for:

- Tension-type headaches

Characteristics of headache:

- Steady ache (not throbbing)
- Located in the forehead, down back of head, or over left eye
- Made worse by touch and motion
- Worse in hot rooms
- May be accompanied by nausea and constipation

Individual's characteristics while ill:

- Intolerant of motion
- Irascible
- Prefers to be alone and in cool areas

Gelsemium

Indicated for:

- Tension-type headache

Characteristics of headache:

- Located in back of head, or band around the head
- Triggered by anxiety or nervousness

Individual's characteristics while ill:

- Weak and heavy
- Drooping eyelids
- Seeks out warmth to relieve possible chills

Iris

Indicated for:

- Migraine

Characteristics of headache:

- Aura
- Right side of forehead
- Recurrent on a predictable basis

Individual's characteristics while ill:

- May feel nauseated
- Headache not relieved by vomiting

Kali Bichromium

Indicated for:

- Sinus-related headaches

Characteristics of headache:

- Accompanied by thick, stringy mucus
- Pain or pressure above the root of nose

- Pain in forehead or over one eye
- Made worse by bending, motion, and cold weather

Individual's characteristics while ill:

- Listless and indifferent

Natrum Muriaticum

Indicated for:

- Migraine
- Hormone-related

Characteristics of headache:

- Acute pounding
- Triggered by emotional upset
- Worse in the late morning, early afternoon

Individual's characteristics while ill:

- Emotionally sensitive
- Difficulty expressing feelings
- Rattled by sudden noises
- Craves salt

Nux Vomica

Indicated for:

- Hangover headache
- Tension-type headache

Characteristics of headache:

- Accompanied by stomach upset
- Triggered by cold
- Worse in the morning

Individual's characteristics while ill:

- Hard-driving, goal-oriented
- Irritable from overwork

Pulsatilla

Indicated for:

- Sinus headache
- PMS-related symptoms

Characteristics of headache:

- Worse at night
- Accompanied by nausea or indigestion

Individual's characteristics while ill:

- Weepy
- Moody
- Depressed

Sanguinaria

Indicated for:

- Right-sided migraines
- Hormone-related migraines
- Cluster headache

Characteristics of headache:

- Sharp, intense
- May begin in back of head and progress to right side or eye
- Accompanied by nausea, vomiting
- Made worse by motion
- Predictable pattern

Individual's characteristics while ill:

- Tense and nervous

Sepia

Indicated for:

- Left-sided migraine with nausea

Characteristics of headache:

- Left-sided
- Accompanied by nausea
- Aggravated by heat or sweets
- Triggered or aggravated by menstruation

Individual's characteristics while ill:

- Lackluster, sluggish
- Withdrawn and apathetic, even with loved ones

SIDE EFFECTS AND WARNINGS

While conventional medicine may have many beefs with the homeopathic community, safety is not one of them. There is little dispute
that at such infinitesimal doses, homeopathic remedies are very safe.
*However, it is vital that you rule out any possibly dangerous or life-
threatening causes of headache before trying homeopathy or any alternative treatment.*

Though considered a therapeutic effect, symptoms may worsen at
the beginning of a homeopathic treatment before they get better. Since
symptoms reflect the body's fight against disease, homeopaths see this
phenomenon as a good sign that the body is engaging more actively in
the battle against the underlying problem.

WHAT TO EXPECT

If you go to a homeopath, you can first expect to answer an extensive
list of questions, which help give the practitioner a profile of all symptoms (down to the most minute detail) and of your emotional makeup.
This can take upward of an hour. Then, possibly with the aid of a
computer program, your homeopath will recommend a remedy in an
effort to uncover the similum—the right remedy for you as an individual.

Finding your similum may be a trial-and-error process, during which
time you will keep in contact with your homeopath about any changes
in your symptoms. If your symptoms worsen, for example, you may be
asked to ride it out for a day or two to see whether it is a function of
your body gearing up for a fight against the disease that causes the
symptoms (a good sign) or whether the remedy has no effect and your
condition is simply worsening.

You may also find that other symptoms arise as the old ones fade,
which may be physical, mental, or emotional. This trend is expected by
homeopaths—and may require fine-tuning of your remedy.

In addition your symptoms may shift in location, another expected
phenomenon that shows the remedy is working.

However, once you and your homeopath find the similum, you will not need to stay on it for very long—just long enough for the remedy to set your own healing abilities in motion.

Depending on the background of your homeopath, he or she may also make lifestyle recommendations or suggest other treatments to help you cope with your problem.

FINDING A RELIABLE HOMEOPATH

The licensing requirements for homeopathic practice vary from state to state. Homeopathic practitioners can be found among M.D.'s, D.O.'s, dentists, naturopaths, chiropractors, and nurse practitioners, as well as others. Three states have licensing boards: Arizona, Connecticut, and Nevada. There are many schools to train doctors and laypeople. See "Resources" for organizations that may help in locating a homeopathic practitioner or physician near you.

QUESTIONS AND ANSWERS

• *Does homeopathy work as fast as drugs?* It depends on your illness. You may have very fast relief with homeopathy. However, since homeopathy theoretically works by triggering the body's own healing powers, homeopathic treatments may take some time to create an effect. And even then, other symptoms may become apparent.

• *How do homeopaths explain why remedies work at such high dilutions?* In general only small amounts of the actual agent are needed because the goal is not to wipe out symptoms but to stimulate the body's innate ability to heal itself. Some homeopaths explain the effects in terms of "new physics," suggesting that the medications exert an electromagnetic energy. They also theorize that the dilution and shaking process changes the structure of the water and alcohol molecules that contain the active ingredient—so although there is no evidence remaining of the original substance, the carriers are altered in such a way that they exert therapeutic benefit.

• *Can children take homeopathic remedies?*   Yes, but it is best to have treatment guided by a homeopath.

• *Is homeopathy covered by medical insurance?*   If you buy the remedies on your own based on self-diagnosis, probably not. On the other end of the spectrum, homeopathic consultations by a physician, nurse, osteopathic physician, dentist, or other health care professional are quite likely to be covered. Check with your insurance carrier.

Glossary

ACEPHALGIC MIGRAINE. See *migraine equivalents*.

ACUPOINTS. Acupressure and acupuncture points throughout the body along meridians.

ACUPRESSURE. The application of pressure to energy-releasing trigger points of the body to enhance the flow of energy; employed traditionally by Japanese and Chinese medical systems.

ACUPUNCTURE. An ancient method of Chinese medicine that employs hair-thin needles to stimulate specific points of the body along *meridians* (pathways) to encourage the flow of vital energy.

ACUTE. Sharp, severe; having a sudden onset and short course; not chronic.

ALLERGEN. Any substance that causes an allergic reaction; some allergens are thought to trigger headache.

ALLOPATHIC. System of treating disease by inducing a physiological reaction that is antagonistic to the disease being treated; for example, giving antibiotics to treat bacterial infection.

AMINE. Substance found in the body and some foods that is vital to the functioning of the brain and blood vessels.

ANALGESIA. Pain relief.

ANALGESIC. An agent (drug or nondrug) or method that produces pain relief.

ANEURYSM. An abnormality of a blood vessel in the head that can rupture, causing a stroke; rare cause of headache.

ANTIGEN. A natural substance that can identify cells that belong to or are foreign to the body.

AURA. Neurological symptoms, such as flashing lights, shapes, or blind spots, numbness, muscle weakness, or slurred speech that, in some people, may precede a migraine headache by ten to thirty minutes but can occur without head pain as well.

AUTOGENIC TRAINING. A relaxation technique that focuses on repeating positive statements to oneself regarding specific parts of the body (for example, "My shoulder muscles are relaxed").

AUTONOMIC NERVOUS SYSTEM. The part of the nervous system that regulates involuntary functions (e.g., heartbeat, breathing).

B CELLS. White blood cells, or lymphocytes, produced by the bone marrow that in turn create antibodies.

BEHAVIOR MODIFICATION. A psychological technique for changing behavioral habits by way of awareness and specific exercises.

BIOFEEDBACK. Method used to help individuals willfully (consciously) control involuntary activities of the body.

CBC. Complete blood count.

CHELATION. Forming of molecules; used to change a biological reaction by removing an ion.

CHI. See *qi*.

CHIROPRACTIC. Discipline of healing based on the belief that diseases emerge from changes in the skeletal structure.

CHRONIC. Continuous or intermittent over a long time.

CHRONIC PAROXYSMAL HEMICRANIA. Clusterlike headaches characterized by attacks that are more frequent and shorter in duration.

CLINICAL STUDY. A formal method of evaluating the effects of a drug or procedure. According to modern Western medicine, the best-designed studies are nonbiased. To avoid biases, the studies should have the following characteristics:

- Studies should be large-scale. The study segment should be large enough to represent a good cross-section of the general population for whom the procedure or drug (herb, remedy) would be given. For people with headaches, this would include both men and women, young and old, and so forth. Due to the many possible variables, oftentimes studies focus on one segment of the population, such as women, the elderly, or individuals with a similar level of disease severity.
- Studies should be comparative if possible. The effectiveness of any treatment is best gauged against a standard. In many cases the standard is a *placebo* (see page 337). In other situations the standard is a similar type of treatment.

- Studies should be double-blind—that is, neither the subject nor the investigator knows which treatment was given.
- Studies should be randomized—that is, subjects in the study are relegated to different study groups at random.
- Studies should be "crossover" if possible: After taking one treatment then they cross over to the other treatment.

CLUSTER HEADACHE. Severe headaches on one side of head that occur in clusters over a limited period of time.

COMPLICATED MIGRAINE. Migraine characterized by symptoms that continue at least twenty-four hours after head pain ends.

CRANIAL ARTERITIS. See *giant cell arteritis*.

CRANIOSACRAL. Relating to the cranium and the sacrum.

DIETETICS. The study of diet.

DOSHAS. The three fundamental energy types, or constitutional types, in Ayurvedic medicine.

DOUBLE-BLIND. Relating to clinical trials or experiments whereby neither the subject nor the researcher knows which individuals are receiving which treatment.

DYSMENORRHEA. Painful menstruation.

ELECTROMAGNETIC FIELD. Force associated with electromagnetic interactions.

ENDORPHINS. Natural substances produced by the body to relieve pain or elevate mood.

ENKEPHALIN. A natural substance produced by the body to relieve pain or increase the ability to endure pain.

EPIDEMIOLOGY. The study of populations to determine the incidence and distribution of diseases.

EPISODIC. Not constant; occurring every once in a while, either regularly or irregularly.

ETIOLOGY. The study of the causes of disease.

FAITH HEALING. Recovery due to belief in a healer's ability or other power.

FASCIA. The layer of fibrous tissue surrounding the body beneath the skin; encloses muscles and joints.

GIANT CELL ARTERITIS. Inflammation of the arteries of the head causing headaches and occasionally blindness.

HOMEOSTASIS. The condition of balance in the body; physiological well-being.

HYDROTHERAPY. Treatment of conditions with water.

HYPERTENSION. High blood pressure.

HYPOGLYCEMIA. Low blood sugar; a possible headache trigger.

IATROGENIC. Injury or illness caused by physician or healer.

ICE-PICK HEADACHE. Acute, severe stabbing pain on the head's surface, lasting two to three seconds.

IDIOPATHIC. A condition with no known cause.

IMMUNOGENIC. Used to describe any substance or factor that causes an immune response.

INFLAMMATION. Swelling and heat in response to a stressor, such as infection or nerve irritation.

INNATE INTELLIGENCE. The body's own ability to react to changing conditions.

KAPHA. One of the three Ayurvedic *doshas.*

KI. Japanese term for *qi.*

LEUKOCYTES. Also known as white blood cells, active in fighting off disease.

MANIPULATION. Use of manual force to heal; often used by chiropractic and osteopathic practitioners to adjust or influence the body's structure.

MATERIA MEDICA. Listing of drugs used for treatment, especially in homeopathy.

MENINGES. Tissues that cover the brain and spinal cord, composed of three layers.

MENINGITIS. Inflammation of meninges.

MERIDIAN. Also known as channel: in traditional Oriental medicine, fourteen channels that connect major organs to other body parts, and channel *qi* (energy) throughout the body.

MIGRAINE EQUIVALENTS. Migraines characterized by symptoms besides headache.

MIGRAINE HEADACHE. A headache, usually present on one side of the head, sometimes preceded by aura; often accompanied by nausea, vomiting, and sensitivity to noise and light.

MIGRAINEUR/MIGRAINEUSE. A term used to describe people with migraine.

MIGRAINE WITH AURA. A type of migraine preceded by an aura, occurring in 10 percent of people with migraine.

MIGRAINE WITHOUT AURA. A type of migraine that is not preceded by aura, seen in 90 percent of people with migraine.

MOBILIZATION. The process of making a stiff or fixed part of the body movable; also used to describe methods that use passive manipulations to achieve mobility (e.g., Feldenkrais).

MONOSODIUM GLUTAMATE (MSG). A flavor-enhancer found in some foods (particularly Chinese foods), commonly thought to trigger headaches.

MUSCLE CONTRACTION HEADACHE. See *tension-type headache.*

MYOFASCIAL. Relating to the fascia and muscles.

NATUROPATHIC MEDICINE. A multidisciplinary approach to healing that emphasizes prevention of disease through ongoing health maintenance.

NEUROLOGICAL. Pertaining to the nervous system, or neurology.

NEUROLOGY. The study of the nervous system, or a medical specialty in the study and care of diseases of the nervous system.

NEURONS. Cells of the nervous system.

NEUROTRANSMITTER. A naturally produced chemical that transports messages from one neuron to the next.

NITRITES. Preservatives used often in meats and processed foods that may cause headache.

NONLOCAL HEALING. Healing that occurs at a distance (e.g., prayer).

NONORGANIC HEADACHES. Known as primary headache disorders, these conditions have their own causes and mechanisms; migraine, tension-type headache, and cluster headache are examples.

NONSPECIFIC. In disease diagnosis, it refers to symptoms that could be seen in other conditions.

ORGANIC. Also known as secondary disorders, these conditions are symptoms of underlying medical problems; with regard to headache, these include serious causes such as aneurysm, meningitis, or sinus infection.

OSTEOPATHIC. Medical discipline that focuses on body mechanics and manipulation.

OXIDATION. Adding oxygen.

PATHOGEN. A disease-causing substance.

PATHOGENESIS. The origin and development (genesis) of a pathology (disease condition).

PATHOLOGY. The condition caused by a disease, or the study of disease-causing changes.

PHOTOPHOBIA. Sensitivity to light.

PITTA. One of the three *doshas,* or constitutional biotypes, described in Ayurvedic medicine.

PLACEBO. A "dummy" pill or treatment that is outwardly indistinguishable from an actual treatment but has no physiological effect. Used as a comparison to test the effects of a treatment.

PLACEBO EFFECT. Improvement in a disease or condition when taking a placebo. In clinical trials approximately one third of individuals taking a placebo can be expected to show improvement.

PLATELETS. Disk-shaped particles in the blood that function mainly to coagulate blood; one theory holds that individuals with migraine are prone to overaggregation (clumping) of platelets, which releases serotonin and causes headache.

PMS. See *premenstrual syndrome.*

POSTTRAUMATIC HEADACHE. Head pain resulting from head injury.

PREMENSTRUAL SYNDROME. A grouping of symptoms that occur in some women before menstruation, such as headache, irritability, and bloating.

PREMONITORY SYMPTOMS. See *prodrome.*

PRODROME. A combination of symptoms that occur from minutes to days before a headache; symptoms of the migraine prodrome may include mood changes and decreases/increases in appetite and energy, among others.

PROSTAGLANDIN. Hormonelike substances thought to contribute to headache.

PSYCHOGENIC. Relating to effects produced by psychic or mental factors.

QI. In Oriental medicine and metaphysics, the vital life energy that permeates the universe and every living being (also known as *ki* and *chi*).

REFERRED PAIN. Pain that occurs in one part of the body caused by injury or stress in another part.

SACRUM. The five vertebrae of the backbones that connect with the pelvis.

SCINTILLATIONS. Perceived flashing lights or lines seen by some people during the aura before a migraine.

SCOTOMA. A blind spot, sometimes occurring during aura.

SEROTONIN. An amine found in the body and some foods (e.g., bananas) that regulates blood vessels and pain perception; found in individuals with migraine and cluster headaches, as well as depression.

SOMATIC. Relating to the body, versus the mind.

SUBLUXATION. Term used by chiropractors to describe the disturbance of two linked joint vertebrae, producing dysfunction in those joints or related body systems.

SUBSTANCE P. A natural substance that aids in the biological process of inflammation.

SYMPATHETIC NERVOUS SYSTEM. Part of the nervous system responsible for involuntary muscle actions (e.g., blinking and breathing) and for some sensory activities (e.g., sight and smell).

SYNAPSE. The interface or connection between neurons.

SYNCOPE. Short periods of loss of consciousness, or fainting.

SYNDROME. The signs and symptoms of a specific illness.

SYSTEMIC. Referring to symptoms or diseases that affect the entire body versus those that are localized to a specific part of the body.

TEMPOROMANDIBULAR JOINT (TMJ) DISORDER. Jaw dysfunction that may cause headache pain in some people.

TENSION-TYPE HEADACHE. Sometimes called just tension headache, or muscle tension headache; characterized by bandlike steady pain; unlike migraine, there is no aura, nausea, or sensitivity to light or sound.

THALAMUS. An oval-shaped tissue that sits at the base of the brain, which is responsible for receiving and relaying almost all sensory stimuli (sight, sound, etc.) except smell.

TINNITUS. Ringing or pounding sound in the ear.

TRANSCUTANEOUS ELECTRICAL NERVE STIMULATION (TENS). Electrical stimulation of the nerves through the skin; for headache, directed at specific areas to block the transmission of pain.

TRIGEMINAL NERVES. Nerves leading from the base of the skull to the head.

TRIGGER. Any stressor that sets off a headache; could be physical (such as diet or allergen) or emotional (such as stress).

TYRAMINE. Substances found in many foods (e.g., citrus fruits, chocolate, wine, and aged cheese), which possibly trigger headache.

VASCULAR. Pertaining to blood vessels or other channels for body fluids.

VASCULAR HEADACHE. Headaches caused by constriction or dilation of the blood vessels near the brain.

VASOACTIVE SUBSTANCES. Drugs or foods that exert activity on the blood vessels, either by dilating or by constricting them.

VASOCONSTRICTION. Narrowing or constriction of the blood vessels.

VASODILATION. Opening or widening of the blood vessels.

VATTA. One of the three Ayurvedic *doshas,* or constitutional biotypes.

VERTIGO. Spinning sensation

Resources and Selective Bibliography

We offer here a selective list of organizations, books, and other resources that can provide more in-depth information about the issues we have covered in this book, and guide you toward practitioners of alternative methods in your region.

ACUPRESSURE

Acupressure Institute
1533 Shattuck Avenue
Berkeley, CA 94709
800-442-2232
510-845-1059
Provides catalog of literature, as well as training in acupressure, shiatsu, reflexology, and other bodywork skills, as well as operating a clinic.

American Oriental Bodywork Association
6801 Jericho Turnpike
Syosset, NY 11791
516-364-5533
Provides information on Oriental bodywork (e.g., acupressure, shiatsu), as well as referrals.

National Commission for the Certification of Acupuncturists
1424 16th Street NW, Suite 501
Washington, DC 20036
202-232-1404
Administers testing for certification in acupuncture and Chinese herbology; offers directories listing acupuncturists and Chinese herbologists who either have passed the exam or met requirements to take the exam (e.g., formal education, apprenticeship, or substantial number of years in practice). For referrals, write to the above address, and enclose a $3 check for the state directory or a $24 check for the national directory.

Books and Other Resources

Acupressure's Potent Points, by Michael Reed Gach, Ph.D. (Bantam).

The Complete Book of Shiatsu Therapy, by Toru Namikoshi (HarperCollins).

ACUPUNCTURE

Organizations

American Academy of Medical Acupuncture
800-521-2262
Provides acupuncture training for *physicians* and offers a list of referrals.

American Association of Acupuncture and Oriental Medicine
433 Front Street
Catasauqua, PA 18032
610-266-1433
Fax: 610-264-2768
National organization that provides general information on acupuncture and Oriental medicine, literature about specific disease conditions, and referrals to qualified practitioners who have undergone national certification and, where required, state licensure.

American Foundation of Traditional Chinese Medicine
505 Beach Street
San Francisco, CA 94133
415-776-0502
National referral resource for classes and programs in Chinese medicine.

National Commission for the Certification of Acupuncturists
1424 16th Street NW, Suite 501
Washington, DC 20036
202-232-1404
Administers testing for certification in acupuncture and Chinese herbology; offers directories listing acupuncturists and Chinese herbologists who either have passed the exam or met requirements to take the exam (e.g., formal education, apprenticeship, or substantial number of years in practice). For referrals write to the above address and enclose a $3 check for the state directory, or a $24 check for the national directory.

Books

Acupuncture, by Michael Nightingale (Charles E. Tuttle Company, Inc.).

Acupuncture: Is It for You? by J. R. Worsley (Harper & Row).

The Chinese Art of Healing, by S. Palos (Bantam Books).

The Healing Power of Acupuncture, by Michael Nightingale (Javelin Books).

ALEXANDER TECHNIQUE

Organizations

North American Society of Teachers of the Alexander Technique (NASTAT)
P.O. Box 517
Urbana, IL 61801
800-473-0620
Information and referrals to instructors in your area and general background.

Books

The Alexander Technique, by Wilfred Barlow (Alfred A. Knopf).

The Alexander Technique: The Essential Writings of F. Matthias Alexander, edited by Edward Maisel (University Books, Carol Communications).

The Alexander Technique Workbook, by Richard Brennan (Element Books, Ltd.).

Back Trouble: A New Approach to Prevention and Recovery, by Deborah Caplan (Triad Publishing Company).

Body Awareness in Action, by Frank Pierce Jones (Pantheon Books).

The Use of the Self, by F. Mathias Alexander (Centerline Press).

ALLERGY

(See "Diet" and "Environmental and Chemical Sensitivity.")

ALTERNATIVE MEDICINE (GENERAL)

Organizations

Office of Alternative Medicine
National Institutes of Health
Information Center
6120 Executive Boulevard, Suite 450
Rockville, MD 20892-9904
301-402-2466

The U.S. government's research branch into alternative therapies. In addition to research, the OAM acts as a clearinghouse of information for the general public. It publishes a number of free fact sheets, available from the address above, as well as a growing number of programs aimed at public education.

Books and Other Resources

Alternative Medicine: Expanding Medical Horizons (Washington, D.C.: U.S. Government Printing Office). A comprehensive report from the Office of Alternative Medicine to the National Institutes of Health about the state of alternative-medicine research and future directions. Includes contributions from more than two hundred researchers and practitioners of alternative medicine. An excellent general resource about a wide range of alternative therapies. For information call the Government Printing Office at 202-512-1800.

Alternative Medicine: The Definitive Guide, compiled by the Burton Goldberg Group (Future Medicine Publishing). Also an excellent seminal resource for background on alternative therapies in general and their application to different types of illness.

Alternative Medicine Yellow Pages: A Comprehensive Guide to the New World of Health (Future Medicine Publishing). A good but incomplete listing of resources for a variety of alternative therapies.

Free Yourself from Headaches: The Natural, Drug-Free Program for Prevention and Relief, by Jan Stromfeld and Anita Weil (Upledger Institute).

Natural Therapies: The Complete A–Z of Complementary Health, by Margot McCarthy (Thorsons). Written for a United Kingdom audience, provides good information about alternative therapies.

Planet Medicine, by Richard Grossinger (North Atlantic Books). A theoretical exploration of alternative therapies, written in a very academic style—good background.

Smart Medicine for a Healthier Child: A Practical A–Z Reference to Natural and Conventional Treatments for Infants and Children, by Janet Zand, L.Ac.; Rachel Walton, R.N.; and Bob Rountree, M.D. (Avery Publishing Group). Good background for parents seeking natural therapies for children with chronic and acute illness.

Your Inner Physician and You, by John E. Upledger (North Atlantic Books).

Alternative Medicine Digest
Future Medicine Publications, Inc.
5009 Pacific Highway
Puyallup, WA 98424
Bimonthly newsletter describing advances in alternative medicine.

Journal of Alternative and Complementary Medicine: Research on Paradigm, Practice and Policy
Mary Ann Liebert, Inc., Publishers
1651 Third Avenue
New York, NY 10128
Quarterly journal reviewing and setting standards for clinical studies on alternative medical therapies.

Townsend Letter
911 Tyler Street
Pt. Townsend, WA 98368
206-385-6021

Though written for doctors, contains much useful information for laypeople about alternative healing.

APPLIED KINESIOLOGY AND TOUCH FOR HEALTH

Organizations

International College of Applied Kinesiology
6405 Metcalf Avenue, Suite 503
Shawnee, KA 66202-3929
913-384-5336

Provides information, a newsletter, and referrals to practitioners of applied kinesiology.

Touch for Health Association
6955 Fernhill Drive
Malibu, CA 90265
310-457-8342
800-466-8342

A membership organization dedicated to self-help approaches related to applied kinesiology and Oriental principles of meridian therapy. Provides a quarterly newsletter, a national directory of Touch for Health practitioners, and educational materials.

Books

Kinesiology Balanced Health, by Brian Butler (TASK Publications).

Kinesiology: Muscle Testing and Energy Balancing for Health and Well-being, by Ann Holdway (Element).

You'll Be Better: The Story of Applied Kinesiology, by George Goodheart (A. K. Printing).

AROMATHERAPY

Organizations

International Federation of Aromatherapists
Room 8, Department of Continuing Education
Royal Masonic Hospital
Ravenscourt Park, London W6 OTN

National Association for Holistic Aromatherapy
P.O. Box 17622
Boulder, CO 80308
Provides training nationwide in aromatherapy, publishes a magazine, and offers a directory of aromatherapists.

Pacific Institute of Aromatherapy
P.O. Box 6842
San Rafael, CA 94903
415-479-9121

Books and Other Resources

Aromatherapy: A Complete Guide to the Healing Art, by Kathi Keville and Mindy Green (Crossing Press).

Aromatherapy: An A to Z, by Patricia Davis.

The Aromatherapy Book: Applications and Inhalations, by Jeanne Rose (North Atlantic Books).

The Aromatherapy Guide, by Susan Hollick (Vencom Publishing, Inc.)
24 Hanover Road #2205

Brampton, Ontario
Canada L6S 5K8
905-799-2108
Resource guide to aromatherapy books, services, videos, products, education centers, and associations.

Aromatherapy Quarterly
P.O. Box 421
Inverness, CA 94937
415-663-9519

Aromatherapy Product Sources

Floralis
P.O. Box 40233
Washington, DC 20016
617-861-6142
Essential oils and supplies for aromatherapy, as well as expert guidance to the use of aromatherapy.

Ledet Oils
P.O. Box 2354
Fair Oaks, CA 95628
Catalog of supplies for aromatherapy.

ASTON-PATTERNING

Organizations

Aston-Patterning
P.O. Box 3568
Incline Village, NV 89450
702-831-8228
Provides training, referrals to practitioners, and educational information about Aston-Patterning.

AYURVEDIC MEDICINE

Organizations

Ayurvedic Institute
P.O. Box 23445
Albuquerque, NM 87192
505-291-9698

A nonprofit educational corporation to promote knowledge of Ayurveda. Offers instruction (at the institute and by correspondence courses), as well as a catalog of educational materials.

The College of Maharishi
Ayur-Veda Health Center
P.O. Box 282
Fairfield, IA 52556
515-472-5866

Trains practitioners, disseminates educational information to the public, and provides referrals to Ayurvedic and other health centers for Ayurvedic treatment.

Books and Other Resources

Ageless Body, Timeless Mind, by Deepak Chopra, M.D. (Harmony Books).

Ayurveda: Life, Health and Longevity, by Robert E. Svoboda (Penguin Books).

Ayurveda: The Ancient Indian Healing Art, by Scott Gerson, M.D. (Element Books)

Ayurveda: The Gentle Health System, by Hans H. Rhyner (New York: Sterling Publishing, Inc., 1994).

Ayurveda: The Science of Self-healing, by Vasant Lad (Lotus Press).

The Ayurvedic Cookbook, by Amadea Morningstar with Urmila Desai (Lotus Press).

Perfect Health, by Deepak Chopra, M.D. (Harmony Books).

Prakruti: Your Ayurvedic Constitution, Robert Svoboda (Geocom Ltd.).

The Yoga of Herbs: An Ayurvedic Guide to Herbal Medicine, by Dr. Vasant Lad and David Frawley (Lotus Press).

Ayurvedic News
P.O. Box 188
Exeter EX4 5AB
United Kingdom
Newsletter about Ayurvedic practices.

Quantum Publications
P.O. Box 598
South Lancaster, MA 01561
800-858-1808
508-368-1810
Catalog of books and videotapes by Deepak Chopra, M.D.

Products

Ayurvedic Institute
P.O. Box 23445
Albuquerque, NM 87192-1445
505-291-9698
Catalog of Ayurvedic products (herbs, oils, etc.) and publications, videotapes, and audiotapes.

BEHAVIORAL THERAPY, COGNITIVE RESTRUCTURING, AND PSYCHOTHERAPY

Organizations

American Association for Marriage and Family Therapy
1133 15th Street NW, Suite 300
Washington, DC 20005
800-374-2638
Referrals to therapists with special training in marriage and family counseling—especially useful for children with chronic health problems.

American Psychological Association
750 First Street, NE
Washington, DC 20002
202-336-5700
Governing organization for psychologists, also offers educational information and referrals to local organizations that can direct you to therapists with background in behavioral therapy.

Center for Cognitive Therapy
The Science Center, Room 754
3600 Market Street
Philadelphia, PA 19104
215-898-4102
Offers referrals to therapists trained in cognitive therapy.

National Association of Social Workers
750 First Street, NE, Suite 700
Washington, DC 20002
202-408-8600
Governing organization for therapists who have earned a master's degree in social work (M.S.W.), also offers educational information and referrals to local organizations that can direct you to therapists with background in behavioral therapy.

Books

The Consumer's Guide to Psychotherapy, by Jack Engler and Daniel Goleman (Fireside/Simon & Schuster).

Feeling Good: The New Mood Therapy, by David D. Burns (New American Library/Dutton).

Health and Optimism, by Christopher Peterson and Lisa M. Bossio (Macmillan).

BIOFEEDBACK

Organizations

Biofeedback Certification Institute of America
Association for Applied Psychophysiology and Biofeedback
10200 West 44th Avenue, #304
Wheat Ridge, CO 80033-2840
303-422-8436
800-477-8892
Will send a list of local chapters, from which you can obtain referrals for certified biofeedback practitioners.

Books

Biofeedback: An Introduction and Guide, by David G. Danskin and Mark Crow (Mayfield Publishing).

CHELATION THERAPY

Organizations

American Board of Chelation Therapy
1407B North Wells
Chicago, IL 60610

312-787-2228

Original standard-setting organization for chelation therapy; provides referrals of physicians for the public.

American College of Advancement in Medicine
23121 Verdugo Drive, Suite 204
Laguna Hills, CA 92653
800-532-3688

Establishes certification standards for the practice of chelation. Provides referrals to ACAM-certified physicians and information on the basics of chelation for the public.

Books

The Chelation Way, by Morten Walker, D.P.M. (Avery).

The Healing Powers of Chelation Therapy, by John Towbridge, M.D., and Morten Walker, D.P.M. (New Way of Life, Inc.).

CHEMICAL SENSITIVITY

(See ''Diet'' and ''Environmental and Chemical Sensitivity.'')

CONVENTIONAL WESTERN MEDICINE

Organizations

American Council for Headache Education
875 Kings Highway, Suite 200
West Deptford, NJ 08096

Publishes a quarterly newsletter, ''ACHE,'' devoted to describing and answering questions about headache. Also referral resource for over forty local support groups. Underwritten by Glaxo Pharmaceuticals, so it is not likely that information about alternative treatments will be cautionary.

National Headache Foundation
428 West St. James Place, 2nd Floor
Chicago, IL 60614
312-878-7715
800-843-2256

Nonprofit membership organization committed to research and information about headache. An informational resource, the NHF publishes a newsletter, *National Headache Foundation Newsletter,* and offers several hundred "information sheets" about different types of headache and treatment approaches (alternative and not). For referrals to more than fifteen hundred board-certified M.D.'s and D.O.'s who are members of NHF, send a self-addressed, stamped envelope. Also a referral resource for headache support groups.

Books

Conquering Headache, by Alan Rapoport, M.D., and Fred Sheftell, M.D. (Empowering Press).

The Headache Book, by Seymour Solomon and Steven Fraccaro (Consumer Reports, 1991).

Headache Relief: A Comprehensive, Up-to-Date, Medically Proven Program That Can Control and Ease Headache Pain, by Alan M. Rappaport, M.D., and Fred Sheftell, M.D. (Simon and Schuster).

The Hormone Headache, by Seymour Diamond, M.D.; Bill Still; and Cynthia Still (Macmillan).

Migraine: Beating the Odds, by Richard B. Lipton, M.D.; Lawrence C. Newman, M.D.; and Helene MacLean (Addison-Wesley Publishing Company).

Newsletters

Chronic Pain Letter
P.O. Box 1303 Old Chelsea Station
New York, NY 10001

CHIROPRACTIC

Organizations

Chiropractic is licensed in all fifty states. Chiropractors who are members of the the Orthopractic Society focus on manipulations to improve joint mobility and do not adhere to the concept of subluxations. For referrals and more information, contact these organizations at:

American Chiropractic Association
1701 Clarendon Boulevard
Arlington, VA 22209
703-276-8800
The American Chiropractic Association is the governing organization for chiropractors who view themselves as the equivalents of primary-care physicians—treating a wide range of conditions. Provides educational background information about chiropractic, as well as referrals.

International Chiropractors Association
1110 North Glebe Road, Suite 1000
Arlington, VA 22201
703-528-5000
The original chiropractic organization, members focus on relieving subluxation. Provides educational information and referrals.

National Association for Chiropractic Medicine
Send a self-addressed, stamped envelope to:

15427 Baybrook Drive
Houston, TX 77062
713-280-8262
Members of the National Association of Chiropractic Medicine generally focus on musculoskeletal problems. Provides educational information and referrals.

Books

The Chiropractor's Adjuster, by Daniel David Palmer (Palmer Press).

Migraine Headache Disease, by Charles W. Theisler (Aspen Publications).

Today's Health Alternative, by Raquel Martin (America West Publishers).

CRANIOSACRAL THERAPY

Organizations

American Osteopathic Association
142 East Ontario Street
Chicago, IL 60611
800-621-1773
In Illinois: 312-280-5800
Provides information about osteopathy, osteopathic medical manipulations, and craniosacral therapy, as well as referrals.

The Cranial Academy
8606 Allisonville Road #130
Indianapolis, IN 46250
317-594-0411
Referrals to osteopathic physicians with training in cranial therapy.

The Upledger Institute
11211 Prosperity Farms Road
Palm Beach Gardens, FL 33410
407-622-4334

A comprehensive educational and therapeutic resource center that integrates conventional health care with complementary techniques, including craniosacral therapy. Write or call for referrals to practitioners, information about the on-site clinic, as well as background information on craniosacral therapy and headache.

Books

Your Inner Physician and You, by John E. Upledger (North Atlantic Books).

Also a wide range of books and articles about craniosacral therapy is available through the Upledger Institute.

DIET

(See also "Macrobiotics," "Naturopathic Medicine," "Traditional Oriental Medicine," and "Ayurvedic Medicine.")

Organizations

American Association of Naturopathic Physicians
2366 Eastlake Avenue, Suite 322
Seattle, WA 98102
206-323-7610

Provides educational information and referrals to naturopathic practitioners.

American College of Advancement for Medicine
P.O. Box 3427
Laguna Hills, CA 92654

714-583-7666

Directory of physicians with training in nutritional medicine. Also offers printed information on nutrition.

American Dietetic Association
Nationwide Nutrition Network
800-366-1655
Weekdays 9 A.M.–4 P.M. central time
Provides referrals to registered dietitians in different regions who can help you create a diet that meets your needs.

American Natural Hygiene Society
P.O. Box 30630
Tampa, FL 33630
813-855-6607
The oldest existing vegetarian society, offers literature on lifestyle and diet.

Center for Science in the Public Interest
1875 Connecticut Avenue, NW, Suite 300
Washington, DC 20009
202-332-9110
Publishes *Nutrition Action Newsletter* and provides information about legislation and issues relating to public nutrition policy.

International Academy of Nutrition and Preventive Medicine
P.O. Box 18433
Asheville, NC 28814
704-258-3243
Refers to physicians who practice orthomolecular medicine and provides information.

Price Pottenger Nutrition Foundation
P.O. Box 2614
La Mesa, CA 91943-2614
619-574-7763

Provides referrals to naturopathic physicians. Also offers a wide variety of books about natural approaches to nutrition.

Books and Other Resources

An Alternative Approach to Allergies, by Randolph G. Theron and Ralph W. Moss (Bantam Books).

The Complete Guide to Health and Nutrition, by Gary Null (Dell).

Coping with Your Allergies, by Natalie Golos and Francis Golbita (Simon & Schuster).

Food and Healing, by Annemarie Colbin (Ballantine).

Healing with Whole Foods: Oriental Traditions and Modern Nutrition, by Paul Pitchford (North Atlantic Books).

Migraine and the Allergy Connection, by John Mansfield, M.D. (Healing Arts).

The Nutritional Desk Reference, by Robert H. Garrison, Jr., M.A., R.Ph.; and Elizabeth Somer, M.A., R.D. (Keats Publishing).

The PDR Family Guide to Nutrition and Health (Medical Economics).

Prescription for Nutritional Healing, by James F. Balch, M.D., and Phyllis A. Balch, C.N.C. (Avery Publishing Group).

Prince Wen Hui's Cook: Chinese Dietary Therapy, by Bob Flaws and Honora Wolfe (Paradigm Publications).

Tao of Nutrition, by Maoshing Ni, D.O.M., Ph.D., L.Ac.; and Cathy McNease (Seven Star Communications).

Vegan Nutrition—Pure and Simple, by Michael Klaper, M.D. (Gentle World).

Nutrition Action Newsletter
Center for Science in the Public Interest
(See address, page 358.)

Nutrition and Healing newsletter
P.O. Box 84909
Phoenix, AZ 85701
Monthly newsletter covers nutritional supplements.

Sources for Organic Foods

Organic Trade Association
P.O. Box 1078
Greenfield, MA 01302
413-774-7511
Write with a self-addressed, stamped envelope for a directory of mail-order resources for organic foods.

ENVIRONMENTAL AND CHEMICAL SENSITIVITY

Organizations

American Academy of Allergy and Immunology
611 East Wells Street, Suite 400
Milwaukee, WI 53202
800-822-2762
In Wisconsin: 414-272-6071
Provides referrals to board-certified allergists.

American Academy of Environmental Medicine
4510 West 89th Street, Suite 110
Prairie Village, KS 66207
Offers referrals to doctors (mostly allergists) who specialize in environmental medicine. Produces a quarterly newsletter, *The Environmental Physician,* and conducts conferences—geared toward physicians and laypeople.

Chemical Injury Information Network (CIIN)
P.O. Box 301
White Sulphur Springs, MT 59645
406-547-2255

A nonprofit, charitable organization that offers a variety of services for members (membership is free), including referrals to doctors specializing in chemical injury, peer counseling, and educational materials. For people engaged in legal problems with employers, CIIN also offers referrals to expert witnesses and doctors. Send a self-addressed, stamped envelope.

Human Ecology Action League (HEAL)
P.O. Box 49126
Atlanta, GA 30359
404-248-1898

In addition to a quarterly magazine, offers information about products for people with chemical sensitivities, brochures about legal rights, including a brochure describing the American Disability Act of 1990, and tips for creating an environmentally safe home and office. Offers a comprehensive reading list.

National Center for Environmental Health Strategies
1100 Rural Avenue
Voorhes, NJ 08403
609-429-5358

Advises organizations on ways to improve work environment, clearinghouse of information on national policy, increases public and legislative awareness of issues relating to chemical sensitivity. Offers physician recommendations. Send a self-addressed, stamped envelope with inquiry.

National Foundation for the Chemically Hypersensitive
1158 North Huron Road
Linwood, MI 48634
517-697-3989

Nonprofit organization offers referrals to physicians who specialize in chemical sensitivity, phone counseling, information on disability and workman's compensation, reading lists, and brochures. Send a self-addressed, stamped envelope.

National Organization of Legal Advocates for the
Environmentally Injured
P.O. Box 29567
Atlanta, GA 30329
404-264-4445

A nonprofit organization that dispenses legal information to support the rights of people who have suffered environmental injuries on their jobs.

Share, Care, Prayer
P.O. Box 2080
Frazier Park, CA 93225

Nonprofit Christian organization includes more than three thousand members with chemical and/or food sensitivity. Offers newsletter, tape lending library, informational brochures, and social directory. Send a self-addressed, stamped envelope with inquiries.

Books

An Alternative Approach to Allergies, by Randolph G. Theron, M.D., and Ralph W. Moss (Bantam Books).

Chemical Exposures: Low Levels and High Stakes, by Nicholas A. Ashford and Claudia S. Miller (Van Nostrand Reinhold).

Clean and Green: The Complete Guide to Nontoxic and Environmentally Safe Housekeeping, by Annie Berthold-Bond (Ceres Press).

The Healthy Home: An Attic-to-Basement Guide to Toxin-Free Living, by Linda Mason Hunter (Rodale Press).

Less Toxic Living, by Carolyn Gorman (Environmental Health Strategies). (See page 361 for address.)

Migraine and the Allergy Connection, by John Mansfield, M.D. (Healing Arts).

The Pulse Test, by Arthur F. Coca, M.D. (Barricade Books, Inc.)

Rapid Guide to Hazardous Chemicals in the Workplace, 2d edition, by Richard J. Lewis, Sr. (Van Nostrand Reinhold).

Treating Sinus, Migraine and Cluster Headaches: An Allergist's Approach to Headache Treatment, by William E. Walsh, M.D., F.A.C.A. (ACA Publications).

Product Resources

Allergy Control Products
96 Danbury Road
Ridgefield, CT 06877
800-422-DUST
Will send a brochure with information and products of FDA-registered products that help keep allergens, particularly dust mites and pet dander, under control in the home.

Allergy Research Group
400 Preda Street
San Leandro, CA 94577
800-545-9960
Staff nutritionist will answer questions regarding allergy and food sensitivity over the telephone. Also sells for and provides information about hypoallergenic food supplements and at-home tests for intestinal permeability and liver function.

Fisher Henney Naturals
1-800-3HENNEY
Organic cotton clothing.

Healthy House Catalog
Environmental Health Watch
4115 Bridge Avenue

Cleveland, OH 44113
800-222-9348
A national directory of indoor pollution resources.

Natural Lifestyles Supplies
16 Lookout Drive
Asheville, NC 28804
794-254-9606
Resource for books and supplies for people with environmental sensitivity.

Natural Nouveax
P.O. Box 97856
Las Vegas, NV 89193-7856
702-222-1919
Facial, body, and hair-care products for chemically sensitive people. Send self-addressed, stamped envelope.

Safer Alternatives
546 Olympic Street
Redding, CA 96003
916-243-1352
Free catalog of household and personal products for chemically sensitive people, including air purifiers, pillows, radiant heaters, soaps, and paints.

SelfCare Catalog
P.O. Box 182290
Chattanooga, TN 37422
800-520-9924
Sells many health-enhancing products, including those for people with sensitivities.

FELDENKRAIS METHOD

Organizations

The Feldenkrais Guild
P.O. Box 489
Albany, OR 97321-0143
800-775-2118
Referals to practitioners in your area as well as background information.

Books and Other Resources

Feldenkrais Resources
P.O. Box 2067
Berkeley, CA 94702
800-765-1897
In California: 510-540-7600
Call or write for a catalog of books, audiotapes, and videotapes about the Feldenkrais Method.

Awareness Through Movement: Health Exercises for Personal Growth, by Moshe Feldenkrais (Harper & Row).

Mindful Spontaneity, by Ruthy Alon (North Atlantic Books).

The Potent Self: A Guide to Spontaneity, by Moshe Feldenkrais (Harper & Row).

HELLERWORK

Organizations

Hellerwork International
406 Berry Street
Mount Shasta, CA 96067

916-926-2500
Provides training, education, and referrals to Hellerwork practitioners.

Books

Body-wise: Introduction to Hellerwork, by Joseph Heller and William Henkin (Wingbow Press).

HERBAL THERAPY

Organizations

American Association of Naturopathic Physicians
2366 Eastlake Avenue, East, Suite 322
Seattle, WA 98102
206-323-7610
Provides educational information and referrals to naturopathic practitioners.

American Botanical Council
P.O. Box 201660
Austin, TX 78720
Nonprofit organization that aims to educate the public about beneficial herbs and plants. Disseminates information, conducts research, publishes quarterly newsletter, offers catalog of literature.

Council of Acupuncture and Oriental Medicine
8403 Colesville Road, Suite 307
Silver Spring, MD 20910
301-608-9175

Herb Research Foundation
1007 Pearl Street, Suite 200
Boulder, CO 80302
800-748-2617

Nonprofit research and educational organization dedicated to educating the public about herbs. Offers research services, information packets on 170 popular topics, access to information specialists.

National Commission for the Certification of Acupuncturists
1424 16th Street NW, Suite 501
Washington, DC 20036
202-232-1404

Administers testing for certification in acupuncture and Chinese herbology; offers directories listing acupuncturists and Chinese herbologists who either have passed the exam or met requirements to take the exam (e.g., formal education, apprenticeship, or substantial number of years in practice). For referrals write to the above address, and enclose a $3 check for the state directory, or a $24 check for the national directory.

Books

An Elder's Herbal: Natural Techniques for Promoting Health and Vitality, by David Hoffmann (Healing Arts Press).

Green Pharmacy: The History and Evolution of Western Medicine, by Barbara Griggs (Healing Arts Press).

Handbook of African Medicinal Plants, by Maurice M. Iwu (CRC).

Healing Wise, by Susun Weed (Ash Tree).

The Herb Book, John Lust (Bantam).

Herbs of Choice: The Therapeutic Use of Phytomedicines, by Varro E. Tyler (Hawthorn Press).

Herbs That Heal: Prescription for Herbal Healing, by Michael . Weiner, Ph.D. and Janet Weiner (Quantum Books).

The Honest Herbal: A Sensible Guide to the Use of Herbs and Related Remedies, by Varro E. Tyler, Ph.D. (Hawthorn Press).

The New Age Herbalist, Richard Mabey (Collier/Macmillan).

Potter's New Cyclopedic of Botanical Drugs and Preparations, by Saffron Walden (C. W. Daniel Co., Ltd.).

Catalogs and Herbal Products

American Herbal Products Association
Box 2410
Austin, TX 78768
512-320-8555
Establishes standards for and provides public with information about herb quality.

American Herb Association
Box 353
Rescue, CA 95672
Catalogs of herbal books, herb products, and schools that train in herbology.

Herbal Green Pages 1995–1996
Herb Growing & Marketing Network
P.O. Box 245
Silver Springs, PA 17575
717-393-3295
Comprehensive listing of herb suppliers and information resources.

The Herb Companion Wishbook and Resource Guide, by Bobbie McRae
Interweave Press
Box 49770
Austin, TX 78765-9770
Lists resources for herbs.

The Information Sourcebook of Herbal Medicine, edited by David Hoffman (The Crossing Press). Includes information on accessing herbal information, summaries of articles, and scientific resources for herbal information, newsletters, and books.

Jean's Greens
R.R.1 Box 55J
Hale Road
Rensselaerville, NY 12147
518-239-TEAS
Mail-order resource for quality herbs.

Northwind Farm Publications
R.R.2 Box 246
Shevlin, MN 56676-99535
Resource for herbs and books, including the annual *Herb Resource Directory,* which includes entries listed by state for herb products, gardens, nurseries, and growing supplies.

Ya-ka-ama
Indian Education and Development, Inc.
6215 Eastside Road
Forestville, CA 95436
Indian-controlled, nonprofit corporation and educational program, including herb sources.

Newsletters and Tapes

Gaia Herb Education Seminars
P.O. Box 57
Swan's Island, ME 04685
Audiotapes and seminars on herbs for women.

HerbalGram Magazine
Published by the American Botanical Council and Herb Research Foundation (see address, page 366). Reviewed by professional advisory board of the HRF.

The Roots of Healing: The New Medicine audiotape
New Dimensions Tapes
P.O. Box 410510
San Francisco, CA 94141
415-563-8899
Three-part National Public Radio series, cohosted by Michael Toms and Andrew Weil.

HOMEOPATHY

Organizations

Foundation for Homeopathic Education and Research
2124 Kittredge Street
Berkeley, CA 94704
Extensive educational and product resource for homeopathic information and products.

International Foundation for Homeopathy
P.O. Box 7
Edmonds, WA 98020
206-776-4147
Nonprofit organization devoted to promoting public awareness of classical homeopathy. Professional courses, information, research, and bimonthly magazine, *Resonance.*

Books and Other Resources

Boiron Research Foundation
1208 Amosland Road
Norwood, PA 19074
Suppliers of homeopathic products and educational information.

The Consumer's Guide to Homeopathic Medicines, by Dana Ullman

(Tarcher/Los Angeles). Includes background on homeopathy as well as specific recommendations for headache and other conditions.

Homeopathic Medicines for Women, by Trevor Smith (Healing Arts).

Homeopathic Remedies for Our Infants and Children, by Dana Ullman (Tarcher).

HYDROTHERAPY

(See ''Naturopathic Medicine.'')

HYPNOTHERAPY

Organizations

American Institute of Hypnotherapy
16842 Von Karman Avenue, Suite 475
Irvine, CA 92714
714-261-6400
Trains and certifies hypnotherapists. Resource for books and tapes on hypnotherapy, and provides referrals.

American Society of Clinical Hypnotherapy
2200 East Devon Avenue, Suite 291
Des Plaines, IL 60018
708-297-3317
Membership organization for M.D.'s and dentists who are trained in hypnotherapy. Provides referrals with self-addressed, stamped envelope.

International Medical and Dental Hypnotherapy Association
4110 Edgeland, Suite 800
Royal Oak, MI 48073
313-549-5594

800-257-5467
Certifies and trains M.D.'s, dentists, and hypnotherapists in hypnotherapy. Offers referrals.

Books and Other Resources

Hypnosis, Acupuncture and Pain, by Maurice Tinterow (Bio-
Communications Press).

American Institute of Hypnotherapy
(See address, page 371.)
Resource for books and tapes on hypnotherapy.

IMAGERY

Organizations

Academy for Guided Imagery
P.O. Box 2070
Mill Valley, CA 94942
800-726-2070
Certifies health professionals in the use of guided imagery, accredited by the American Psychological Association. Provides referrals and
a catalog of books and tapes.

International Imagery Association
P.O. Box 1046
Bronx, NY 10471
Nonprofit organization dedicated to the study and application of
mental imagery. Produces two publications, *Journal of Mental Imagery*
and *Imagery Today* newsletter.

Books and Other Resources

Healing Yourself: A Step-by-Step Program for Better Health Through Imagery, by Martin L. Rossman (Walker).

Imagery in Healing: Shamanism and Modern Medicine, by Jeanne Achterberg and G. Frank Lawlis (Shambala: New Science Library).

Imagination and Healing, edited by Anees A. Sheikh (Baywood).

Man and His Symbols, by Carl Jung (Doubleday).

Minding the Body, Mending the Mind, by Joan Borysenko (Reading).

The Imagery Store
P.O. Box 2070
Mill Valley, CA 94942
700-726-2070
Free catalog of books and tapes about imagery and healing.

MACROBIOTICS

Organizations

Kushi Institute
Leland Road
Becket, MA 01223
413-623-5741
Devoted to studies and practical application of macrobiotics; also offers referrals to macrobiotic counselors.

Books

Cooking with Rachel, by Rachel Albert (Ohsawa Macrobiotic Foundation).

Macrobiotic Cooking for Everyone, by Wendy Esko and Edward Esko (Japan Publications).

Natural Healing Through Macrobiotics, by Michio Kushi (Japan Publications).

Practical Guide to Far-Eastern Macrobiotic Medicine, by George Ohsawa (Ohsawa Macrobiotic Foundation).

The Unique Principle: The Philosophy of Macrobiotics, by George Ohsawa (Ohsawa Macrobiotic Foundation).

MASSAGE

Organizations

American Massage Therapy Association
820 Davis Street, Suite 100
Evanston, IL 60201
708-864-0123
Provides information, conducts research, and offers referrals to accredited, approved programs for massage therapists. Establishes standards for accreditation and ethics in massage therapy; membership includes more than 22,000 massage therapists.

Associated Bodywork & Massage Professionals
28677 Buffalo Park Road
Evergreen, CO 90439-7347
303-674-8478
800-458-2267
A network organization of many bodywork methods; provides referrals to certified or licensed bodyworkers.

International Association of Infant-Massage Practitioners (IAIMP)
5660 Clinton Street
Elma, NY 14059

800-248-5432
716-684-3299
Provides training for and referrals to massage therapists with expertise in infant and child massage.

Books

Good Hands, by Robert Bahr (New American Library).

The Massage Book, by George Downing (Random House).

Massage for Common Ailments, by Sara Thomas (Fireside).

MEDITATION AND PRAYER

(See also "Yoga" and "Traditional Oriental Medicine.")

Organizations

Himalayan Institute of Yoga, Science and Philosophy
R.R.1 Box 400
Honesdale, PA 18431
717-253-5551
800-822-4547
Provides instruction and an extensive catalog of educational materials, as well as referrals to classes around the country.

Maharishi International University
1000 North 4th Street
Fairfield, IA 52556
515-472-5031
Information and referrals for Transcendental Meditation instruction.

The Stress Reduction Clinic
University of Massachusetts Medical Center
55 Lake Avenue, North

Worcester, MA 01655
508-856-8332
Teaches mindfulness meditation for stress reduction. Offers programs in eleven different cities around the country.

Books and Other Resources

Fire in the Soul, by Joan Borysenko (Warner Books).

Full-Catastrophe Living: Using the Wisdom of Your Mind and Body to Face Stress, Pain and Illness, by John Kabat-Zinn (Delacorte Press).

How to Meditate, by Lawrence LeShan (Bantam).

Minding the Body, Mending the Mind, by Joan Borysenko (Addison-Wesley).

Prayer and Temperament: Different Prayer Forms for Different Personality Types, by Monsignor Chester P. Michael and Marie C. Norrisey.

Theory and Practice of Meditation, Rudolph M. Balantine (Himalayan Institute).

The Tibetan Book of Living and Dying, by Sogyal Rinpoche (HarperSanFrancisco).

Zen Mind, Beginner's Mind, by Shunryo Suzuki (Weatherhill).

Stress Reduction Tapes
P.O. Box 547
Lexington, MA 02173
Mindfulness meditation audiotapes from Jon Zabat-Zinn of the University of Massachusetts Medical Center's Stress Reduction Clinic.

MIND-BODY MEDICINE (GENERAL)

(See also "Biofeedback," "Hypnotherapy," "Meditation and Prayer," "Reiki," "Relaxation," "Therapeutic Touch.")

Books

Full-Catastrophe Living: Using the Wisdom of Your Mind and Body to Face Stress, Pain and Illness, by Jon Kabat-Zinn (Delacorte Press).

The Healer Within: The New Medicine of Mind and Body, by Steven Locke and Douglas Colligan (E. P. Dutton).

Healing Words: The Power of Prayer and the Practice of Medicine, by Larry Dossey, M.D. (HarperCollins).

Health and Healing, by Andrew Weil, M.D. (Houghton Mifflin).

Love, Medicine and Miracles, by Bernie S. Siegel, M.D. (HarperPerennial).

Mind/Body Medicine: How to Use Your Mind for Better Health, by Daniel Goleman, Ph.D., and Joel Gurin (Consumer Reports Books).

Prayer: Finding the Heart's True Home, by R. J. Foster (HarperSanFrancisco).

Quantum Healing, by Deepak Chopra, M.D. (Bantam Books).

Unconditional Life: Mastering the Forces That Shape Personal Reality, Deepak Chopra (Bantam).

MYOTHERAPY

Bonnie Prudden Pain Erasure
7800 East Speedway
Tucson, AZ 85710
520-529-3979
800-221-4634

Training and information resource on Myotherapy. Provides a number of books, audiotapes, and videotapes, including a tape about relieving headache with Myotherapy.

NATUROPATHIC MEDICINE

Organizations

American Association of Naturopathic Physicians
2366 Eastlake Avenue East, Suite 322
Seattle, WA 98102
206-323-7610
Disseminates information about naturopathic approaches and provides referrals to naturopathic physicians (N.D.'s). In addition offers educational material including a newsletter and brochures on different health topics. For information and a directory of naturopathic physicians, send $5 to the address above.

National College of Naturopathic Medicine
11231 Southeast Market Street
Portland, OR 97216
503-255-4860
In addition to offering schooling in naturopathic medicine, distributes a listing of naturopathic physicians.

Books and Other Resources

Encyclopedia of Natural Medicine, by Michael T. Murray, N.D., and Joseph E. Pizzorno, N.D. (Prima Publishing Co.).

Natural Medicine Update Newsletter
Vital Communications
15401 SE 54th Court
Bellevue, WA 98006
800-488-0753

Edited by naturopathic physician and author Michael T. Murray, focuses on nutritional research and some herbs.

OSTEOPATHIC MEDICINE

Organizations

American Academy of Osteopathy
3500 DePauw Boulevard, Suite 1080
Indianapolis, IN 46268
317-879-1881
Member organization for doctors of osteopathy (D.O.'s) who perform osteopathic manipulations and, through the Cranial Academy (see below), D.O.'s who perform cranial manipulations. Provides referrals.

American Osteopathic Association
142 East Ontario Street
Chicago, IL 60611
800-621-1773
312-280-5800
Governing organization that sets standards for accreditation of osteopathic medical schools. Also distributes information about osteopathic medicine and provides referrals to doctors of osteopathy (D.O.'s).

The Cranial Academy
8606 Allisonville Road #130
Indianapolis, IN 46250
317-594-0411
Referrals to osteopathic physicians with training in cranial therapy.

Books

Osteopathic Self-treatment, by Leon Chaitow, D.O. (Thorsons).

With Thinking Fingers, by Ada Strand Sutherland (The Cranial Academy).

PHYSICALMIND THERAPY

PhysicalMind Institute
1807 Second Street #28/29
Santa Fe, NM 87505
505-988-1990

POLARITY THERAPY

American Polarity Therapy Association
P.O. Box 44-154
Somerville, MA 02144
617-776-6696

QIGONG

Organizations

American Taoist Healing Center, Inc.
396 Broadway, Suite 502
New York, NY 10013
A comprehensive treatment clinic that also publishes a quarterly newsletter devoted to qigong and traditional Chinese medicine.

Health Action
243 Pebble Beach
Santa Barbara, CA 93117
805-682-3230
Offers treatment, as well as books, audiotapes, and videotapes about qigong and traditional Chinese medicine.

International Qi Gong Directory and Body-Energy Center
2730 29th Street
Boulder, CO 90301
303-442-3131
Provides referrals to qigong practitioners and masters nationwide.

National Commission of Certification
of Acupuncturists
1424 16th Street NW, Suite 501
Washington, DC 20036-2211
202-232-1404
Governing agency that sets standards for schools in all facets of Oriental medicine. Provides referrals to accredited schools.

Qigong Institute
East West Academy of Healing Arts
450 Sutter Street, Suite 2104
San Francisco, CA 94108
Promotes research, training education, and clinical study of Chinese healing arts, including a qigong database of studies related to qigong.

Books and Other Resources

Qigong for Health: Chinese Traditional Exercise for Cure and Prevention, by Masaru Takahashi and Stephen Brown (Japan Publications).

Health Action Press
243 Pebble Beach
Santa Barbara, CA 93117
805-682-3230
An excellent source of books, audiotapes, and videotapes about traditional Chinese medicine, including *Qigong: The Most Profound Medicine,* by Roger Jahnke, O.M.D. Write or call for catalog.

Qigong Magazine
Pacific Rim Publishers, Inc.

P.O. Box 31578
San Francisco, CA 94131
Quarterly magazine about qigong for practitioners and interested general public.

Qi: The Journal of Traditional Eastern Health and Fitness
Insight Graphics
P.O. Box 18476
Anaheim Hills, CA 92817
800-787-2600
Quarterly magazine devoted to disseminating information about traditional Oriental healing methods.

YMAA Publication Center
38 Hyde Park Avenue
Jamaica Plains, MA 02130
800-669-8892
Catalog of books, videotapes, clothing, and music relating to qigong and martial arts.

REFLEXOLOGY

Organizations

International Institute of Reflexology
P.O. Box 12642
St. Petersburg, FL 33733-2642

Books

Body Reflexology: Healing at Your Fingertips, by Mildred Carter (Parker Publishing).

Feet First: A Guide to Foot Reflexology, by Laura Norman (Simon & Schuster).

Hand Reflexology: Key to Perfect Health, by Mildred Carter (Parker Publishing).

How to Heal Yourself Using Hand Acupressure (Hand Reflexology), by Michael Blate (Falkynor Books).

REIKI

Organizations

Center for Spiritual Development
Center for Reiki Training
29209 Northwestern Highway, #592
Southfield, MI 48304
800-332-8112
In Michigan: 810-948-8112

The Reiki Alliance
P.O. Box 41
Cataldo, ID 83810-1041
208-682-3535
Training and resources for the general public, and referrals to Reiki Masters throughout the world.

Reiki Outreach International
P.O. Box 609
Fair Oaks, CA 95628
916-863-1500
Provides referrals to trained Reiki instructors.

Books and Other Resources

The Reiki Alliance
(See address and phone number above.)
Offers a number of books, audiotapes, and videotapes about Reiki methods.

A Complete Book of Reiki Healing, by Brigitte Muller and Gunther Hort (Life Rhythm).

Empowerment Through Reiki, by Paula Horan (Lotus Light Publications).

Reiki in Everyday Living, by Earlene Gleisner, R.N./R.M. (White Feather Press), available by writing to White Feather Press, P.O. Box 1209, Laytonville, CA 95454.

Reiki Plus Publications
Rte. 3 Box 313
Celina, TN 38551
615-243-3712
Offers several books about Reiki by Reiki Master, David G. Jarell.

RELAXATION

Organizations

Center for the Improvement of Human Functioning
3100 North Hillside Avenue
Witchita, KA 67219
316-682-3100
In addition to research and clinical course, offers support groups and programs for people with chronic illness.

The Mind/Body Institute
Division of Behavioral Science
New England Deaconess Hospital
Harvard Medical School
185 Pilgrim Road
Boston, MA 02215
617-732-9530
Training and research center for professionals and clinical programs for people with stress-related illness. Also offers relaxation audiotapes.

Books and Other Resources ·

Beyond the Relaxation Response, by Herbert Benson, M.D. (Times Books).

Relaxation and Stress Workbook, edited by Matthew McKay, Martha Davis, and Elizabeth R. Eshelman (New Harbinger).

The Relaxation Response, by Herbert Benson, M.D. (Outlet Books).

The Wellness Book: The Comprehensive Guide to Maintaining Health and Treating Stress-Related Illness, by Herbert Benson, M.D., and Eileen M. Stuart (Carol).

The Mind/Body Clinic at New England Deaconess Hospital
(See address, page 384.)
Offers workbooks and audiotapes on relaxation response.

ROLFING (STRUCTURAL INTEGRATION)

Organizations

Rolf Institute of Structural Integration
P.O. Box 1868
Boulder, CO 80306
800-530-8875
Governing organization for certification in the methods of Structural Integration. Provides referrals to trained Rolfers, offers pamphlets, books, and videotapes on Rolfing and Rolfing Movement Integration.

Books and Other Resources

Rolf Institute of Structural Integration
(See address above.)
Offers a catalog of books, tapes, and brochures about Rolfing Structural Integration and Movement Integration.

Ida Rolf Talks About Rolfing and Physical Reality, edited by Rosemary Feitis (Harper & Row).

Rolfing: The Integration of Human Structures, by Ida Rolf (Harper & Row).

SUPPORT GROUPS

American Self-Help Clearinghouse
Northwest Covenant Medical Center
25 Pocono Road
Denville, NJ 07834
201-625-7101
Maintains a national directory of support groups and other self-help clearinghouses for a wide range of conditions. In addition, provides information on starting your own support group.

National Headache Foundation
(See address and phone number, page 354.)

Books

The Healing Web: Social Networks and Human Survival, by Marc Pilisuk and Susan H. Parks (University Press of New England).

Living Beyond Limits, by David Spiegel (Times Books).

THERAPEUTIC TOUCH

Organizations

Nurse Healers Professional Associates
P.O. Box 444
Allison Park, PA 15101
412-355-8476

A network of health care professionals with interest in Therapeutic Touch and other complementary healing methods.

Books

The Therapeutic Touch, by Dolores Kreiger (Prentice Hall).

TRADITIONAL ORIENTAL MEDICINE

(See also "Acupressure" and "Acupuncture.")

Organizations

American Academy of Medical Acupuncture
800-521-2262
Provides acupuncture training for *physicians* and offers a list of referrals.

American Association of Acupuncture and Oriental Medicine
433 Front Street
Catasauqua, PA 18032
610-266-1433
Fax: 610-264-2768
National organization that provides general information on acupuncture and Oriental medicine, literature about specific disease conditions, and referrals to qualified practitioners who have undergone national certification and, where required, state licensure.

American Foundation of Traditional Chinese Medicine
505 Beach Street
San Francisco, CA 94133
415-776-0502
National referral resource for classes and programs in Chinese medicine.

East West Academy of Healing Arts
450 Sutter Street, Suite 2104
San Francisco, CA 94108
Promotes research, training education, and clinical study of Chinese healing arts and maintains the most extensive U.S. database of studies related to qigong.

National Commission for the Certification of Acupuncturists
1424 16th Street NW, Suite 501
Washington, DC 20036
202-232-1404
Administers testing for certification in acupuncture and Chinese herbology; offers directories listing acupuncturists and Chinese herbologists who either have passed the exam or met requirements to take the exam (e.g., formal education, apprenticeship, or substantial number of years in practice). For referrals, write to the above address, and enclose a $3 check for the state directory, or a $24 check for the national directory.

Books

Between Heaven and Earth: A Guide to Chinese Medicine, by H. Beinfield and E. Korngold (Ballantine Books).

The Web That Has No Weaver: Understanding Chinese Medicine, by Ted Kaptchuk (Contemporary Books).

Catalogs

Blue Poppy Press
1775 Linden Avenue
Boulder, CO 80304
800-487-9296
Publishes a wide range of books on traditional Chinese medicine, including *Migraine and Traditional Chinese Medicine,* by Bob Flaws. Write or call for free catalog.

Health Action Press
(See address and phone number, page 380)

Insight Publishing
Box 18476
Anaheim Hills, CA 92817
800-787-2600
Catalog of books on traditional Chinese medicine.

Seven Star Communications
1314 Second Street
Santa Monica, CA 90401
310-576-1901
Catalog of books and tapes about Taoist practices and philosophy.

YMAA Publication Center
38 Hyde Park Avenue
Jamaica Plains, MA 02130
800-669-8892
Catalog of books, videotapes, clothing, and music relating to qigong
and martial arts.

Publications

East-West Medical Digest Newsletter
American Institute of Chinese Herbs
16 Almond Tree Lane
Irvine, CA 92715
714-786-0828
Though a technical publication, easy to understand for laypeople.
Provides information on herb research.

TRAGER WORK

Trager Institute
21 Locust Avenue
Mill Valley, CA 94941
415-388-2688
Contact for background books on Tragerwork, training, and a directory of practitioners nationwide.

YOGA

Organizations

Himalayan Institute of Yoga, Science and Philosophy
R.R.1 Box 400
Honesdale, PA 18431
717-253-5551
800-822-4547
Provides classes and an extensive catalog of educational materials, as well as referrals to classes around the country.

International Association of Yoga Therapists
109 Hillside Avenue
Mill Valley, CA 94941
415-383-4587
A nonprofit organization emphasizing education and research for yoga and yoga therapy, IAYT provides referrals to schools, institutions, and associations that offer yoga-teacher certification.

Iyengar Yoga
2404 27th Avenue
San Francisco, CA 94115
415-753-0909
In addition to instruction and teacher training, this organization of-

fers referrals to yoga instructors and a mail-order catalog of educational materials.

Kripalu Center
P.O. Box 2218
Lenox, MA 01240
800-967-7279

Kripalu is a form of yoga; the Kripalu Center is the largest residential yoga and health facility in North America. Yoga and meditation retreats, including instruction, and complementary medical care and bodywork, are available. Kripalu By Mail offers books and videotapes for instruction in the Kripalu approach.

Samata Yoga and Health Institute
4150 Tivoli Avenue
Los Angeles, CA 90066
301-306-8845

Specializes in reducing stress and improving back problems.

Books and Other Resources

Easy Pregnancy with Yoga, by Stella Weller (Thorsons/HarperCollins).

Light on Yoga, by B.K.S. Iyengar (Schoken Books).

Relax and Renew: Restful Yoga for Stressful Times, by Judith Lassater (Rodmell Press); 800-841-3123.

The Yoga Back Book, by Stella Weller (Thorsons/HarperCollins).

Yoga for Common Ailments, edited by Nancy Ford-Kohne (Simon & Schuster).

Yoga Therapy, by Stella Weller (Thorsons/HarperCollins).

Bodhi Tree Bookstore
800-825-9798

Offers catalog of books, audiotapes, and videotapes.

Himalayan Institute of Yoga, Science and Philosophy
(See address and phone number, page 390.)
An extensive catalog of educational materials—books, audiotapes, and videotapes—as well as referrals to classes around the country.

Integral Yoga Distribution
Yogaville
Buckingham, VA 23921
800-262-1008
Extensive catalog of books about yoga as well as other alternative-health practices and spirituality.

Kripalu By Mail
(See address and phone number, page 391.)
Catalog of instructional books, videotapes, and audiotapes as well as products for yoga practice.

References

Introduction
1. Eisenberg, D. M., et al. "Unconventional medicine in the United States: Prevalence, costs, and patterns of use." *The New England Journal of Medicine,* 1993; 328:246–252.

Chapter 1
1. Moyers, B. D. *Healing and the Mind.* New York: Doubleday, 1993.
2. Beecher, H. K. "The powerful placebo." *JAMA* 1955; 268:1334–1338.
3. Moyers, *Healing and the Mind.*
4. Benson, H. *The Relaxation Response.* New York: Morrow, 1975.
5. Weed, S. *Healing Wise.* Woodstock: Ash Tree, 1989.
6. Janssen, GWHM. "The application of Maharishi Ayur-Veda in the treatment of ten chronic diseases: a pilot study." *Nederlands Tijdshrift Voor Integrale Geneeskunde,* 1989; 5:586–594.

Chapter 2

1. Dubois, E., and Wallace, D. J. "Clinical and laboratory manifestations of systemic lupus erythematosus." In *Dubois' Lupus Erythematosus*. 3d ed, eds. D. J. Wallace and E. Dubois. Philadelphia: 1987; pp. 317–469.
2. Hack, G. D., Robinson, W. L., and Koritzer R. T. "Previously undescribed relation between muscle and dura." Presented at the American Association of Neurologial Surgeons and the Congress of Neurological Surgeons, February 14–18, 1995.
3. Matthew, N., et al. Fifth International Headache Congress, Washington, DC, 1991.

Chapter 3

1. Diamond, S. "Diet and headache." *Nutr Rep,* 1987 5:12–13.
2. De Belleroche, J., et al. "Erythrocyte choline concentration and cluster headache." *British Medical Journal,* 1988; 288:268–270.
3. O'Banion, D. R., et al. "Dietary and stress management in tension headache treatment." *Clinical Ecology,* 1982; 1:75–83.
4. Seltzer, S. "Foods, and food and drug combinations, responsible for head and neck pain." *Cephalalgia,* 1982; 2:111–124.
5. Shirlow, M. J., and Mathers, D. C. "A study of caffeine consumption and symptoms: indigestion, palpitations, tremor, headache and insomnia." *International Journal of Epidemiology,* 1985; 14:239–248.
6. Silverman, K., Evans, S. M., et al. "Withdrawal syndrome after the double-blind cessation of caffeine consumption." *The New England Journal of Medicine,* 1992; 327:1109.
7. "Food Allergies and Intolerances." *Nutritional Fact Sheet.* National Center for Nutrition and Dietetics, American Dietetic Association, 1994.
8. Mauskop, A., Altura, B. T., Cracco, R. Q., and Altura, B. M. "Intravenous magnesium sulfate relieves migraine attacks in patients with low serum ionized magnesium levels: a pilot study." *Clinical Science,* 1995; 89:633–636.
9. Sarchielli, P., Coata, G., Firenze, C., et al. "Serum and salivary magnesium levels in migraine and tension-type headache. Results in a group of adult patients." *Cephalalgia,* 1992; 12:21–27.

10. Mauskop, A., Altura, B. T., Cracco, R. Q., and Altura, B. M. "Intravenous magnesium sulfate relieves cluster headaches in patients with low serum ionized magnesium levels." *Headache,* 1995; 35 (10):597–600.

11. Altura, B. T., and Altura, B. M. "Withdrawal of magnesium causes vasospasm while elevated magnesium produces relaxation of tone in cerebral arteries." *Neurosci Lett,* 1980; 20:323–327.

12. Weglicki, W. B., and Phillips, T. M. "Pathophysiology of magnesium deficiency: a cytokine/neurogenic inflammation hypothesis." *Am J Physiol* 1992; 263:R734–R737.

13. Bic, Z., Bliz, G. G., Hopp, H. P., et al. "Influence of low dietary fat intake on incidence and severity of migraine headache." In publication.

14. Harrison, D. "Copper as a factor in the dietary precipitation of migraine." *Headache,* 1986; 26:248–250.

15. Garrison, R. H., and Somer, E. *Nutrition Desk Reference.* New Canaan, CT: Keats Publishing, Inc., 1990.

16. Garrison, et al. *Nutrition Desk Reference.*

17. *Environmental Nutrition Newsletter,* July 1995.

18. Weglicki and Phillips. "Pathophysiology of magnesium deficiency."

19. "Food Allergies and Intolerances," *Nutritional Fact Sheet.*

20. Walsh, W. E., "Treating sinus, migraine and cluster headaches: an allergist's approach to headache treatment." St. Paul: ACA Publications, Inc., 1993.

Chapter 4

1. Chemical Injury Information Network, 1994.

2. Wallace, L., et al. U. S. Environmental Protection Agency. "Identification of polar volatility of organic compounds and common microenvironments." 84th Annual Meeting and Exhibition of the Air and Waste Management Association. Vancouver, British Columbia: June 16–21, 1991.

Chapter 5

1. Altura, B. T., and Altura, B. M. "Withdrawal of magnesium causes vasospasm while elevated magnesium produces relaxation of tone in cerebral arteries." *Neurosci Lett,* 1980; 20:323–327.

2. Weglicki, W. B., and Phillips, T. M. "Pathophysiology of magnesium deficiency: a cytokine/neurogenic inflammation hypothesis." *Am J Physiol,* 1992; 263:R734–R737.

3. Mauskop, A., Altura, B. T., Cracco, R. Q., and Altura, B. M. "Intravenous magnesium sulfate relieves migraine attacks in patients with low serum ionized magnesium levels: a pilot study." *Clinical Science,* 1995; 89:633–636.

4. Facchinetti, F., Sances, G., Borella, P., et al. "Magnesium prophylaxis of menstrual migraine: effects per intracellular magnesium." *Headache,* 1991; 31:298–301.

5. Premarin Package Insert. In *Physicians' Desk Reference.* 49th ed. Oradell, NJ: Medical Economics Company, Inc., 1996.

6. Loestrin 21 Package Insert. In *Physicians' Desk Reference.* 49th ed. Oradell, NJ: Medical Economics Company, Inc., 1996.

7. Cady, R., and Farmer, K. *Headache Free.* New York: Bantam Books, 1996.

Chapter 6

1. "Food Allergies and Intolerances." *Nutritional Fact Sheet.* National Center for Nutrition and Dietetics, American Dietetic Association, 1994.

2. Egger, J., Carter, C. M., et al. "Is migraine food allergy? A double-blind controlled trial of oligoantigenic diet treatment." *The Lancet,* 1983; 2:865.

3. Carter, C. M., Egger, J., and Soothill, J. F. "A dietary management of severe childhood migraine." *Hum Nutr: Appl Nutr,* 1985; 39A:294–303; and Egger, J., Carter, C. M., et al. "Is migraine food allergy?"

4. Mauskop, A., Altura, B. T., Cracco, R. Q., and Altura, B. M. "Intravenous magnesium sulfate relieves migraine attacks in patients with low serum ionized magnesium levels: a pilot study." *Clinical Science,* 1995; 89:633–636.

5. Facchinetti, F., Sances, G., Borella P., et al. "Magnesium prophy-

laxis of menstrual migraine: effects per intracellular magnesium.''
*Headache,*1991; 31:298–301.

6. Mauskop, A., Altura, B. T., Cracco, R. Q., and Altura, B. M. ''An open trial of magnesium supplementation for the treatment of migraines and symptoms of premenstrual syndrome in premenopausal women. Effect on serum ionized magnesium levels.'' *Neurology,* 1997; 48 (3 suppl.):A260.

7. Peikert, A., Wilimzig, C., and Kohne-Volland, R. ''Prophylaxis of migraine with oral magnesium results from a prospective, multi-center, placebo-controlled and double-blind randomized study.'' *Cephalalgia,* 1996; 16:257–263.

8. Schoenen, J., Jacquy, J., Lenaerts, M. ''High-dose riboflavin as a novel prophylactic antimigraine therapy: results from a double-blind, randomized, placebo-controlled trial.'' *Cephalalgia,* 1997; 17:244.

9. Werbach, M. R. ''Headache.'' In *Nutritional Influences on Illness: A Sourcebook of Clinical Research.* Tarzana, CA: Third Line Press, Inc. 1988.

10. Dupois, S. ''A comprehensive approach to treatment of intractable headaches.'' *Townsend Letter for Doctors,* November 1990; 740–744.

11. De Belleroche, J., et al. ''Erythrocyte choline concentration and cluster headache.'' *British Medical Journal,* 1984; 288:268–270.

12. Mauskop, A., Altura, B. T., Cracco, R. Q., and Altura, B. M. ''Intravenous magnesium sulfate relieves cluster headache in patients with low serum ionized magnesium levels.'' *Headache,* 1995; 35:597–600.

Chapter 7

1. Puustjarvi, K., Airaksinen, O., and Pontinen P. J. ''The effects of massage in patients with chronic tension headache.'' *Acupunct Electrother Res,* 1990; 15:159–162.

2. Ghan, Zhen-yuan, et al. ''Treatment of 31 cases of migraine by penetrating Xuan Lu, Tai Yang towards Shuai Gu.'' *Chinese Acupuncture and Moxibustion,* 1983; 3:4.

3. Carlsson, J., Augustinsson, L. E., Blomstrand, C., and Sullivan, M. ''Health status in patients with tension headache treated with acupuncture or physiotherapy.'' *Headache,* 1990; 30:593–599.

4. Millman, B. "Acupuncture: context and critique." *Annual Review of Medicine,* 1977; 27:223–236.

5. Jahnke, R. *The Most Profound Medicine.* Santa Barbara, CA: Health Action Publishing, 1991.

6. Achterberg, J., Dossey, L., Gordon, J. S., et al. "Mind-body interventions, in Alternative Medicine: Expanding Medical Horizons." Report to the National Institutes of Health on Alternative Medical Systems and Practices in the United States; prepared under the auspices of the Workshop on Alternative Medicine, Chantilly, Virginia, September 14–16, 1992.

7. Monro, R., Ghosh, A. K., and Kalish, D. "Yoga research bibliography, scientific studies on yoga and meditation." Yoga Biomedical Trust, Cambridge, England, 1989.

8. Weinberg, R. S., Hunt, V. V. "Effects of structural integration on state trait anxiety." *Journal of Clinical Psychology,* 1979; 35:319–322.

9. Chapman-Smith, D. "Chiropractic management of headache." *The Chiropractic Report,* 1991; 5:1–6.

10. Wight, J. S. "Migraine: a statistical analysis of chiropractic treatment." *ACA J Chiro,* 1978; 15:S63–S67.

11. Jaret, P. "You don't have to sweat to reduce your stress." *Health,* November/December, 1995: 83–88.

12. Vijayan, N. *Headache,* 1993; 33:40–42.

Chapter 8

1. Gutkin, A. J., Holborn, S. W., Walker, J. R., and Anderson, B. A. "Treatment integrity of relaxation training for tension headaches." *J. Behav Ther Exp Psychiatry,* 1992; 23:191–198.

2. Blanchard, E. B., Nicholson, N. L., Taylor, A. E., et al. "The role of regular home practice in the relaxation treatment of tension headache." *J Consult Clin Psychol,* 1991; 59:467–470.

3. Turk, D. C., and Nash, J. M. "Chronic pain: new ways to cope." In Goleman, D., and Gurin, J. eds. *Mind Body Medicine.* New York: Consumer Reports Books, 1993; 111–130.

4. Engel, J. M., Rapoff, M. A., and Pressman, A. R. "Long-term follow-up of relaxation training for pediatric headache disorders." *Headache,* 1992; 32: 152–156.

5. Bannerman, R. H., Burton, J., and Wen Chieh, C., eds. *Traditional Medicine and Health Care Coverage.* Geneva, Switzerland: World Health Organization, 1983.

6. Spiegel, H., and Spiegel, D. *Trance and Treatment: Clinical Uses of Hypnosis.* Washington, DC: American Psychiatric Press, 1987.

7. Achterberg, J., Dossey, L., Gordon, J. S., et al. "Mind-body interventions, in Alternative Medicine: Expanding Medical Horizons," Report to the National Institutes of Health on Alternative Medical Systems and Practices in the United States. Prepared under the auspices of the Workshop on Alternative Medicine, Chantilly, Virginia, September 14–16, 1992.

8. Rossman, M. L."Imagery: learning to use the mind's eyes." In Goleman, G., Gurin, J., eds. *Mind Body Medicine.* New York: Consumer Reports Books, 1993; 291–300.

9. Kabat-Zinn, J. *Full Catastrophe Living: Using the Wisdom of Your Body to Face Stress, Pain, and Illness.* New York: Delacorte Press, 1990.

10. Hatch, J. P., Fisher, J. G., and Rugh, J. D. *Biofeedback: Studies in Clinical Efficacy.* New York: Plenum, 1987.

11. Grazzi, L., Leone, M., Fediani, F., and Busone, G. "A therapeutic alternative for tension headache in children: treatment and one-year follow-up results." *Biofeedback Self Regul,* 1990; 15:1–6.

12. Cott, A., Parkinson, W., Fabich, M., et al. "Long-term efficacy of combined relaxation: biofeedback treatments for chronic headache." *Pain,* 1992; 51:49–56.

13. Grazzi, L., Bussone, G. "Effect of biofeedback treatment on sympathetic function in common migraine and tension-type headache." *Cephalalgia,* 1993; 13:197–200.

14. Turk, D. C., and Nash, D. M. In Goleman, G., Gurin, J., eds. *Mind Body Medicine.* New York: Consumer Reports Books, 1993; 111–130.

15. Dossey, L., *Healing Words,* San Francisco: HarperSanFrancisco, 1993.

16. Keller, E., and Bzkek, V. M. "Effects of therapeutic touch on tension headache pain." *Nurs Res,* 1986; 101–104.

Chapter 9
1. Farnsworth, N. R., et al. "Medicinal plants in therapy." *Bulletin of the World Health Organization,* 1985; 63:965–981.
2. Mark, D. R., et al. "A double-blind, placebo-controlled trial of intranasal capsaicin for cluster headache." *Cephalalgia,* 1993; 13:114–116.
3. Faivelson, S. "Fruit extract checks cluster headaches." *Medical Tribune,* July 25, 1991.
4. Johnson, E. S., Kadam, N. P., Hylands, D. M., and Hylands, P. J.: "Efficacy of feverfew as prophylactic treatment of migraine." *Br Med J,* 1985; 291:569–573.
5. Makheja, A. M., and Bailey, J. M. "The active principle in feverfew." *The Lancet ii,* 1981; 1054.
6. Göbel, H., Heinze, A., Dworschak, M., et al. "Oleum menthae piperitae significantly reduces the symptoms of tension-type headache and its efficacy does not differ from that of acetaminophen." In *Headache Treatment: Trial Methodology and New Drugs,* eds. J. Olesen and P. Tfelt-Hansen. Philadelphia: Lippincott-Raven, 1997; 169–174.

Chapter 10
1. Eisenberg, D. M., Kessler, R. C., Foster, C., et al. "Unconventional medicine in the United States." *New England Journal of Medicine,* 1993; 246–252.
2. Bouchayer, F. "Alternative medicines: a general approach to the French situation." *Complementary Medical Research,* 4:4–8.
3. Kishore, J. "Homeopathy: the Indian experience." *World Health Forum,* 1983; 4:105–107.
4. Kleijnen, J., Knipschild, P., and terRiet, G. "Clinical trials of homeopathy." *British Medical Journal,* 1991; 302:316–323.
5. Brigo, B., and Serpelloni, G. "Homeopathic treatment of migraines." *The Berlin Journal on Research in Homeopathy,* 1991; 1:98–106.

Index